Eat Like You Love Yourself

A modern guide to Ayurvedic cooking and living

For Matt, Scarlett & Zev
My greatest loves, my kitchen dancing partners, my co-creators in this delicious life!

EAT LIKE YOU LOVE Yourself

A Modern Guide to Ayurvedic Cooking and Living

Cover & Back cover images by: Wanda Chin
Book design by: Chara Caruthers and Chiara Pennella
Recipe Consulting chef: Jessica Harris

Table of Contents

Introduction

Origins of a lifelong love affair with eating...

"There is no love sincerer than the love of food."
George Bernard Shaw

Since as long as I can remember, I've had this crazy love affair with food. The type of relationship that is a bit clandestine, deep, and definitely complicated. Some of my first and fondest memories are of my mother's freshly baked, warm chocolate chip cookies waiting on the countertop as I came home from school. Rising early the night after one of my dad's poker parties to dive head first into bowls of stale potato chips and pretzels, abandoned by the party-goers.. The "bone soup" served by the sisters who ran the Catholic preschool my sister and I attended (I hated that soup, who would have guessed it'd become such a fad decades later!).

As a kid of newly divorced parents, my teenage years were colored with bad food choices and experimentation in the kitchen. I discovered cookbooks (those were the pre-internet days), cooking shows (my faves were Julia Child, Jacques Pepin, and Justin Wilson - just for the laughs), and the joys of making things from scratch. But even as my interest and skills in cooking were blossoming, the food I chose and consumed most often served a pretty singular purpose...comfort.

At the time I didn't realize it so much, but looking back I can see very clearly the origins of emotional eating that started with huge pancake breakfasts (my sister and I loved making pancakes), deep fried burritos, french fries, burgers, pizza (gotta love school lunches), and bowl after bowl after bowl of cereal (Frosted Flakes were a favorite). I did my level best to drown my teen angst in meat, fat and sugar and learned to bake my anxieties into batches of cookies.

Even then I was somehow tuned in to the value of the process of cooking. I knew nothing other than to cook with love, driven by a passion for the process and the promise of enjoying the results. While other kids played outside after school, I pored over cookbooks while eating bowls of popcorn in front of the television, The Frugal Chef, anyone?

When I look back I can clearly see that cooking...and eating have been an important part of who I am. Back then, it filled a hole in my life and provided the love, stability, comfort, ,and confidence (like making clam chowder from scratch and it was actually good) that was missing in my mind, body and life. **And so more than just filling my belly, food made me feel whole.**

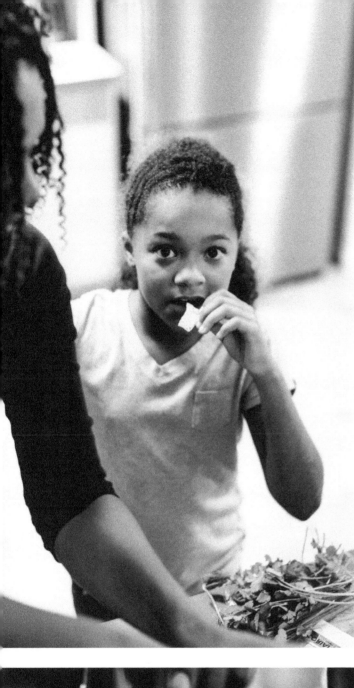
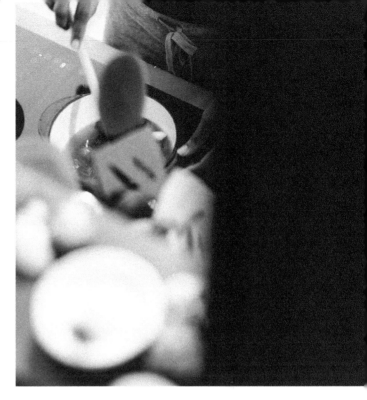
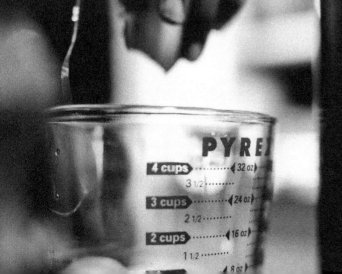
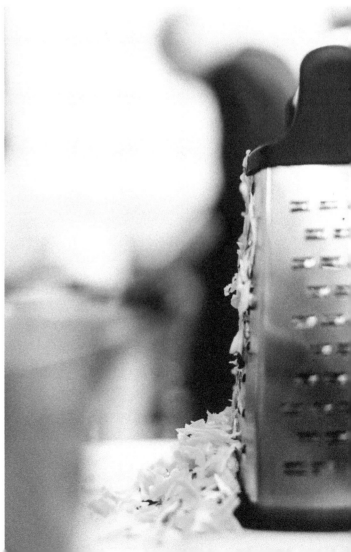

What I know now, as mother, wife and wellness professional, is that my story isn't all that unique. Many of my clients, students, and friends cite food moments as some of their first and fondest memories. Family dinners and picnics by the shore, road trips with drippy ice cream cones and camping vacations cooking hot dogs and s'mores over an open fire.

In many ways, food is the teller of our life's story. It's our sole constant companion as we move through the highs and lows that define our paths of self-discovery and growth. Our relationship with what we consume is one of the most powerful and vital partnerships that we'll have during our time on this earth. But, these days, by the time most children reach adulthood, their relationship with food has become dysfunctional at best, with more and more experiences taking a turn towards destructive. What's more is that as our anxiety (it's actually more like a mania) around food (how healthy is it, does it have all the right nutrients, how much fat, sugar, preservatives, or gluten are in it?) deepens, we're beginning to see the signs of strain showing up in the relationship that children at younger and younger ages are forging with their diets and their bodies.

It is my belief that the way out ISN'T more scrutiny of our diets. It isn't more analysis of the chemical makeup and nutrient composition of every piece of food we might dare to put into our mouths. It isn't the toxin fearmongering or designation of "organic" being the only healthy option. It's not deleting fat, sugar, meat or grains from your culinary vocabulary in the name of keeping up with the unnaturally fit, tanned, skinny, or otherwise "beautiful" people. It also isn't glorifying being obesely overweight as a healthy mental "choice". I believe that the ONLY way of repairing our relationship with food is to fix our relationship with ourselves.

We need a new way of looking at this vital partnership. One that initiates from the inside instead of from the outside. One that begins and ends with a single, powerful, eternal principle… LOVE.

We also need to acknowledge that no matter what or how much we're consuming, whether it's convenience store tacos, home-cooked mac and cheese or filet mignon, each experience of feeding ourselves shares a singular purpose; To give the body-mind what it needs to shine. But every individual experiences food (choosing, preparing, eating) as a series of complex transactions that carry the weight of our entire life history right up to the point that we put down the fork.

Eating is complicated. And when you consider how many different diets, rules, guidelines, studies, warnings, and disclaimers are associated with it these days, I think we can all

agree that it's only getting more convoluted...
and scary.

But who we are as a species hasn't changed
much in the hundreds of thousands of
years of our existence on this earth. In form
and function we are much the same as our
prehistoric counterparts, but for the fact that
we're experiencing one of the most unhealthy
times in recent history. Lifestyle diseases
like diabetes, obesity and heart disease have
grown to epidemic levels, affecting individuals
and children at ever-younger ages.

As a culture deeply invested in body image,
many of the messages we experience every
day about the connections between what we
eat and who we are, are unhealthy at best,
and, at worst, deadly.

As a parent, wellness educator, and child of a
mother who has dieted nearly her entire life
(something I never took up with much gusto),
I feel a responsibility to examine my hangups,
beliefs and habits around food as a matter of
integrity.

And it's only now, in the last decade or so as
I've begun to really look at my relationship
with it that I can embrace my food history with
more clarity (and less judgement). I can see
how even my earliest food choices (and those
of my parents and friends) have shaped who
I am today, and even who my children are. I
can feel how the dietary foundation that was
laid at childhood supports, and sabotages me
throughout the day and the year.

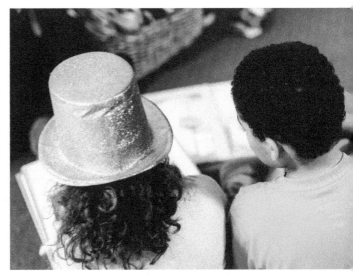
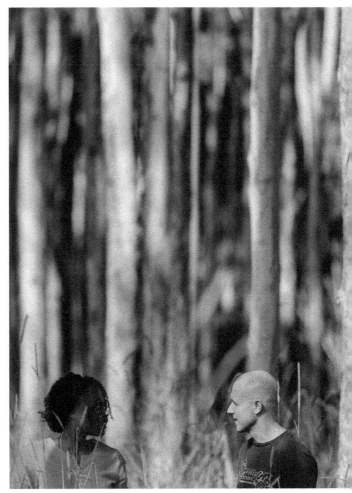

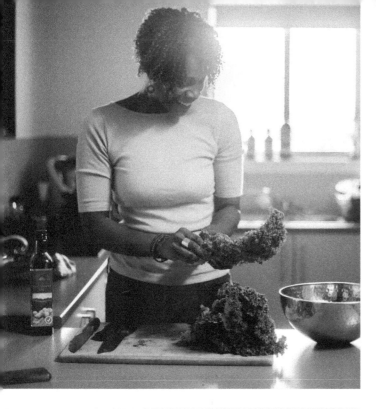
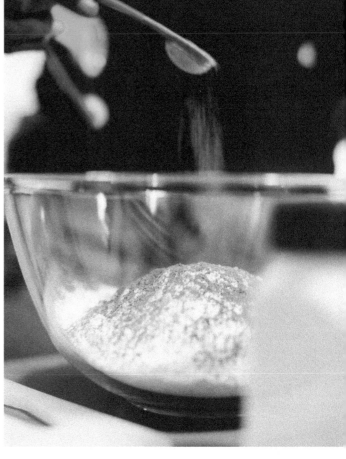
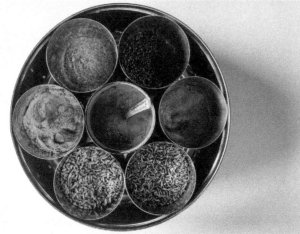
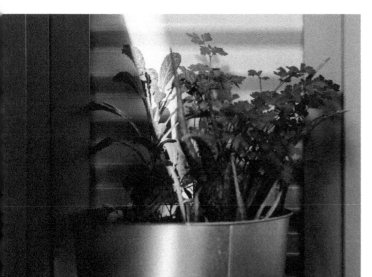
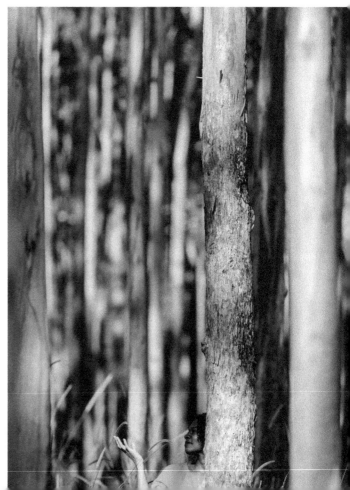

It's only since embracing the ancient wisdom of Ayurveda that I've begun to feel more empowered and expressive in my relationship with food. The confusion about what is genuinely healthy for me, and what's not, has faded. The guilt or anxiety that came from eating fat, sugar, wheat, meat and all other "non-healthy" foods has subsided considerably, and something closer to a feeling of conscious awareness and relative balance has sprung up in its place. With that has also come body awareness, balance, and confidence.

Food is SO much more powerful than we give it credit for. In yoga we call the physical body the annamaya kosha or "food sheath," owing to the idea that "we are what we eat." Ayurveda refines that idea even further with the statement that "we are what we digest and assimilate." Within these pages, we'll take a closer look at these concepts and discover how our food defines who we are and shapes who we can be in the moment and in our lives.

With this book my goal is to enlighten, excite, and empower you, to see your experiences with food as more than just entertainment, intoxication, or sustenance. My hope is to incite you to look within your own relationship with food to discover the healthy and not-so-healthy ways that you interact with it and take action toward creating a partnership with it that nurtures every aspect of your being and provides a foundation of support for your authentic wellness.

So I encourage you to explore the writings and recipes with a deep love and a curiosity for discovering how your food can give you the freedom to truly BE yourself. I also hope to inspire you to let that love flow through every step of the ritual and the process of your cooking, so that ultimately you'll learn to...

Eat like you love yourself.

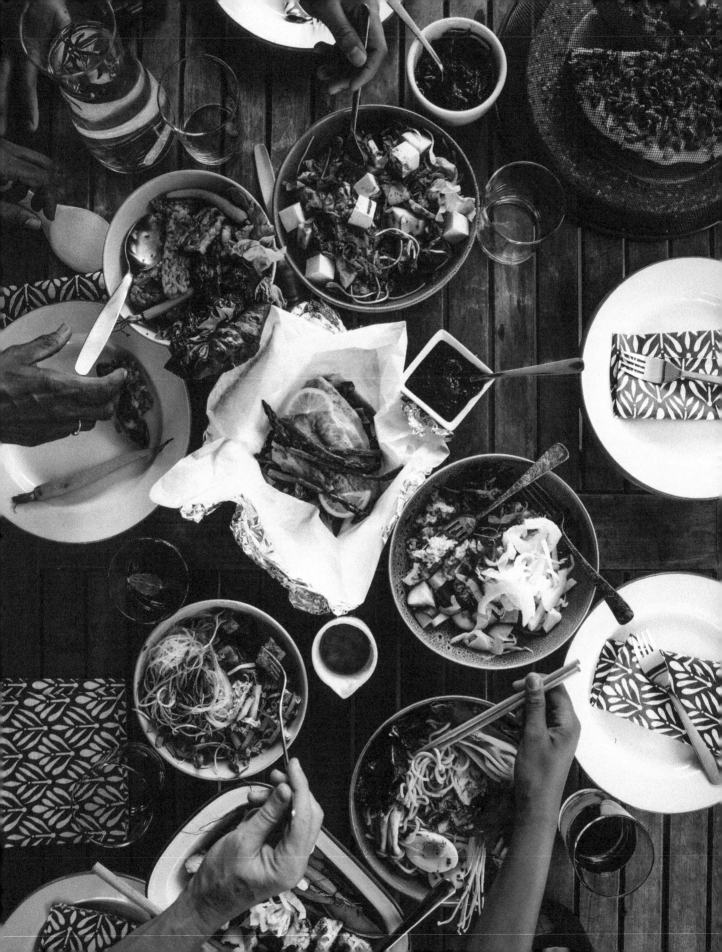

Chapter 1

Discovering your food truth.

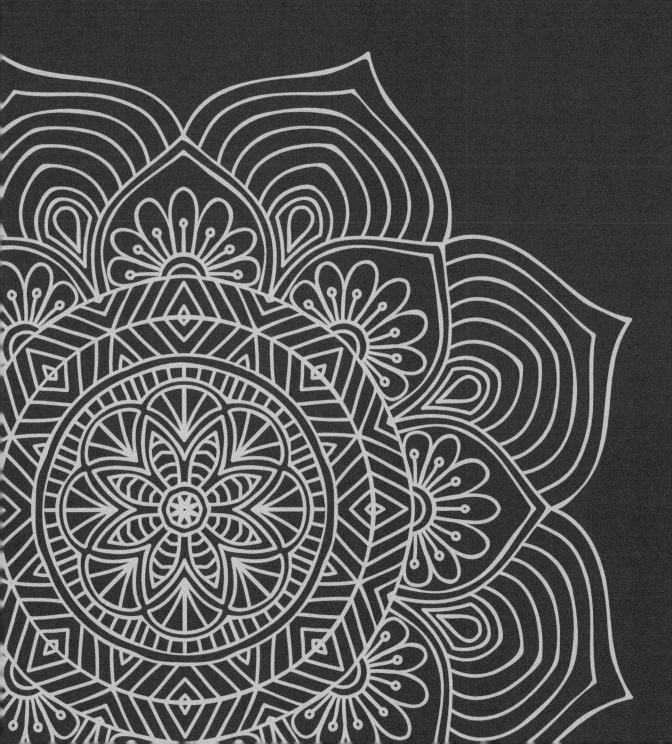

"Tell me what you eat, and I shall tell you what you are." – Jean Anthelme Brillat-Savarin

I've got a question for you... What if eating made you feel good...always? Yes, what if every bite of food you consumed felt like a joyous step towards creating your best self?

Sounds like some kind of crazy dream, doesn't it? Largely because you know as well as I do that rather than nourishing them, we often punish our bodies with the foods that we eat. We smother our emotions and our physical realities with the dizzying onslaught of sugar, salt, and man-made additives on a regular basis. We quiet our inner knowing by overindulging with foods that offer very little in the way of value for our physical, mental, and emotional wellbeing.

And that can be said about the "healthiest" people among us, including the weight loss and fitness gurus, the green juicers, and paleo provocateurs. So many of us have given up listening to our bodies and have given our power to know ourselves over to the "experts" who stand ready with a "one-size-fits-all", approach to making eating easier, more convenient, and well suited to supporting the busy, disconnected lives that are slowly killing us anyway.

Most people these days have NO idea what's healthy for them, or how that might change from day to day or season to season. And the reason for this is that we've stopped listening to our inner voice. The reality is that we're afraid to take responsibility for the health of our minds and bodies, because we think, "**What do I know?**"

Everything I thought I knew about everything (including health and nutrition),changed when I started studying Ayurveda. Food was no exception.

By the time I started learning about Ayurveda, I'd been living my beliefs about food for decades. The relationship with food that I'd established at a young age was playing out in my mind, body, and choices. And my understanding of what's good, what's not so good, what's healthy, and what's not so healthy was, like many people growing up in the 80s and 90s, almost constantly being toppled and redefined by the latest scientific research.

So by the time I arrived at Ayurveda's door in my late thirties, I felt confused, disenfranchised and distrustful of the non-stop stream of new "wisdom" emerging from the world of wellness.

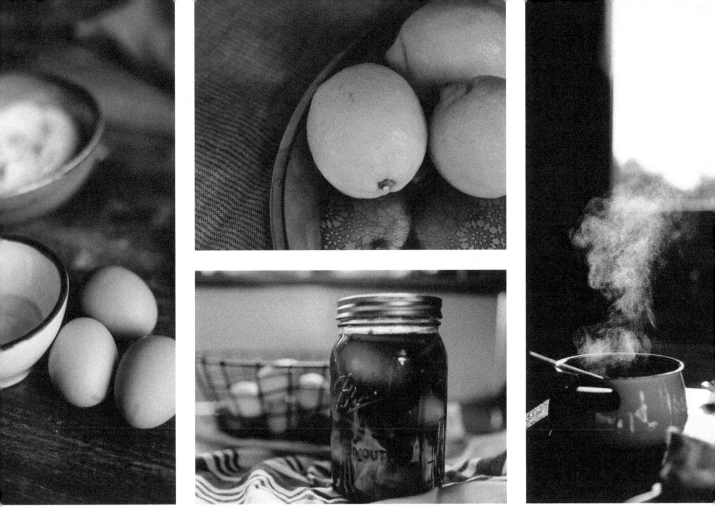

Ayurveda actually made things simple. And in a world of 24/7 news, endless social media, the exploding global marketplace, and more choices than anyone could ever need, the beautiful simplicity of the Ayurvedic approach to everything sang to me like a favorite tune on the radio.

The best part about it,though,was that as I began to follow it, I could feel its effects in my mind and body. And it became clear to me why it's endured, nearly unchanged, for these many thousands of years. Ayurveda feels like truth because it is.

So Ayurveda and I want you to understand that you know yourself better than anyone else ever could. You have the power to listen for and sense what you need. You can even feel if you've made the right choice. But like most people, you've probably lost the boldness that it takes to back yourself.

And that's why, more than anything else, eating like you love yourself requires courage. It asks us to make choices from a deep and dedicated connection to our own truth. And like anything that we approach in this heart-centered way, it rewards us for our trouble.

As someone who has struggled with food and had the priveledge of being a support to others in their struggles to know and love themselves, I've witnessed the emotional roller coaster that healthy eating has become -- the guilt, the excitement, the self-loathing, and the craving that food creates in our bodies and minds. And the many ways that it impacts our relationships and our interactions.

I want nothing more than for everyone to feel empowered about what they're eating, always. That joy that comes from cooking with love in your heart and eating with an even greater joy born from knowing that you're actually nourishing yourself on so many levels, I want that to replace the guilt and confusion that sometimes shows up before, during, or after the average meal eaten in or outside the home.

So my aim (and my dharma) is to educate and empower myself, my family, my community, and the world. I want people to understand that there's another way to do this food thing, one that feels good,but that no one is really talking about.

"Food is NOT the saviour." – Dr. Claudia Welch

Chapter 2
How to use this book...

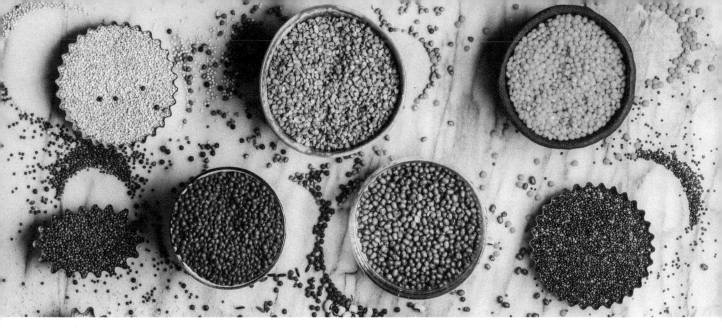

"The most creative act you will ever undertake is the act of creating yourself." – **Deepak Chopra**

A toolkit for taking inspired action

Ayurveda is an ancient, vast and beautiful science. Its wisdom spans the whole of life and living, and just like your mother-in-law, it's got advice to offer on just about every subject under the sun.

But our focus for this book is to **motivate, educate, and inspire** you to feed yourself, and those you love, in ways that will make it possible for you to experience what it feels like to be your best self.

So I've targeted the information in this book to achieve that goal and to leave you happier, healthier, more confident, and informed about yourself and the world around you. I've also created it as a handy, user-friendly reference of practical Ayurvedic wisdom including only what you need to know to seek balance in a way that is natural and individually you!

Inside this book you'll find...

- Recipes for healthy go-to meals that create mind body balance throughout the year and throughout your life!

- Guidelines for seasonal living and suggestions for how to incorporate self care and healthy eating into your day.

- Ayurvedic insights into some of your favorite ingredients and recipes for healing common issues with food.

- Lists and guidance for setting up your own Ayurvedic pantry and what to restock it with from season to season.

- Quizzes and questionnaires to help you discover your true nature and current states of mind- body balance.

- LIVE links and scannable QR codes to instantly connect you to video tutorials, further resources and the Eat Like You Love Yourself community.

Making sense of the recipes & information

The recipe section (Chapter 13) has been broken down by season and course (i.e. breakfast, lunch, dinner, etc.) to assist you in the process of planning for and creating balance throughout the year. Each recipe includes a few personal insights and guidance for how it can be used to manage the doshas, i.e. $\pm V \pm P \pm K$, where:

> "**-**" means, the recipe has a balancing effect on the dosha*
> "**+**" means the recipe has an aggravating effect on the dosha*
> "**=**" means the recipe has a neutral effect on the dosha.*
> *I'll explain what dosha means in further chapters.*

My hope is that this book will become a resource that you come back to again and again as your knowledge of yourself, and what works for YOU, comes to light and evolves. And that it will inspire you (as writing it has me) to honor and transform your relationship with yourself and the world around you, one meal at a time.

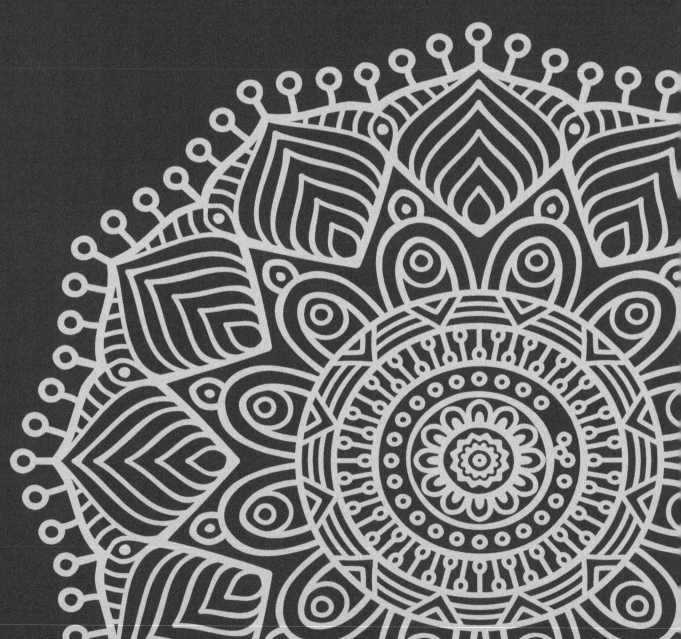

Chapter 3
Welcome to the World of Ayurveda...

"Ayurveda is about discovering what feeds you."
Chara Caruthers

Imagine for a moment life without judgment or criticism, where everything is simplified, clear and authentic. You recognize what makes you happy, sad, anxious, or blissful and why. You embrace everything about who you are and who you're not. You live in harmony with the environment around you, understanding and appreciating where you fit into it and how it changes. You accept that your health and happiness rely on your ability to see things as they truly are. You know your truth by how it feels and you live it. This is you + Ayurveda.

What IS Ayurveda?

Ayurveda is one of the oldest systems of health and healing in the world. At more than 5,000 years old, it is often referred to as the "Mother of all Medicine" and the "Science of Living." It comes from the same traditions as yoga so they're often called sister sciences, but the singular focus of Ayurveda is the health, healing, and rejuvenation of the mind and body.

Four simple principles of Ayurveda.

We are more than just a body being driven by a brain: Ayurveda recognizes that as individuals we're more than just a sack of muscles, bones, and organs. And as such there's more to being happy and healthy than how we eat and exercise. Ayurveda helps us to connect the dots between the way we move, eat, and think, our relationships, our environments and even our weather, and how we look, feel, and express ourselves in the world. It's all connected. Health is not a zero sum game, meaning eat this or exercise in this way and all will be well. There are many more pieces to the puzzle than we've been led to believe. Research into mindfulness techniques like meditation and things like epigenetics or the impacts of our environment on who we are support many of the principles of Ayurveda.

We change as the world around us changes: Have you ever noticed how the way you feel, think, and even the way your body looks changes throughout the year? Well, imagine a tree. They change quite a bit from season to season and not just the way they look on the outside. Even the way they metabolize and process nutrients, sunlight, and other environmental inputs changes slightly from winter, to spring, to summer. Things speed up and slow down and trigger other process and expressions. Ayurveda would say that we're the same. But as human beings capable of manipulating our environments, it can be easy to forget this simple, powerful truth.

We are completely unique: You've heard the quote "Comparison is the thief of joy"? If so, you've likely come to understand that comparison steals so much more than that! It takes our motivation, our enthusiasm, our self-worth and our sense of responsibility to ourselves, our communities, and those we love. One of the key principles of Ayurveda is that we are each unique, totally unique. We're made up of the same stuff, but our combination of it is completely unique to each individual. The implications of this are both simple and complex, but the simplest part to get your head around is that what works for someone else won't necessarily work for YOU and vice versa. In other words, even if your diet and exercise routine are exactly the same as that supermodel or rocket scientist, your mind, body, and experience of life, as a result, will be completely your own. There's something liberating and motivating about freeing yourself from the confines of comparison. And what it means is that the real focus, the only thing worth any of your time and energy is discovering and loving who YOU are, and forging your own unique path to what you want. Embracing this simple idea is the beginning of everything!

Prevention is the best medicine there is: According to the CDC (Centers For Disease Control)

> *"Chronic diseases and conditions such as heart disease, stroke, cancer, diabetes, obesity, and arthritis are among the most common, costly, and preventable of all health problems. Half of all American adults have at least one chronic condition, and almost one in three have multiple chronic conditions."*

We have the knowledge and insight to prevent the most common diseases and conditions. But our systems of medicine and health care emphasize treatment (or more correctly put "symptoms management") over prevention of illnesses in the first place. This is in part because prevention is far less lucrative (fear and money go hand in hand). And it's

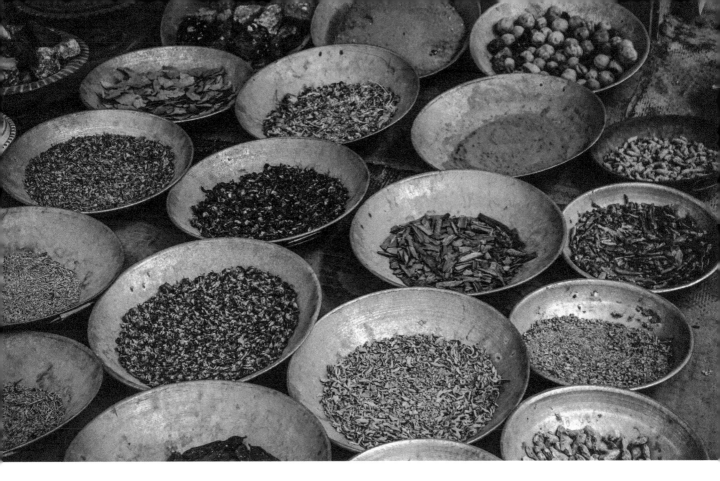

also because prevention involves something our culture finds uninspiring, unsexy, and in some cases totally unfathomable...personal responsibility and self love. I sum up the Ayurvedic view in this way: we have to love ourselves enough to be aware and take steps to create balance in our minds, bodies and lives before ANYTHING goes wrong, before we experience any pain or discomfort. Before diagnoses, blowups or meltdowns.

Why balanced living is a conversation

Ayurveda teaches us that everything we come into contact with has the potential to support or sabotage our well-being. Every idea, experience, interaction, emotion or piece of food or information is a single-dot point of reference that influences (in some small or not-so-small way) who you are and who you're able to be in the moment and beyond.

It's only when you can connect these dots, i.e. notice the effect that your last meal had on the quality of your skin, organs and digestion or the impact that your favorite song on the radio has on your mind, mood, or choices, that you can truly begin to influence your health and happiness in ways that are proactive, practical and sustainable (yay, no more yo-yo dieting or yo-yo living, for that matter).

The secret to owning your wellness

The bottom line is that Ayurveda recognizes the potential in everyone to live life to the fullest. And to that end, it is dedicated to increasing our awareness of the natural intelligence that we were born with, and how we can use it to create balance and harmony inside and out.

Because we each have our own unique path in life and are motivated, inspired, and transformed in different ways, the road to health and happiness will look different for everyone. There is no such thing as a "one size fits all approach" to wellness. And more than anything, Ayurveda wants us to embrace that..

What this means is that to apply and benefit from the wisdom of Ayurveda, you've got to create your own relationship with it! And that starts with a willingness (and curiosity) to know yourself and the world around you better.

Learning the language of self love...

Applying Ayurveda to your living, thinking, and eating can be a little like learning a new language. It gives you a framework for looking at things you've already known, loved or disliked for years (e.g. apples, oil, early mornings, spices), in ways that will reveal the truth about how you can interact with them to bring you happiness, energy, clarity and healing throughout the year and the rest of your life.

But one of the most powerful things to know about Ayurveda is that it wants us to understand and embrace change. In part, because it's change in some area of our lives that causes us to deviate from or abandon our healthy choices (anyone who's ever made a New Year's resolution knows this). And it's our conscious or subconscious resistance to change that defines or amplifies our struggle to maintain healthy weight, escape stress and overwhelm, build stronger bodies and relationships and ultimately live our bliss.

What's important to know and embrace (lovingly) is that change is the only thing in our lives that is constant. It is happening in every moment. In every second, we are being recreated as new people relative to the weather outside, the temperatures inside, the experiences we've had most recently, the relationships, and interactions that we're engaged in now and, of course. the food we've most recently eaten or are about to consume.

So, in many ways, Ayurveda is a language of self love that will help you understand and navigate the changes that are happening inside and outside of you,and inform your choices for food, exercise, self-care, and mindset along YOUR individual path to greatness.

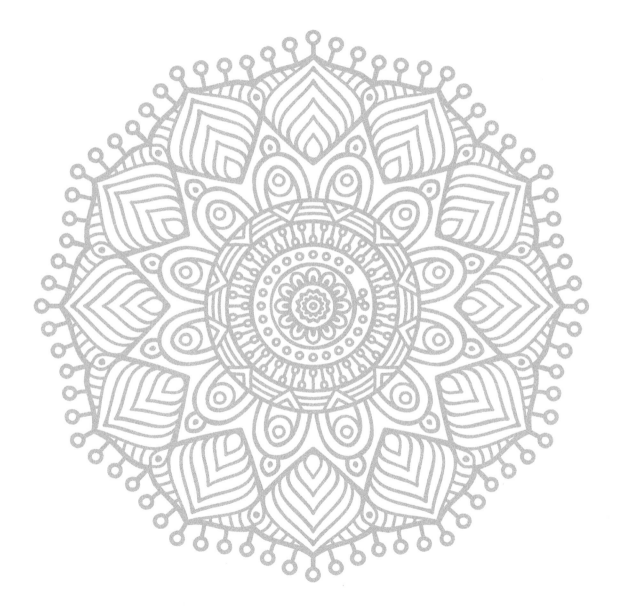

Chapter 4

Seeing your world through
Ayurveda-colored glasses...

"You are made of the same things as the stars...and your ham sandwich." – *Chara Caruthers*

In order to see ourselves, our world, and our food in the simplest and truest terms, Ayurveda suggests that we lift the veil of our thinking and tune into the qualities and energies that define our experience.

Ayurveda is often described as a science. Thinking about it in this way gives you a sense of the vastness and depth of its wisdom, but it can also make it seem more complicated and less accessible as a tool for everyday living than it is. In reality, as I mentioned in the previous chapter, Ayurveda is more like a language.

It provides a context to describe the physical, mental, and emotional interactions and experiences that define our current state of balance and our overall capacity for health and wellness. To do this, it simplifies how we see ourselves and everything around us, including our food, to give us a more clear understanding of how our choices impact the way we look, feel, and act. I've come to see the language of Ayurveda as a clear and simple expression of a truth that we're not always willing to embrace (because it means looking at ourselves honestly), but that will set us free.

Our elemental truth...

When it comes down to it, cooking is all about science. There are actions and reactions, mixtures, properties, and the application of qualities like heat, cold, moisture, and dryness to expand, contract, and transform.

Ayurveda reminds us that the same things occur within our minds and bodies in every moment of every day. So for many of us, cooking was our first foray into the beautiful chemistry that is who we are. And just like making a loaf of bread, understanding the constituent ingredients, and how they interact with each other, and their environment is the key to creating the most authentic and delicious expression of you.

Ayurveda makes it easy by teaching us that everything we experience (including ourselves and our food) is made up of just five ingredients, known as the five great elements (*panchamahabhutas* in Sanskrit): **space (ether), air, fire, water, and earth.**

SPACE: Is the container for everything. It's pure possibility and potential. It feels like stillness, freedom, awareness. It supports and fuels transformation by providing a place for the magic to happen.

Physically, space is present in the body wherever there is a cavity like in the nostrils, mouth, ears, throat, lungs, and stomach. Emotionally and psychologically, it represents awareness, intuition, presence, and acceptance.

The qualities of space are: Cold, light, dry, subtle, smooth, clear. Space is silent, infinite, and all-encompassing..

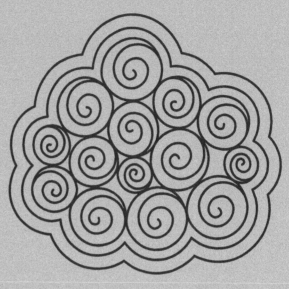

AIR: Is movement, expansion, and lightness. The breath in and out of the body, the opening and contraction of the muscles and the mind. Like wind, the element of air gives us rhythm, grace, mobility, and a sensation of mental and physical openness. Air fuels the body and stokes the fire of inspiration.

Physically, air is present in all movement in the body, including expansion, contraction, and suppression (e.g. lungs, heart and digestive tract). Emotionally and psychologically, it represents agility, clarity, wisdom, and dynamism.

The qualities of air are: Cold, dry, light, subtle, mobile, sharp, rough, clear. Air is expanding, drying, activating, moving, tightening.

FIRE: Is discipline, transformation, inspiration. The fire in our thinking and being is experienced as insight, intensity, and abundance. The processes of digestion and assimilation of food, ideas, thoughts, and emotions are driven by the fire (agni) inside each of our cells and nerve impulses.

Physically, fire is present in the metabolic activity of every cell, and is responsible for the warmth of the body. It is associated with our sense of sight so you'll also find fire in the light of the eyes and of intelligence. Emotionally and psychologically, it represents radiance, inspiration, vitality, exuberance, energy, and passion.

The qualities of fire are: Hot, dry, light, subtle, mobile, sharp, rough, clear. Fire is: heating, transforming, purifying, stimulating, expanding, intensifying.

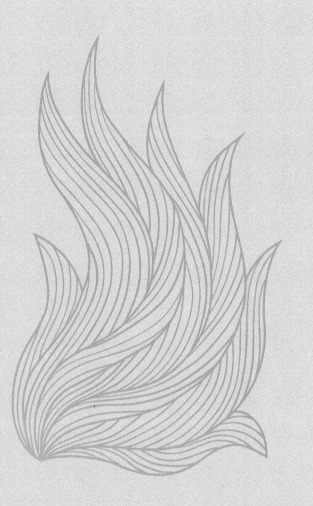

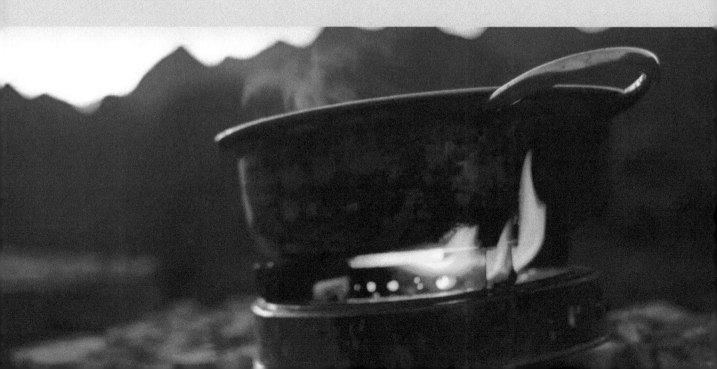

WATER: Is fluidity, connection, adaptability. It shows up in our ability to consciously hold on and let go at the same time. It fuels our thinking and being with compassion and resilience that return to us as fluid movement, supple muscles, agile minds.

Physically, water is present in the body in the fluids of life: plasma, blood, mucus, and saliva, urine, and sweat. It's associated with the sense of taste and makes tasting possible. Emotionally and psychologically, it represents fearlessness, sympathy, yielding, tranquility, and truth.

The qualities of water are: Cool, heavy, wet, soft, gross (as in touchable), smooth. Water is lubricating, softening, nourishing, cohesion, and stability.

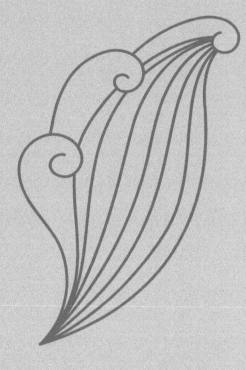

EARTH: Is home. It's structure, cohesion, foundation. It's the centered, grounded, and authentic expression of you (and everything around you). Earth is the sensation that we want to return to, the physical stillness that creates mental and emotional stillness (and vice versa).

Physically, earth represents all the solid structures within and around us: bones, flesh, skin, tissues, and hair. It is related to the sense of smell. Emotionally and psychologically it represents determination, patience, equanimity, stability and groundedness.

The qualities of earth are: Cold, dry, heavy, solid, hard, stable. Earth is form, stability, firmness, cohesion, maintaining, grounding and doing.

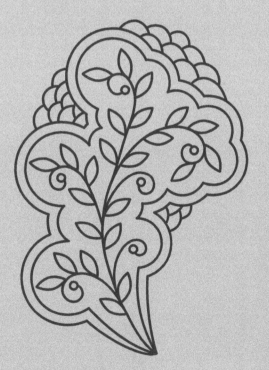

The most beautiful thing about these five elements, different to most of the elements on the periodic table, is that we have an immediate recognition of them. Over the course of our lives, as we've become familiar with ourselves and the world, we've created a relationship with all of them through our experiences of flying a kite on a windy day or feeling the breath in the body; the stinging, soothing warmth of the sun on your face or an open fire; the strong, soft, calming and cooling experience of being near the sea, or a cool drink on a warm day; the solid earth beneath your feet and yielding sand between your toes. Each element has qualities that impact us on all levels of our being and gives us clues about how to interact with it in healthy ways that support who we are.

Ayurveda-colored glasses...

In a world of ever-increasing complexity, it's nice to be able to cut through the clouds of misinformation and confusion and see things for what they truly are. Ayurveda gives us that gift by inviting us to notice and embrace the simple truth in everything (ourselves, our food, our weather, our loved ones).

Seeing your food, for example, stripped of the layers of judgement, cultural conditioning, media messaging, self-limiting beliefs, anxiety, and fear creates a kind of clarity that makes choosing between an apple and a slice of apple pie a la mode SO much easier. One is light, dry, cold, and clarifying; the other is warm, moist, heavy and grounding. Knowing which one is healthiest on any given day will come down to recognizing these qualities and how they can be used as a tool to resolve the challenges you're facing.

I call this wearing your "Ayurveda-colored glasses," and Ayurveda gives us the code to doing this by identifying a set of twenty attributes, qualities, or gunas (in Sanskrit) that can be applied to the things we see and interact with.

Ayurveda glasses strip away the pretense and give us the ability to see the reality of the things we surround ourselves with, allowing us to make clear, powerful and compassionate choices to engage with what nourishes and balances us.

The Gunas: The personality of everything!

The qualities of matter (or *gunas* in Sanskrit) are a simple shorthand for understanding your relationship with everything! Each can be recognized in some part of your everyday experience and each has an action (karma) or impact on you physically, mentally, or emotionally.

There are twenty gunas; ten sets of opposite physical qualities that can very simply define or characterize our mental, emotional, or sensory (physical) experience. They are:

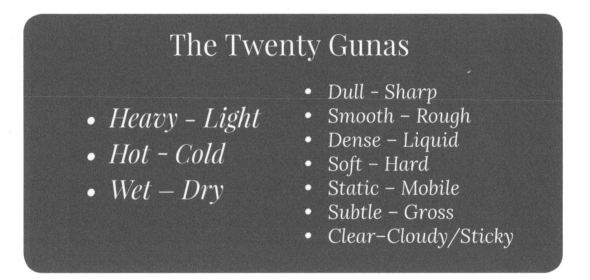

The Twenty Gunas

- *Heavy – Light*
- *Hot – Cold*
- *Wet – Dry*

- *Dull – Sharp*
- *Smooth – Rough*
- *Dense – Liquid*
- *Soft – Hard*
- *Static – Mobile*
- *Subtle – Gross*
- *Clear–Cloudy/Sticky*

But the good news is that for the most part (and for the purposes of the rest of this book), we can focus our attention on just six qualities on the left: the first three sets of opposites, known as the **upakarmas**. These are the primary qualities used to describe energetics, temperature, moisture, and weight, something most people are pretty familiar with.

To give you a sense for the power and reach of these qualities, check out the table below for some examples of how you might experience them in your everyday living. What does your world look like through the lens of Ayurvedic glasses? How would you use these attributes to characterize your thoughts, emotions and physical sensations?

Check out the charts in the appendix for a breakdown of the qualities of your favorite foods.

The Twenty Gunas (Qualities)

Quality (Guna)	Action (Karma)	Thing/Object	Food	Emotion
Heavy (Guru)	Adds weight, builds tissues, condenses, stabilizes,	boulder, water	yogurt, meat, cheese, sugar, oil	sadness, groundedness, stability
Light (Lagu)	lightens,catabolic, activates, easy to digest	feather, wind	popcorn, rice, ginger, coffee	fear, insecurity, anxiety
Hot (Ushna)	heats, stimulates, activates, expanding	fire, acid, radiation, sunlight	chili pepper, alcohol, eggs	anger, envy, irritability
Cold (Shita)	cools, calms, reduces, slows digestion	snowflake, rock, water	mint, wheat, milk	fear, insensitivity, consciousness
Wet/Moist/Oily (snigdha)	moistens, nourishes, fills, lubricates	nuts, oil, water	oil ,cheese, avocado	love, compassion
Dry (Ruksha)	dehydrates, tightens, tones, constipates	fire, wind	quinoa, rye, dry cereal, crackers, popcorn	Isolation, separation, rejection, lonelines
Dull (Manda)	slows, impedes, calms, stabilizes	mud, mucus,	tofu, yogurt, meat	calm, relaxed, sluggishness
Sharp (Tikshna)	quickens, intensifies, stimulates,	light, laser, glass	peppers, ginger, mustard, coffee	intelligence, inspiration, contempt, condescension, hate.
Slimy/Smooth (Shlakshna)	lubricates, moistens, calms, eases roughness, binds	flower, glass, silk	oil, ghee, yogurt	satisfaction, maliciousness
Rough (Khara)	dries, dehydrates, makes brittle, scrapes/scratches	tree bark, sand	salad, popcorn, raw veggies	insensitivity, indifference

Quality (Guna)	Action (Karma)	Thing/Object	Food	Emotion
Dense (Sandra)	strengthens, difficult to digest, increases mental resolve	gold, rubber, wood	meat, cheese, tofu	strong, grounded
Liquid (Drava)	binds, lubricates, moistens	lava, saliva, tears	juices, water, milk	compassion, cohesiveness
Soft (Mrudu)	calms, pacifies, reduces hardness/ roughness	flower, skin, water	avocado, ghee, oils	love, tenderness, relaxation
Hard (Kathina)	strengthens, difficult to digest, stabilizes	macadamia nut shell, rock	coconut, almonds	selfishness, rigidity, insensitivity
Stable/static (Sthira)	relaxes, slows, dulls	elephant, tree	ghee, dry grains, dry beans	supportive, stability, healing
Mobile, moving (Chala)	moves, releases	river, wind,	spices, alcohol, oil	restlessness, insecurity, thoughts and feelings
Subtle (Sukshma)	expands, penetrates deep, increases awareness	smoke, steam	ghee, honey, alcohol	spaciness, disconnected, sensitivity
Gross, obvious (Sthula)	difficult to digest, obstructs. slows	rock, elephant	mushrooms, meat, cheese	dull, stubborn, ignorance, complacency
Clear (Vishada)	clarifies, lightens	glass, air, water	freshwater, algae, veggie juice, sprouts, sprouted beans	clarity, confidence, joy, openness
Sticky, Cloudy (Picchila)	heals breaks, binds, reduces clarity	mud, mucus	yogurt, cheese, porridge oats, honey	cohesiveness, unclear, confusion.

"Balance is not something you find, it's something you create" — Jana Kingsford

A formula for creaing balance

Ayurveda says it's important to think about these qualities as you interact with the world, your meals, the things around you, your thoughts, the way you carry yourself. How are these characteristics reflected in the way you live?

We are constantly affected by changes in these qualities both in and around us.

- We change from warm to cold depending on things like the weather, which changes from cloudy to clear to dry.
- We enjoy foods that are oily or rough, which has an impact on how we feel physically or mentally.

The qualities work together in a way that helps us to understand one of THE most important functional principle of Ayurveda; the concept of "Like Increasing Like" and opposites balancing each other.

In order to illustrate this idea, I want you to imagine a spectrum or a line drawn on the ground in chalk.. At one end of the line, imagine you see the word "HOT" and at the other end of the line you see the word "COLD".

At the very center point of the line is a bucket of water. If you dip your finger into the water, you'll notice that it is room temperature, which represents balance between the extremes of hot and cold,

If you were asked to decrease the water's temperature or move it closer to the cold end of the line, you might add something with cold qualities (ice, cold water, etc.), right? The opposite would be true if you were asked to increase the water's temperature. You'd add something hot (hot water, a hot rock, heat from the sun, etc.)

Alternately, if you were dealing with something more extreme, say a bucket of boiling hot water, and needed to cool it down, you'd counter that heat and bring down the temperature by adding something cold or cooler to the water.

This is a simple illustration of the Ayurvedic principle of "Like Increases Like", adding hot to something that's already hot or warm increases the intensity and impact of heat, and moves you closer to an extreme condition of that quality. This same principle applies to all of the gunas: cold, light, heavy, wet, etc.

In the Ayurvedic view, imbalance results from an accumulation or increase of a particular quality or qualities. For example, an increase or buildup of heat in your system, perhaps caused by eating hot chillies, out in the desert, on the hottest day of the year, dressed in a sweater, might show up as anger, inflammation, or diarrhea among other things, because all are symptoms of an excess of heat in the body-mind.

The good news, though, is that we have the power of opposites to balance out the extremes, which means that introducing cold or cooling qualities to something that is hot can move the system or situation closer to a more balanced middle ground and away from the "danger zones" of imbalance.

These are simple and SUPER important concepts to understand and embrace. They form the basis of how Ayurveda can work in your life to help you manage or avoid the imbalances that can lead to illness and disease. They also give you simple insights into how you can blend the qualities of you with the qualities of your food and environment to create an experience of wellness and bliss. .

"We live as ripples of energy in the vast ocean of energy." – **Deepak Chopra**

The doshas - energies of living

The five elements (***panchamahabhutas***) and the twenty gunas are tools to help us understand and experience our material existence. But when you look at a human body, it's not difficult to see that there's A LOT going on. In any given moment within your body, there are countless processes that define the way:

· Matter moves from place to place;
· Physical matter is held together together and broken down;
· Physical matter is rebuilt, cushioned, assimilated and transformed,

and that's just within the walls of a single cell.

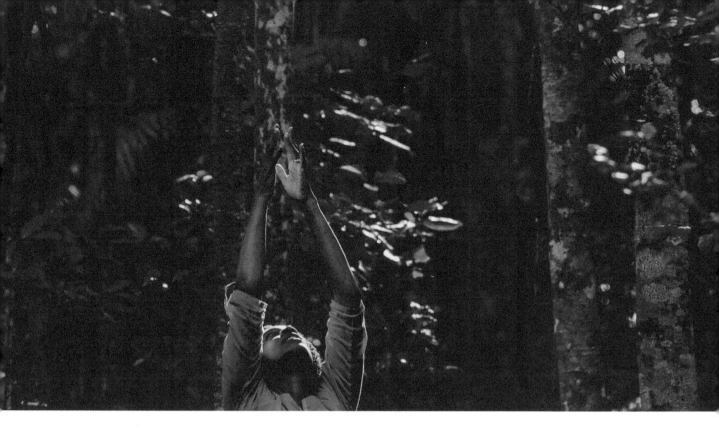

Ayurveda isn't alone in understanding that there's a natural **intelligence that controls all of that.** A form of energy that:

- Moves blood in the veins, converts food into nutrition and nutrition into organs, skin and bones.
- Directs the formation of tissues and fluids to lubricate and cushion our entire bodies from the brain down to the toes.
- Builds us from the inside out, directing the cells to form a wide or thin nose, long or short legs, sharp wit or quiet demeanor.

Ayurveda holds that there are three specific energies that generate these functions within living things. They're commonly referred to as "**Doshas**", a Sanskrit word that means "something that can become imbalanced". The names given to them are: vata, pitta, and kapha. Each is governed by a different combination of the five elements and each serves a different function within the mind and body.

VATA IS... *The energy of movement*

- Combination of Air and space
- All the movement in the body – blood, nerve impulses moving back and forth from the brain, peristalsis, muscle movements – all part of the intelligence of Vata.
- Dry, light, cold, rough, subtle, mobile, clear

PITTA IS... *The energy of transformation, metabolization*

- Combination of fire and water
- All metabolic processes from within each cell to the processes of digestion. Anything to do with heat from body temperature to the function of the sweat glands. It governs hunger, thirst, the quality of skin and visual perception.
- Hot, sharp, light, liquid, mobile, oily/wet

KAPHA IS... *The energy of lubrication, structure and cohesion*

- Combination of earth and water
- Kapha holds the body together. It gives shape and form, governs growth and development, lubricates and protects from the synovial fluid in the joints to the mucus that lines the inside of the body.
- Heavy, slow/dull, cold, oily, liquid, smooth, dense, soft, static, sticky, hard

The Ayurvedic view is that the energies of vata, pitta, and kapha build and run our bodies. They govern the biological and psychological processes of the body, mind, and consciousness, inhabiting the mind in the form of thoughts and ways of thinking and defining everything about our physical appearance and experience, from height and weight to hair color and shoe size. The doshas influence all we are and all we do, and they all exist in all living things.

And **for every living thing, the combination of doshas is completely unique**. My combination of vata, pitta ,and kapha energies is completely different from yours. Your combination of doshas is entirely different to that of anyone else. So even though we are all made up of the exact same stuff, the way you consume, break down, and assimilate food, information, ideas, emotions, nutrients, and experiences is completely unique to you.

We'll dive deeper into the doshas in the next chapter as we explore the Ayurvedic view of what it means to be YOU. But before we do that, I want to introduce you to the tastiest, and arguably most relevant, principle of Ayurveda for this book.

The Six Tastes

In addition to the five elements and twenty gunas, Ayurveda has provided another set of tools designed specifically to help us gain more clarity around our relationship with the foods, herbs, and minerals we consume. The six tastes are a set of attributes that interact specifically with our sense of taste. The help us understand (and experience) the connection between the flavor of our foods (something we're intimately connected with) and the impact it has on our minds and bodies.

Each of the six tastes represents a combination of two of the five elements from which it borrows qualities like hot, cold, light, etc. Understanding these qualities gives us an immediate recognition of how the flavor of food translates to its actions in the mind and body (for example, foods with hot qualities warm and stimulate the mind and body), and more importantly, how our food can be applied as a balancing force to deepen or restore our experience of wholeness.

In my mind, the most beautiful thing about the six tastes is that we know them. From the moment we first tasted the nourishing sweetness of mother's milk, we've built a relationship with **sweet, sour, salty, pungent, bitter, and astringent** that has unconsciously driven every food choice we've made since. Now it's time to discover why.

Doing so will empower us to see the mental and emotional relationship we have with our food more clearly. It will give us the ability to understand, by the way something tastes, how it can impact our experience and state of balance. And, most importantly it will help us to transcend some of the cultural conditioning and mindlessness that unconsciously drives us to choose comfort instead wellness.

The foundation of food as medicine

Wouldn't it be great to intuitively know the best things to eat when you're feeling tired and overwhelmed, or energized and strong, to restore or maintain your well-being? The six tastes are the basis for empowering that ability. Besides flavor, each of the tastes refers to the action of a substance on/in the body-mind. They give you an understanding of how the foods you eat affect the state of your mind and body. Check out the chart below to see what I mean.

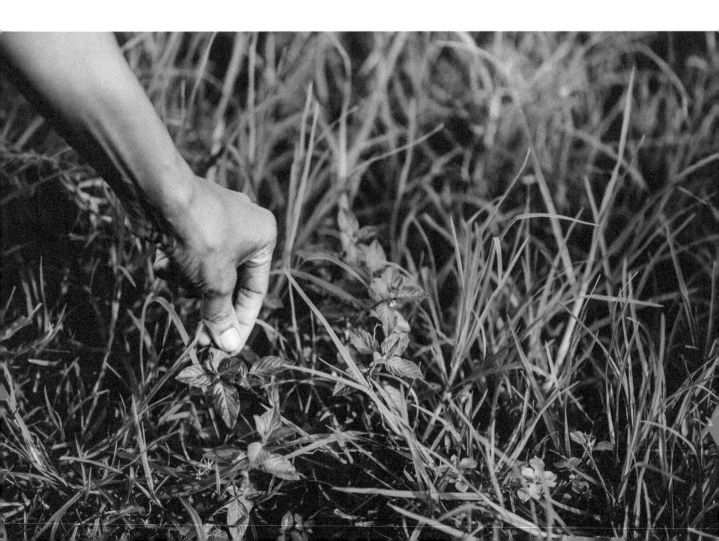

Taste	Qualities	Actions	In excess
Sweet (Madhura)	cold, heavy, wet	builds, strengthens, moistens, calms	slows digestion. promotes heaviness, congestion, mucus, toxins, fungal infections
Sour (Amla)	hot, wet, light	moistens, retains moisture in tissues, stimulates digestion, awakens the mind	increases heat and mucus, aggravates skin and blood issues
Salty (Lavana)	hot, heavy, wet	clears channels, soothes nerves, moistens, stimulates appetite, secretions	irritates digestive tract, increases congestion, water retention, emetic
Pungent (Katu)	hot, light, dry	stimulates digestion and blood flow, dries up fluid and mucus, clears blockages in channels	increases/ aggravates inflammation, dehydration/thirst, reproductive issues.
Bitter (Tikta)	cold, light, dry	cools, promotes bile secretion, stimulates nervous system, clears toxins, parasites, blockages	promotes constipation, excessive dryness, inhibits digestion, dries digestive tract, weakens kidneys, increases anxiety, promotes fatigue, decreased immunity
Astringent (Kashay)	Cold, heavy, dry	dries mucus/fluids, slows appetite, decreases coughs, heals wounds, stops bleeding, tightens tissues	promotes gas, constipation, impairs digestion

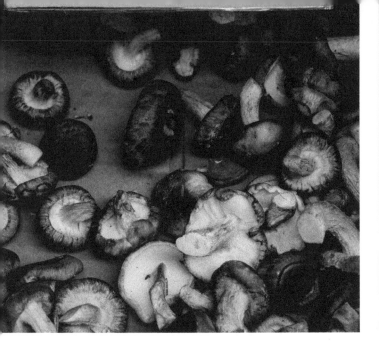
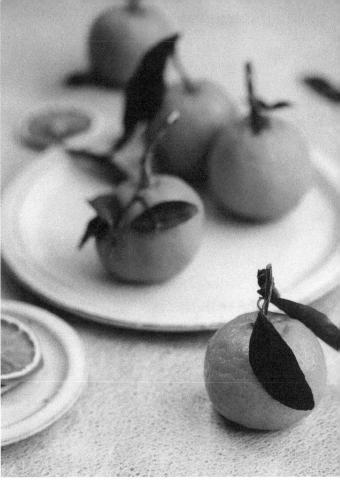
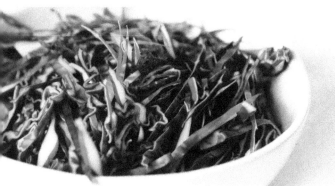
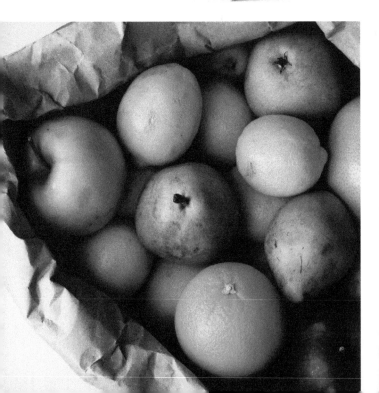
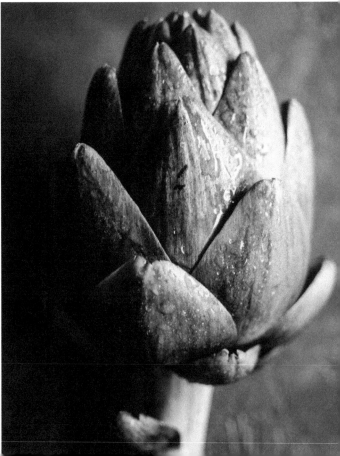

SWEET

Sweet is the taste of love. The first and most desired taste, it is as familiar to every one of us as the feeling of being in our own skin. A ripe mango, a freshly cut, rich and creamy avocado, and even a cool drink of fresh water all have a sweetness that satisfies our deepest need for wholeness.

The sanskrit word for sweet taste is "*madhura*." It is a combination of the earth and water elements. and has **cold, heavy, and moist qualities**. It can be found in fruit sugars, carbohydrates, proteins, and fats.

The sweet taste nourishes, builds and strengthens the body. It also calms the mind, which is a big part of the reason why we might choose a warm slice of apple pie over a salad when we're feeling anxious or in need of calming.

The sweet taste is a predominant quality of most of the foods we eat and can be found in things like grains, root vegetables, fruits, dairy, meats, fish, sugars, and honey. On a subtle level, sweet helps to bolster our vitality and replenish the vital essence of "**ojas**" (a substance that is the subtle essence of vitality), which regulates immunity.

Sweet promotes an experience of love, satisfaction and well-,being. It alleviates the dry lightness that can result in anxiety and cools the heat of anger and aggravation. Overconsumption of sweet foods can result in heaviness, lethargy, depression and an increase in issues like colds, coughs, congestion, and mucus formation. An excess of the sweet taste can also give rise to cravings and greed.

The sweet taste is balancing for vata and pitta dosha but can create an imbalance of kapha dosha. So if you, or someone you know, is suffering from too much heat, dryness, and/or lightness, sweet-tasting foods and herbs could provide an antidote, but it should be avoided in the case of congestion, heaviness, and slow digestion.

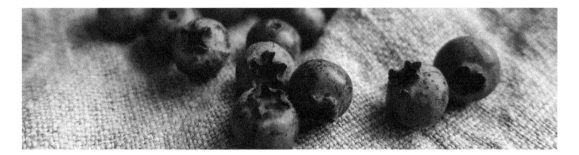

SOUR

Can you imagine the experience and taste of a lemon? That stinging, watery brightness that leaves you hanging in the space between turning away and asking for more, and then you ask for more. This is sour.

Sour, or "*amla*," as it's known in Sanskrit, is a combination of earth and fire elements. It's a predominant taste of citrus fruits, tomatoes, pickles, and fermented food and beverages like wine, cheese, yogurt and sauerkraut.

The sour taste is moderately light, warming, and moist and has that effect on the mind and body. It sharpens the mind and senses and has a cleansing effect on the tissues. It stimulates the appetite and increases the body's ability to absorb minerals.

One of the most important actions of the sour taste is as a digestive. It activates the secretion of saliva and digestive enzymes and stimulates the metabolism. It strengthens the heart, is nourishing to the tissues, and supports healthy liver function.

Sour has moistening and warming qualities that make it a wonderful antidote for cold, dry imbalances like constipation and anxiety. But its lightness and heating nature can create or further aggravate issues that are associated with an excess of heat in the body like diarrhea, psoriasis, or inflammation. In excess, sour can intensify kapha issues like water retention, congestion, cough, and edema. It can also contribute to hyperacidity, dizziness, ulcers, envy, and resentment.

Sour helps increase the flow of bile, which aids in the digestion of fats. Sour fruits are high in vitamin C and tend to be antioxidant, rejuvenating tonics.

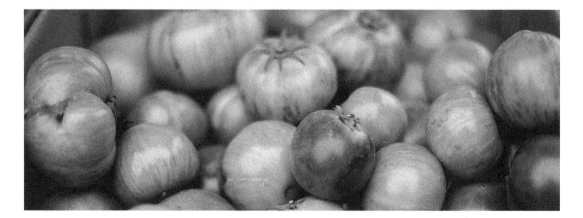

SALTY

The fresh, biting, briny taste of an oyster plucked from the sea brings us back to the very origins of life. The oldest and most perfect flavor enhancer there is, salt awakens and connects us with the promise of what's possible. It's one of the most grounding of the six tastes.

Lavana (*La-vah-nah*), the Sanskrit word for salty, can also be translated to mean "beautiful". Salty is a combination of the water and fire elements and can be found predominantly in sea vegetables (seaweeds), ocean fish and shellfish, sea and mineral salts, soy sauce and vegetables like celery.

Similar to sour, the salty taste stimulates digestion and lubricates and moistens the tissues. It has a soothing effect that calms the nerves and relieves anxiety. As a stimulant, it helps to energize the mind and body, clear and cleanse the channels, and counteract dullness and dryness in the muscles, joints, and attitude.

Used in moderation, it enhances the flavor of foods, but in excess it can raise blood pressure, aggravate skin conditions, promote water retention, and increase pitta conditions like hair loss, hyperacidity, ulcers, and inflammation.

Of all the different forms of salt, the most utilized and revered in Ayurveda is "Himalayan Pink Salt" (*saindhava*), often referred to as rock salt. Different to other salts, it has cooling properties. It's also high in minerals and doesn't cause water retention.

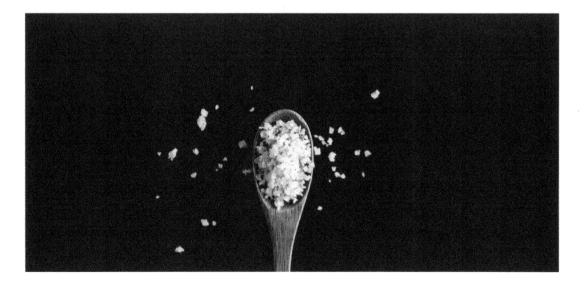

PUNGENT

If you've ever partaken of the fiery, soul permeating effect of fresh wasabi paste or the clarifying sting of a spoonful of Tom Yum soup, you'll have no doubt that these are mind opening, and altering experiences. They are also examples of the power of pungent.

The pungent taste, known as **katu** (*KA-Too*) in Sanskrit, is a combination of fire and air. It is the hottest of the heating tastes, is both dry and light, and can be found in foods like ginger, onions, radishes, chillies, and many herbs and spices.

Pungent has a stimulating effect on the mind, tissues and digestive system. It warms the body, cleanses and clears the mouth and channels, and is one of the most important tastes for supporting detoxification, reducing cholesterol, and eliminating fats from the body. The pungent taste has an invigorating sharpness that penetrates and dries congestion, excess moisture and stagnation.

An excess of the pungent taste can set the mind and body on fire, leading to issues associated with dryness and depletion of tissues (excess vata) like fatigue, constipation, insomnia and heat related (pitta excess) challenges like anger or rage, ulcers, inflammation, diarrhea, and heartburn.

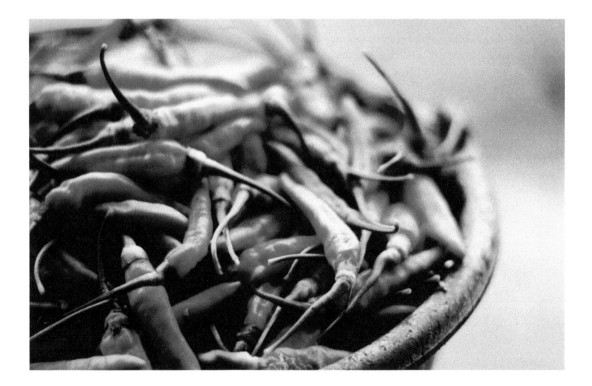

BITTER

Like many "grown up" kids, eating my greens is burned into my memory as one of the lowlights of an otherwise happy childhood, surpassed only by the traumatizing experience of taking medicine. Both have always been met with a cold dread that has lingered, but softened somewhat, into adulthood. Both are my most vivid experiences of the effect of bitter.

Bitter, or *tikta* (*TEEk - Ta,*) as it's known in Sanskrit, is a combination of the space and air elements and has dry, light, and cold qualities. It's a powerful medicinal taste that has detoxifying, antibiotic, and antiseptic properties. And it's most often found in dark leafy greens like kale, dandelion, and spinach, cruciferous veggies like broccoli and cauliflower, foods like beets, coffee, olives, and eggplant, and many healing spices including turmeric.

Being light and rough in nature, the bitter taste increases lightness in the mind and body by scraping away fat, toxins, and congestion. As one of the most cooling tastes, it's great for removing heat (inflammation, infection from the body). It's also a wonderful blood purifier, liver tonic, and digestive stimulant. And if that weren't enough, bitter is brilliant for toning the muscles and skin.

An excess of the dry, light qualities of the bitter taste can dry out the organs and tissues and weaken the bones. It can cause light-headedness or dizziness, constipation and weakness. Too much bitter in the diet can lead to sadness and create an experience of feeling disconnected, ungrounded, or spaced out!

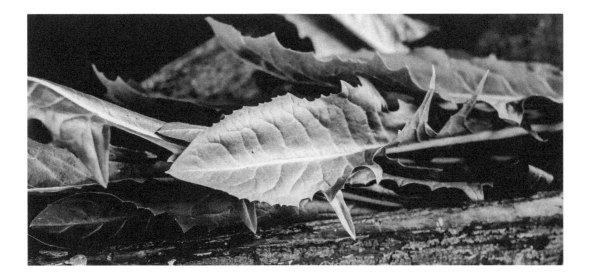

ASTRINGENT

More than a taste, astringent is a very subtle sensation -- the experience of dryness in the mouth when eating a green apple or piece of cucumber, or the more noticeable mouth and body drying experience of red wine. This is what astringent feels like.

The Sanskrit word for astringent is **kashay** (*KAH-shy*). It is a combination of the earth and air elements and has cold, heavy, and dry qualities. Now that you're aware of it, you'll probably start to notice it everywhere! So besides the foods I've already mentioned, you can also experience the astringent taste when eating beans and lentils, cruciferous veggies like broccoli and cauliflower, pomegranates, cranberries, pears, and many herbs and spices.

The astringent taste acts like a sponge, absorbing and drying excess liquids in the body (water, fat, mucus, etc.). It's an important taste in the process of cleansing and detoxification and can improve absorption of minerals and nutrients. Its drying effects are also quite useful in healing wounds, tightening skin, and alleviating diarrhea. But excessive amounts of this cold, heavy taste can slow digestion and elimination, dry out the mouth and eyes and promote gas and bloating. The drying nature of astringent can lead to feeling mentally and emotionally "dry" and without passion, joy, and juiciness!

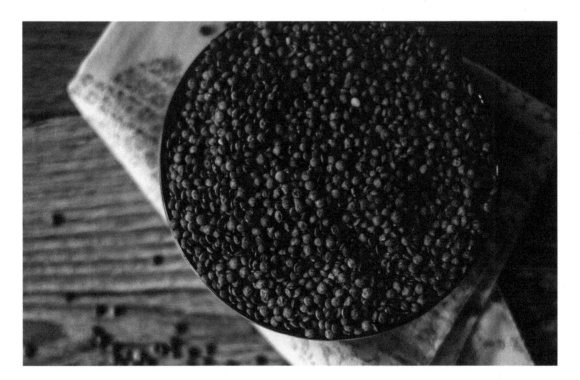

The Six Tastes in your everyday

Every day we come into contact with each of these tastes through our experience with a variety of foods, herbs, spices, minerals ,and even gems and emotions. And given what you now know about each of the tastes and their effects, you can now more clearly tune in to the impacts they have on YOUR energy and state of balance.

Each of the six tastes is associated with certain chemicals, nutrients, and emotions that the mind and body require in order to create an experience of wholeness and well-being:

- **Sweet**: carbohydrates, sugars, fats, amino acids
- **Sour**: organic acids
- **Salty**: salts
- **Pungent**: volatile oils
- **Bitter**: alkaloids, glycosides
- **Astringent**: tannins

Because of this, we say that it's vitally important to include each of the Six Tastes in every meal to ensure that we're eating in a balanced and balancing way. The easiest way to do this, according to Dr. Deepak Chopra, is to fill our plates with a selection of colors from the rainbow and add to the balancing qualities of your meals by using spices!

Now is also the time to consider the power you have to influence your physical, mental and emotional experience through taste.

What does your current diet taste like? What are the predominant tastes that you're eating everyday and how is that showing up in the way that you look, feel, and experience yourself and your wellness?

How can you build a more powerful relationship with the Six Tastes that will fuel your mind, body, and greatness?

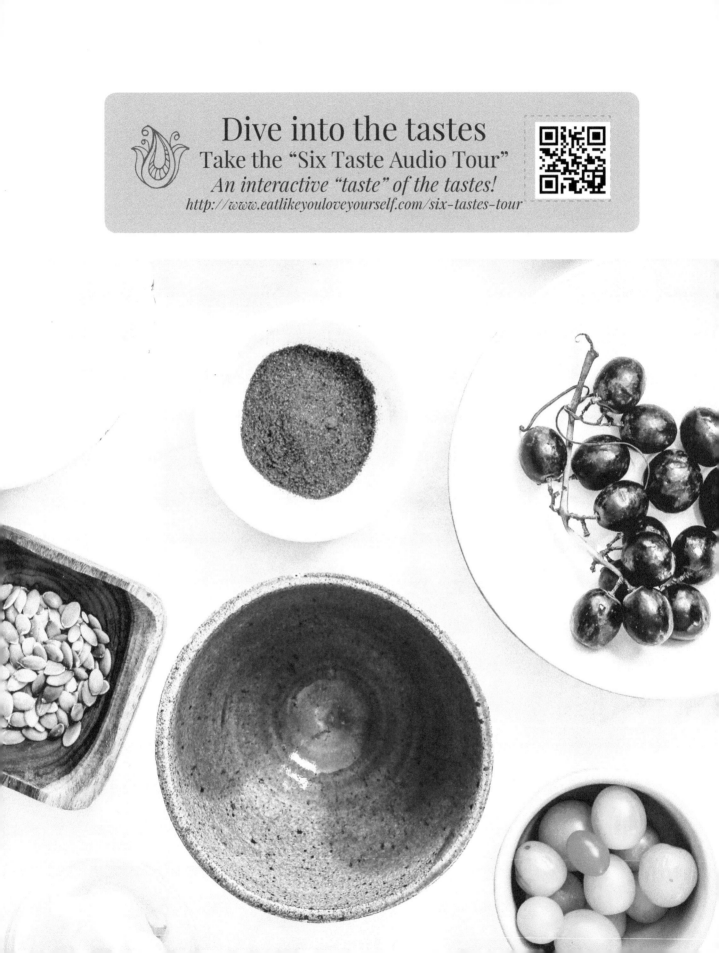

Dive into the tastes
Take the "Six Taste Audio Tour"
An interactive "taste" of the tastes!
http://www.eatlikeyouloveyourself.com/six-tastes-tour

Eating for balance & bliss: THE SIX TASTES OF AYURVEDA

TASTE	ACTIONS	FOODS & SPICES	EFFECTS ON DOSHAS	EFFECTS ON EMOTIONS
Sweet Earth + Water Cold, Heavy, Moist	**Builds, Strengthens, Energizes, Calms the mind.**	Grains, pasta, rice, bread, starchy vegetables, dairy, meat, chicken, fish, sugar, honey, molasses	**Balances:** Vata, Pitta **Aggravates:** Kapha	Promotes love and satisfaction in all **Vata:** Calms anxiety **Pitta:** Cools anger/aggravation In excess: Lethargy, attachment
Sour Earth + Fire Hot, Light, Moist	**Awakens the mind and senses, cleanses tissues, increases absorption of minerals.**	Citrus fruits, berries, tomatoes, pickled foods, sour fruits (cherries, plums, grapes, apples), passion fruits, spinach, chard, yogurt, cheese, sour cream, vinegar, sauerkraut, wine	**Balances:** Vata **Aggravates:** Kapha, Pitta	**Vata:** Sharpens the mind **Pitta:** Increases irritation, anger, manipulative, critical thinking/behavior **Kapha:** In excess creates envy or jealousy
Salty Fire + Water Hot, Heavy, Moist	**Stimulates digestion, lubricates tissues, calms nerves, relieves anxiety.**	Table salt, sea salt, rock salt, soy sauce, salted meats, ocean fish, shellfish	**Balances:** Vata **Aggravates:** Kapha, Pitta	**Vata:** calms anxiety **Pitta:** Stimulates the mind **Kapha:** In excess promotes greed.
Pungent Fire + Air Hot, Light, Dry	**Heating, drying, stimulates digestion/ metabolism, opens the mind.**	Peppers, chilies, onions, garlic, cayenne, black pepper, cloves, ginger, mustard, cumin, cloves, cardamom, turmeric, anise, cinnamon, oregano, thyme, mint, radish	**Balances:** Kapha **Aggravates:** Vata, Pitta	Stimulates all to be more expressive & extroverted **Kapha:** Enlivens the mind **Pitta:** Excites anger, irritability, resentment
Bitter Air+ Space Cold, Light, Dry	**Cleanses, detoxifies tissues, Increases lightness in the mind, antiseptic, antibiotic.**	Green leafy vegetables, green and yellow vegetables, kale, celery, spinach, cabbage, broccoli, sprouts, beets, zucchini, eggplant, turmeric, fenugreek, dandelion root, olives, bitter melon, coffee	**Balances:** Kapha, Pitta **Aggravates:** Vata	**Vata:** In excess promotes grief and depression. **Pitta:** Cools/Calms anger, irritation **Kapha:** Clears foggy mind
Astringent Air + Earth Cold, Heavy, Dry	**Cools, absorbs water, tightens tissues, promotes healing.**	Lentils, beans, grains (rye, buckwheat, quinoa), green apples, cauliflower, broccoli, artichoke, asparagus, turnips, pomegranates, cranberries, pears, dried fruits, turmeric, coffee, tea	**Balances:** Kapha, Pitta **Aggravates:** Vata	**Vata:** In excess promotes fear and insecurity. **Pitta:** Calms arrogance/ Over-confidence **Kapha:** Stops complacency

Chapter 5

Ayurveda and YOU...

"The essence of you is what's capable of lighting up the world AND figuring out what to have for dinner." – **Chara Caruthers**

Understanding how to eat like you love yourself doesn't start with investigating the nutrient content of foods or the optimal combination of daily recommended vitamins and minerals required for the average human being. It doesn't even begin with knowing about the nutritional composition of foods and amounts of proteins, sugars, carbohydrates, and fats in every bite.

Ayurveda says that awareness is our greatest tool for creating genuine health and wellness, and it starts with turning the light inward. Our natural state is a calm, vibrant resilience that reflects balance within and without. And our daily journey is to find our way back to that state of balance. With this in mind, it's easier to understand (and embrace) the simple fact that eating like you love yourself STARTS (and ends) with KNOWING yourself.

So finding the food that feeds your body and soul starts with asking yourself a simple (or not so simple) question -- who are you?

Why who you are matters...

"Who are you?" It might seem like a big question, one that you may never fully have an answer to. That's okay, because the point is NOT to define yourself in any fixed way; it's to acknowledge that who you are can in many ways depend on where you are, when you are, and of course...what you're feeding yourself.

What makes this question so challenging to answer is the fact that we change. If living is a dance with the world around us, we must expand, contract, soften, and intensify our physical, mental, and emotional presence as our environment heats up, cools down, and transforms in its own unique ways. Each and every way we respond defines who we are (and what we need) in the moment.

And if we want to maintain our footing and connection to our best selves, we have to be willing to tune in to the prevailing internal and external states of change and use our deepest inner knowing to make choices that will keep us happily on our feet.

Ayurveda recognizes a number of factors, including your constitution, your state of mind, your season, and your environment, that will determine whether the meal you're eating can actually be considered "healthy" for you.

It sounds like a radical concept in the context of the way most people (including the health and wellness industry) approach diet. But given that diet and lifestyle related diseases are at nearly epidemic proportions around the globe, knowing ourselves a little better, which requires us to seize responsibility for our wellness back from the industries that are profiting from our lack of it, might just be the best place to start.

The Ayurvedic model of you

As an a approach to health and healing, Ayurveda is different to the modern Western medical view that we've all grown up with in a few key ways.

Our Western medical system sees you as a combination of a physical body plus a set of electrical impulses that function to form your mind. We don't know a whole lot more than that, but we're trying to. But the Ayurvedic view of who you are is a bit more expanded. It sees you as a soul plus a mind plus a body plus senses.

Your soul is the center of who you are... It is your individual piece of the natural intelligence that exists all around you. It's your connection to everything. Ayurveda holds that this intelligence seeks health and happiness, the most authentic expression of who you are. It understands your individual path to get there and will give you clues to keep you on that path if you're willing to listen. We commonly refer to it as our intuition. And cultivating a stronger relationship with it, through knowing yourself, is really the key to having everything we want (including a fabulous dinner!).

Your mind calls the shots... it absorbs everything it comes into contact with and maintains that you are separate and different from everything around you, which both serves you and causes you grief. Your mind compares; it wants, it feels, it processes. It also motivates and implements. And sometimes it listens to those messages from the soul – but, for many reasons, including most notably a lack of self trust, we often ignore our inner knowing or refuse to believe that we have the capacity to know ourselves better than anyone else. Because, like every other part of you, the quality and state of your mind can be influenced by where you've been (your past), where you're going (your perceived future), and what you eat in between (the actual foods that you consume!).

Your body is your vehicle for expression and being in the world. It's time to acknowledge your beautiful body as the most powerful and versatile asset you have, not least because it's your tool for communicating what you think and who you are. It's also your greatest (and only) means for living your dharma (your purpose and path). And like any vehicle, it requires care, attention, and feeding, along with a basic understanding of how it works and how it can work for you. The better you understand it, the better chance you have of experiencing it at the highest levels of its ability and potential.

Your senses are the bridge... Touch, taste, hearing, sight, and smell provide information, food and nourishment to the mind, body, and soul. The senses are the bridge between you and the world around you. But more than that, they connect you to yourself. The smell of fresh bread cooking, the taste of bright, juicy lemon, the feel of creamy ice cream on a hot day -- these simple experiences have the power to speak to, and feed our souls, to transport us to happy times and to places we've never been. They also have the power to inspire us to seek out the best in ourselves and those we love.

> *"Everything in the Universe is within you. Ask all from yourself."* – **Rumi**

The energies that run your show...

Okay, so I'm gonna confirm something that your mother has been trying to convince you of for years… Darling, you're not like everyone else! And Ayurveda wants you to love that about yourself!

According to Ayurveda, each of us is 100% unique and different from every other living thing on this planet, AND it believes we should live (i.e. eat, sleep, breathe, exercise, and otherwise interact with the world) from this understanding, which is why Ayurveda advises us to live according to our "True Nature."

Your "True Nature," or "**Prakruti**" in Sanskrit, is a combination of elements and energies that is all yours and no one else's. It's you, as a unique signature in the world. And your combination of biological energies defines everything about you, from the the way you hold your hat to the way you sing off key.

YOUR dose of the doshas...

We all have within us the energies of vata, pitta, and kapha (something we touched on in chapter 4) working to keep us together and moving forward. Most often we find one or two of these energies are predominant in the way we look, think, and act. That (or those) energies are known as YOUR dosha. Understanding your dosha will give you incredible insight into how to look, feel, and be your best throughout the year and your life. It also gives you clues about the best way to interact with your world (i.e. your food, environment, work, relationships, routine, and so on).

The Sanskrit meaning of the word dosha "something that can be made defective" (or as my mom likes to say, "thrown out of whack"), is a reminder that although these three biological energies interact to keep you balanced and healthy, they can also be thrown off balance and wreak havoc, creating everything from crankiness to cancer!

Each of the energies has qualities (remember the Ayurveda colored glasses) that influence our tendencies (anger, anxiety, apathy), our cravings (comfort, solace, control) and the ways we most likely become imbalanced (addiction, hypertension, obesity). Your combination of energies (dosha) is set at conception, before the your parents, environment or cultural conditioning began to have an impact on who you are. So identifying your dosha will give you a view into your purest essence, and can also shed some light on the healthiest ways for you to eat, move and take care of yourself. So it's worthwhile making an effort to discover your dosha. The beautiful thing is that it can be as easy as taking a simple quiz.

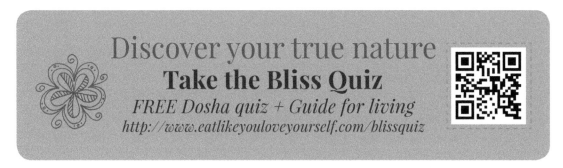

Discover your true nature
Take the Bliss Quiz
FREE Dosha quiz + Guide for living
http://www.eatlikeyouloveyourself.com/blissquiz

So let's take another look at the doshas and how they're most likely to be expressed within you.

Up close and personal with the doshas...

VATA - governs all movement in the body including the activities of the nervous system and the process of elimination. Vata dosha influences the movement and change characteristic of your nature.

The qualities of Vata are: Dry, rough, light, cold, subtle, and mobile

The best words to describe vata are: Active, dynamic, creative, adaptable, and perceptive.

Vata mind is...
Creative; quick to learn and grasp new knowledge, but also quick to forget.

Vata body is...
Slender; unusually tall or short; has tendencies toward cold hands and feet, and discomfort in cold climates. Generally dry skin, dry, frizzy hair, moves erratically, poor circulation, doesn't perspire much.

Vata spirit...
Is excitable, lively, fun; has very changeable moods; has a natural tendency towards irregular daily routine; has high energy in short bursts; tends to overexert and tire easily; is full of joy and enthusiasm when in balance; responds to stress with fear, worry, and anxiety, especially when out of balance; often acts on impulse and has racing, disjointed thoughts.

Vata in living motion...
When vata predominant individuals are at their best and in their flow, they can be unstoppable. Overflowing with ideas and interests; they can be strong and compassionate communicators and wildly perceptive friends, partners, or advisors. They are quick thinking and talking and make naturally good teachers, counselors, performers, consultants, artists ,or healers.

When the wind shifts into a state of imbalance, vatas can be moody and perhaps a little spacey or ungrounded. Their dynamic nature might give way to restlessness, disorganization and oversensitivity. They may even fall prey to addictions of one form or another.

Physically, vatas will find that their digestion is often as variable as their thoughts and that nothing about them tends to be regular and stable, including their appetite (for food and sex). They might be plagued by dryness and internal "wind" (gas and bloating, anyone?) with the vata cold showing up as chilly hands and feet.

The nature of vata is to shake things up and be a vehicle for change and exploration.

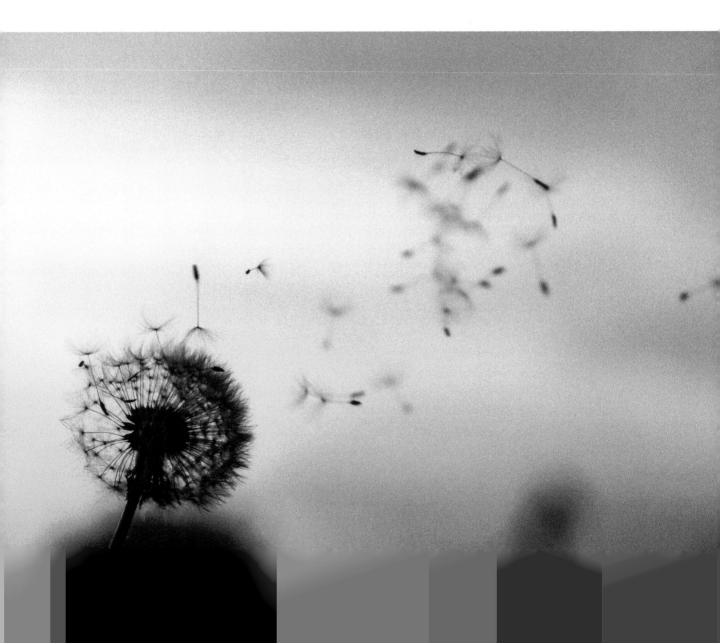

Balanced Vata is...

- Creative
- Artistic
- Lively and Enthusiastic
- Quick moving and fast talkers
- Intuitive
- Spontaneous
- Likes change and variability
- Thinks and acts quickly
- Thin build
- Variable appetite and digestion
- Often tall or short
- Dry stools – prone to constipation
- Light sleepers
- Cold hands & feet

Signs of Vata Imbalance..

- Restlessness/worry/ overly active thinking
- Constipation
- Over sensitivity
- Insomnia
- Dry skin
- Weight loss
- Headaches
- Low back pain
- Arthritis
- Addictions
- Impulsive spending
- Feeling "spacey" or ungrounded
- Lacking confidence, boldness
- Procrastinating
- Moody, emotionally volatile
- Impatience
- Cracking or popping joints
- Bladder/Urinary disorders
- Muscle stiffness
- Dizziness
- Low energy, fatigue

Activities that balance vata:

- Regular routine
- Adding oils, grounding foods to your diet
- Oil massage
- Enjoy warm, cooked foods
- Avoid or limit intake of coffee and alcohol
- Warm environments
- Regular and sufficient sleep
- Slow, strengthening physical exercise
- Listening to calming music
- Hugs
- Grounding yoga practice

Foods that aggravate vata:

- *Dry, light, cold or raw foods*, beans, crackers, cruciferous vegetables, caffeine, overly spicy foods.
- Hot drying spices like chili, cayenne
- Bitter, astringent, pungent tastes

Foods that balance vata:

- *Sweet, warm, moist and heavy foods* (Root vegetables, mangos, oats, meats)
- Warming herbs and spices like ginger, cinnamon, cumin, garlic..
- Hot spiced drinks, room temperature water and juices, warm milk
- Sweet, sour and salty tastes
- **Vata balancing SUPERFOODS:** Sweet potatoes, dates, figs, eggs, mangoes, fennel, amaranth, papaya, beets

A balanced vata plate is:

- 50% Carbohydrates [whole grains, breads, pasta, etc.]
- 20% Protein [nuts, legumes, meat, fish]
- 20% Vegetables [cooked root vegetables, peppers, onions, etc.]
- 10% Fruits [sweet fruits, mainly cooked]
- Generous amounts of dairy and oils

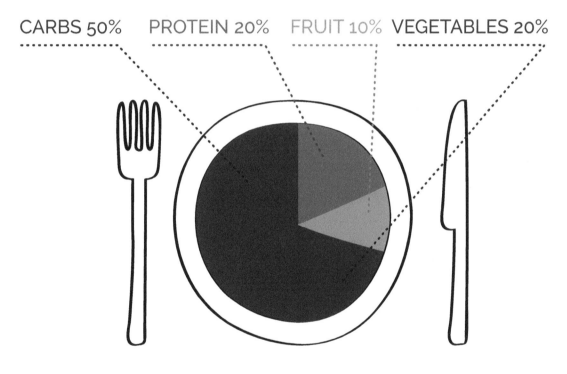

CARBS 50% PROTEIN 20% FRUIT 10% VEGETABLES 20%

Generous amounts of dairy and oils

PITTA - controls digestion, metabolism, and energy production. When a person has a tendency to "overheat," excess pitta is usually the culprit.

Qualities of pitta are: Oily, sharp, hot, light, moving, liquid, and acidic.

The best words to describe pitta are: Smart, focused, engaging, confident, and intense.

Pitta mind is...
Sharp, focused, orderly, confident and competitive.

Pitta body is...
Medium,well-built,and strong; strong appetite and digestion; fair, sensitive skin with freckles; good circulation; tendency to overheat; prone to rashes; tends to perspire a lot.

Pitta spirit is...
Charismatic, engaging, highly intelligent; passionate and romantic; strong sense of duty and focus; joyful, driven and courageous when in balance; responds to stress with anger, irritation, contempt, criticism. Subject to temper tantrums and impatience. Ambitious and geared for success.

Pitta in living motion...
Pittas are the drivers of transformation, the CEOs of getting things done. When the world needs someone to lead the charge, we rely on pittas for their confident wisdom and their ability to organize and motivate. Not only that, but their engaging charm and wicked sense of humor make it hard NOT to love them!

Pittas are fundamentally joyful and driven. Success is in their DNA. Where they go, people will follow, if for no other reason than to bask in the light of their radiance and wit.

When pitta individuals are at their best, they are well and truly ON FIRE, transforming everything in their path with a passion and determination that is unrivaled. They are likely to kick ass at anything they put their minds to, and their natural talent for discernment makes them well suited for careers as entrepreneurs, designers, engineers, politicians, or scientists (you name it really).

When their flames kick up out of control, they can find themselves easily aggravated, hot headed and pissy. That's when the critical streak can rear its ugly head and the intensity jumps up to overload (is it getting hot in here?). They might dig their heels in or take their toys and go home.

Physically, pittas are "hotties"! Their hot nature comes through in body temperature (warm hands and feet), sun sensitive skin and kick butt digestive fire (can you say cast iron gut!). The only thing moderate about a pitta is likely to be their height, weight, and physical features. Everything else, including their appetite (for food and sex) can be intense!

The nature of pitta is to light the fires; to be the driver of AMAZING adventures and projects that inspire us to be better, stronger, and more alive!

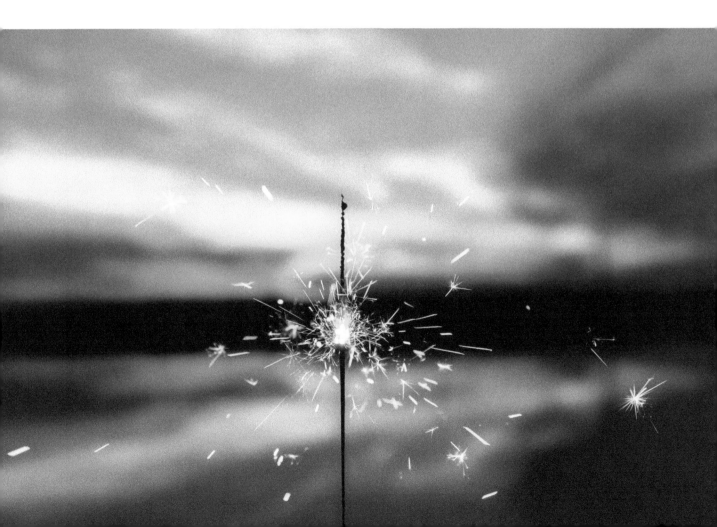

Balanced Pitta is...

- Confident
- Highly Intelligent
- Organized
- Joyful
- Natural leaders
- Sharp memory
- Funny, high achievers
- Sharp and direct
- Willful/Competitive
- Intense – "Type A"
- Articulate
- Medium build/Weight
- Sun sensitive
- Strong appetite
- Delicate, oily skin, acne prone

Signs of Pitta Imbalance..

- Acne/breakouts
- Canker sores
- Heartburn
- Ulcers
- Infections
- Jealousy
- Resentment
- Intense manipulative thoughts, behavior
- Arrogance
- Loud and aggressive
- Controlling of others
- Critical and Judgmental
- Hot flashes
- Hyperacidity
- Skin rashes/psoriasis
- Ulcers
- inflammation
- Diarrhea

Activities that balance Pitta:

- Cool baths
- Regular meals
- Meditation
- Peaceful environments & music
- Volunteer work, random acts of kindness
- Staying hydrated
- Spending time in or around water
- Spending time with good friends/family
- Laughter
- Slow, focused movement
- Nature bathing, moonbathing

Foods that aggravate pitta:

- *Spicy, hot, oily, sour, or fermented foods* (sauerkraut, kimchi, cheese, sour cream)
- Sour fruits and vegetables (tomatoes, tamarind, green mango, lemon, olives, raw onions, and garlic)
- Hot, pungent spices like black pepper, chilli, cayenne, paprika, etc.
- Pungent, sour, or salty tastes

Foods that balance pitta:

- Sweet, cooling fruits & veggies (watermelon, cherries, cucumbers)
- Cooling spices like fennel, coriander/cilantro, cardamom
- Cool, fresh water and juices
- Sweet, bitter, and astringent tastes
- **PItta balancing SUPERFOODS:** Apples, blueberries, dandelion, cabbage, pineapple, tofu, celery, grapes

A pitta balancing plate is:

- 30% Carbohydrates [Whole grains, breads, pasta, etc.]
- 30% Protein [Beans, lentils, tofu]
- 30% Vegetables [Leafy greens, cruciferous, watery roots.]
- 10% Fruits [sweet, cooling fruits, berries]

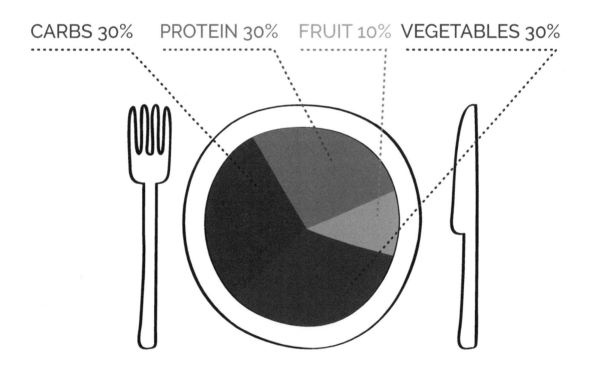

CARBS 30%   PROTEIN 30%   FRUIT 10%   VEGETABLES 30%

Moderate amounts of dairy & oils

KAPHA gives the body physical form, structure, and the smooth functioning of all its parts. It can be thought of as the essential cement, glue, and lubrication of the body in one. The primary function of Kapha is cohesion and protection.

The qualities of kapha are: Moist, cold, heavy, dull, soft, sticky, and static.

The best words to describe kaphas are: Strong, loving, gentle, calm and forgiving.

Kapha mind is...
Easygoing, affectionate and loving; forgiving, compassionate, faithful; slower to learn, but outstanding long-term memory.

Kapha body is..
Physically strong and with a sturdy, heavier build; soft, strong, moist hair and skin; tendency toward weight gain and sluggish digestion.

Kapha spirit is...
Self-sufficient; gentle, and undemanding with steady and enduring energy. physically strong and healthy with a calm nature. Strives to maintain harmony and peace. Responds to stress by closing down emotionally, being possessive (hoarding), depression.

Kapha in living motion...
When at their best and in balance, kaphas are unwavering and true, peaceful community builders, built to go the distance. Their inherent desire to provide and protect makes them natural caretakers, protectors/security, teachers, parents, and healers. And no matter the disturbance or dilemma, they can be relied upon to steady the waters with a calm and loving hand.

When the waters of imbalance rise, kaphas can be rendered immobile, mired by an overwhelming sense of inertia. They're likely to shift into couch potato mode and surround themselves with "things" that make them feel better. Overeating and sleeping, hoarding, and depression are the sometimes results of their natural desire to gather and ground.

Physically (and emotionally), kaphas are resilient. They may have struggled with weight or emotions or their sometimes unhealthy desires to gather and store. But their lighthearted nature can be their saving grace, providing the perspective and buoyancy they need to stay afloat and yet grounded in their cozy sense of self. Their approach to life is slow and steady and this shows up physically in a slower metabolism and steady appetite (for food and sex)

The nature of kapha is to build and nurture, to create a physical and emotional structure for ideas and opportunities to survive and thrive.

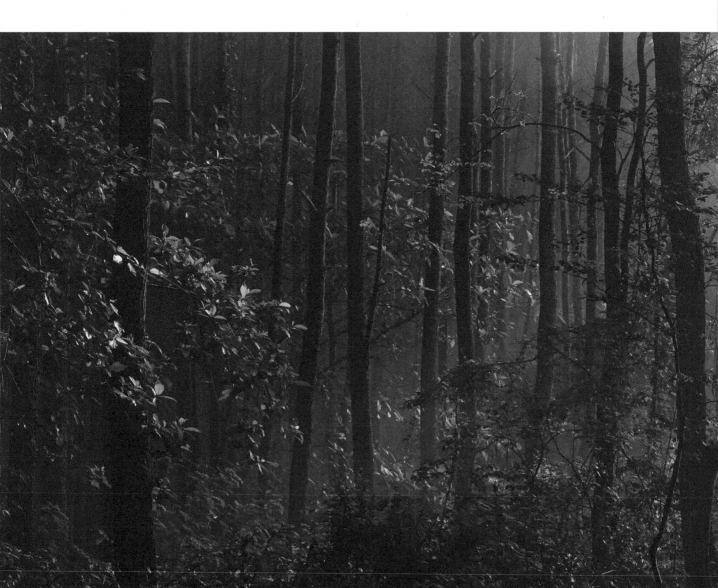

Balanced kapha is...

- Compassionate
- Patient
- Nurturing
- Loyal
- Forgiving
- Strong, heavy set
- Calm, mild mannered
- Strong stamina and endurance
- Romantic
- Oily, smooth skin
- Thick hair
- Cool, clammy hands
- Even tempered
- Good memory
- Deep sleeper

Signs of kapha Imbalance..

- Overeating/emotional eating
- Sinus congestion
- Excessive sleeping
- Allergies
- Hoarding/Possessiveness
- Complacency
- Heart disease
- Anorexia and Bulimia
- Fear of letting go
- Lethargy
- Allergies
- Introversion
- Depression for extended periods
- Complacency
- Inability to say no
- Excess phlegm, mucus
- inability to express themselves
- Obesity
- Diabetes
- Colds & flu, congestion
- Water retention/bloating

Activities that balance kapha:

- Self expression (journalling, talking w/friends)
- Singing
- Laughing
- Dancing
- Avoiding heavy foods and over indulging
- Meditation
- Exercise - running, hiking, vinyasa yoga
- Dry saunas (occasionally)
- Decluttering
- Forgiveness

Foods that aggravate kapha:

- **Sweet, heavy, oily, cold foods** (ice cream, cheese, dairy, meat, fried foods)
- Sweet, watery, cooling fruits & veggies (watermelon, cherries, cucumbers, sweet potatoes, bananas, avocado)
- Salt
- Sweet, sour and salty tastes

Foods that balance kapha:

- Spicy, warm and drying foods (peppers, light grains, beans)
- Astringent fruits (apples, pears, berries, pomegranate, dried fruit)
- Warming spices (ginger, black pepper, cinnamon, cardamom, cumin, etc.)
- Hot spiced drinks, dry wine, herbal teas
- Pungent, bitter, and astringent tastes
- **Kapha balancing SUPERFOODS:** Peppers, corn, spinach, honey, peas, sprouts, dried fruit

A kapha balancing plate is:

- 30% Carbohydrates [Whole grains, breads, pasta, etc.]
- 20% Protein [Beans, lentils, tofu]
- 40% Vegetables [Leafy greens, cruciferous, spring veggies]
- 10% Fruits [light, astringent fruits, pears, apples, dried fruit]
- Sparing amounts of dairy & oils

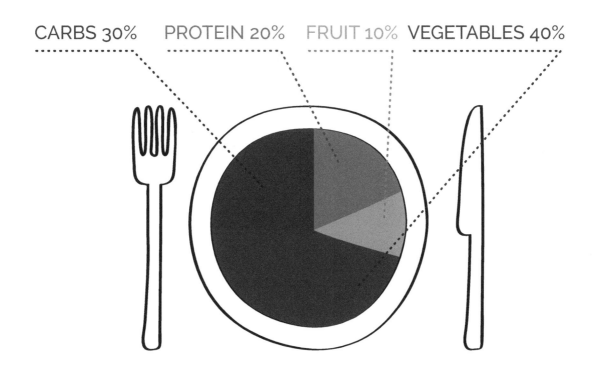

CARBS 30%   PROTEIN 20%   FRUIT 10%   VEGETABLES 40%

Sparing amounts of dairy & oils

State Of Mind = State Of Health...

Ayurveda teaches us that all illness and disease begin in the mind, an idea that feels true but can be hard to get your head around!

Scientific research is diving into this fascinating area and is beginning to understand the deep connection between the mind and body and the resulting power we have to transform our physical well-being by transforming our thoughts. Yoga and Ayurveda provide tools and guidance for becoming aware of and managing our mental state. In essence, these tools empower us to truly own our health and wellness.

> *"the quality of the mind determines the quality of your health and happiness"* – **Chara Caruthers**

Ayurveda recognizes three qualities (gunas) of nature, different to the twenty qualities of matter, which represent our fundamental states of mind. Referred to as the Mahagunas (the Great Qualities) in Sanskrit, they are Sattva, Rajas, and Tamas. Each state characterizes ways of being, thinking, and expression that will influence the choices and actions that define how we live and interact with the world. And as states, they are transitory, dynamic, and often changing from moment to moment and day to day.

The three states of mind

Sattva gives us...

The capacity to create, think, imagine in the purest and most authentic sense. It represents a clear, calm, and focused state, and is expressed as curiosity, fascination, inspiration.

Sattva represents all that is: Illuminating, intelligent, creative, compassionate, and pure.

Sattvic states of mind allow us to:
- Have the greatest freedom from disease.
- Have a harmonious and adaptable nature.
- Strive toward balance and have peace of mind which cuts the psychological root of disease!
- Be considerate of others and take good care of ourselves.

Rajas gives us...

The capacity to act, motivate, organize, implement. It is an active, agitated, and controlling state, and is expressed as movement, action, dominance, outward focus, ego.

Rajas represents all that is: Dynamic, metabolic, hot, restless, attached to outcomes.

Rajasic states of mind bring about...

- Good energy with a tendency to burn out through excessive use of that energy.
- Trying too hard or too much, expecting too much, and overextending ourselves.
- Impatience and inconsistency in dealing with managing health or illness.
- Blaming others for our conditions and wanting others to "fix" us.

Tamas gives us...

The capacity to bring things to an end. It is a heavy, dull, and sluggish state, and is expressed as stubbornness, feeling stuck, apathy, fear, depression, decay.

Tamas represents all that is: Inert, unmoving, dull, unconscious, sluggish, and ignorant.

Tamasic states of mind bring about...

- Chronic diseases, including suppressed emotional conditions.
- Stagnant energy and emotion being caught in a pattern of negativity and self-destruction.
- Refusal to seek proper treatment, help or support.
- Poor hygiene and diet.
- Accepting ill health or disease as fate and unwillingness to seek opportunities to create better life/health.

Each of these mental states is part of our everyday experience. But it doesn't take much to see the benefits of extending your stay in the calm, centered and creative sattvic space. Yoga and meditation are all geared towards making this happen. But even with that on your side, it's important to notice how the quality of the mind affects your experience of living (off the mat or cushion) and what you can do to influence it.

Balance your mood with food

Ayurveda sees food as medicine and holds that what we feed our bodies, we also feed our minds. It understands that the food we eat becomes a part of us and expresses its qualities through us. Our food also has the power to influence the quality of our thinking, perception, and digestion of thoughts and emotions.

So Ayurveda categorizes foods by their impacts on the mind as well as the body, designating everything we eat as either sattvic, rajasic, or tamasic.

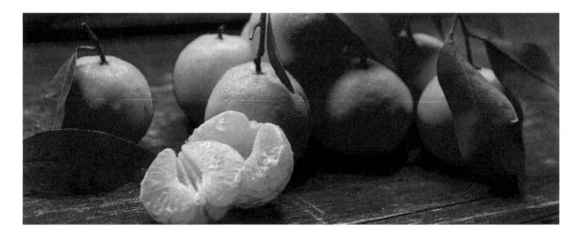

EATING SATTVIC

Sattvic foods are... Fresh, pure, natural, and vibrant. They're free of chemicals and processing, They're light, easy to digest, often sweet (naturally), and nourishing. Sattvic foods help clear the mind. They promote peace, focus, balance, and joy.

Sattvic foods include: most fresh veggies and fruits, honey, fresh milk, butter, whole grains, almonds, cashews, walnuts and macadamia nuts, many beans and lentils, ghee, and fresh yogurt.

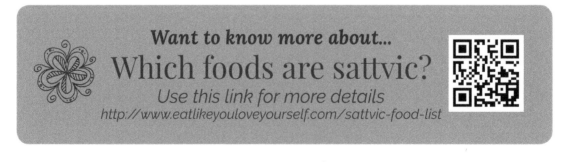

Want to know more about...
Which foods are sattvic?
Use this link for more details
http://www.eatlikeyouloveyourself.com/sattvic-food-list

EATING RAJASIC

Rajasic foods are... Stimulating and agitating to the system, often spicy, sour, salty, or bitter. In moderation, they provide just the right amount of push to keep you motivated and moving, but taken in excess these foods can aggravate your mood (and your digestion) and disturb the balance.

Rajasic foods include: Peppers, garlic, tomatoes, pickles, vinegar, peanuts, citrus fruits, refined sugars, salt, eggs. ghee and fresh yogurt.

EATING TAMASIC

Tamasic foods are... Heavy, dull and devoid of vital energy. In moderation these foods can be grounding, but overdoing it can tend to numb us out, slow us down and even lead to depression.

Tamasic foods include: processed foods, cheese, onions, mushrooms, alcohol, meat, frozen foods, leftovers.

What's the state of YOUR mind...

Thing to remember is that each of these states of mind are vital to maintaining balance. We all need inspiration, motivation, and completion in our lives; the trick is getting the balance right. It starts with knowing that we're empowered with every breath and at every meal to move towards rather than away from who we want and need to be.

What's YOUR current or most common state of mind?
Take this little quiz to find out!

Discovering YOUR state of mind | Which best describes you...

Circle the option which best describes you. Total all the circled items at the bottom to determine your current state of mind.

Your diet is...	Strictly vegetarian	Mostly veggies with a little meat	Probably half and half meat and veggies
Way of speaking	Calm, slow and considered	Slight agitated and fast	Slow, flat and not very engaged.
Attitude toward cleanliness	Like to keep things very clean and tidy	Prefer clean, but don't always get there	Not too worried about keeping things clean
Frequency of Anger	I rarely get angry	I sometimes get angry	I get angry nearly every day
Primary purpose in life	To serve others	To serve myself and my goals	To do as little work as possible.
Your general attitude towards life	Positive, grateful, always seeing the good	Positive, driven, you only get what you work for	Not that interested or engaged.
How easily you forgive	Very easily	Not very easily, but I get there	Rarely do I forgive
Your level of contentment	I'm usually content	I'm somewhat content with life	I rarely feel content with life.
First thing in the morning you...	Express gratitude and meditate	Check my emails	Wish I could go back to sleep.
How open and honest are you...	I am very open and honest with myself and others	I am somewhat open and honest with myself and others	I am rarely open and honest with myself and others
How creative you are	Very creative	Somewhat creative	Not very creative
How often you meditate	Daily	On and off	Not at all
Attitude toward service	Very important, I engage in it regularly	Moderately important, I engage in it sometimes	Not very important, I don't have time for it.
TOTALS	**Sattva**	**Rajas**	**Tamas**

Why digestion is king

Food is one of the most important aspects of who we are. Judging by the sheer number of cooking shows and books, it's definitely clear that food is something that is near and dear to all of our hearts. And when it comes down to it, our food serves a lot of purposes in our lives...

- *Food provides comfort*
- *Food gives us nourishment*
- *Food serves as medicine*

Everyone knows that old saying, "You are what you eat." The Ayurvedic take on it is that you are what you digest and that's because **the food you digest actually becomes who you are**. It's broken down by the body and mind and is absorbed in order to actually become your skin, organs, tissues, bones, and blood. The food that you DIGEST is what gives you the energy to reason, communicate, and connect. So our ability to transform what we consume into nourishment and waste is the key to getting what we need and want in life.

All the energy, focus, strength, and joy that we desire is a function of taking in the right stuff, in the right amounts, and getting rid of what doesn't serve us. When you look at things in this way, it's easy to understand why Ayurveda views digestion as the key to health and wellness. It's also easy to embrace the importance and value of paying attention to how well you're digesting, something that's determined by the state of your agni.

"The body is nothing but fire." – **Robert Svoboda**

Agni: The fire inside

Agni is Sanskrit for the fire of digestion. It cooks, breaks down, assimilates, and metabolizes what you consume in order to separate the nutrients that feed and nourish you from the waste that doesn't.

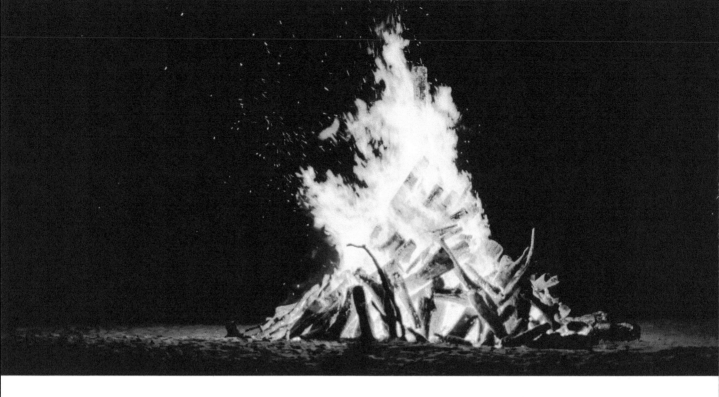

Agni is the fire that keeps the process of nourishing mind and body alive! And just like a campfire, your agni needs to burn at a the right level in order to do its job. If the fire gets too low or too high, your digestion becomes compromised. It might start to feel a bit like:

- Fatigue
- Foggy brain
- Heaviness
- Gas
- Bloating
- Skin issues
- Allergies
- Depression, procrastination, and complacency

A compromised digestive system is a breeding ground for the formation and accumulation of toxins, referred to as "**ama**." Ama is the undigested food, thoughts, and emotions that putrefy in the body and clog the channels. If left untreated, ama (similar to plaque) can accumulate in the tissues and lead to blockages and disease. Regular detoxification is a common way to clear ama from the mind and body, which is why it's recommended at least twice yearly.

But the best cure for ama (and disease) is prevention. The Ayurvedic approach is to start by paying attention to the ways that your mind and body work and respond to environments, situations, thoughts, and beliefs. Tune into your mental and physical traits and tendencies, and use that knowledge of yourself to help you make powerful choices about what's healthiest for you in the moment.

Keeping toxins at bay...

- Include more fresh, organic vegetables, bitter foods, whole grains and easily digested proteins in your diet.

- Eat less fried and heavy foods (aged cheeses, meat, rich desserts)

- Avoid eating or drinking excessive amounts of anything cold.

- Sip warm water throughout the day to.

- Avoid unecessary snacking between meals

- and wait until your previous meal is digested.

- Use warming digestive spices like turmeric, cumin, fennel and coriander to assist the process of digestion.

- Get enough sleep - in bed by 10pm (before pitta time) and up by 6am (before kapha time).

- Daily exercise stimulates digestion and the natural detoxification of the body.

Feeling heavy, tired, or out of sorts?
Check the appendices for a simple quiz to give
you clues to how toxic you are!

How are YOU digesting?

Ayurveda recognizes four types or states of our digestive fire that indicate the level of efficiency with which we're processing and assimilating life (including our food):

Sama Agni - Healthy, balanced digestion
Manda Agni - Slow digestion
Vishama Agni - Variable digestion
Tikshna Agni - Overactive (sharp) digestion

Sama agni or balanced digestion looks like:

- Regular, complet, and consistent elimination
- Feeling light, energetic, and mentally clear and alert after eating
- Clean tongue (no thick white residue)
- Feeling of physical hunger
- Feeling joy, contentment, enthusiasm, and wholeness

Manda Agni or slow digestion most often shows up as:

- Heaviness in the body especially after eating
- Dullness in the mind
- Lack of appetite
- Weight gain, even when you're not eating much
- Congestion in the body or in the mind, like a lack of clarity and lightness

* Kaphas will often experience digestive slowdowns as their kapha becomes imbalanced.

How to avoid/manage manda agni:

- Boost digestion with digestive herbs and spices before meals
- Take small sips of warm water during meals
- Avoid overeating
- Avoid cold drinks and heavy foods
- Take a walk after meal

Vishama Agni or variable digestion often looks like:

· Irregular appetite

· Indigestion, constipation, or bloating

· Gurgling in your belly or the intestines

· And even feeling a bit heavy after meals

* Often related to transitions or times in your life where there's an excess of movement (vata), change, stress, or even travel.

How to avoid/manage vishama agni:

· Eating meals at regular times

· Meditation or relieving stress with yoga and pranayama

· Add a little ghee with meals to stoke the digestive fire

· Include spices with your meals and drinks

*Vishama agni is common amongst vatas, but is not considered to be a balanced state.

Tikshna Agni, or sharp or fast digestion/metabolism, can be related to your constitution (are you a pitta?), hot weather or summer season, or the result of some other imbalance. It often shows up as:

· Strong appetite

· Tendency to get hangry when you skip meals

· Acid indigestion

· Heartburn

· Loose stools or diarrhea

· And even a tendency towards anger, aggressiveness and gastritis

*Tikshna agni is common amongst pittas, but is definitely not considered balanced!

How to manage your tikshna agni:

· Avoid spicy foods

· Eat regularly

· Keep your cool - do your best to avoid tense and stressful situations

· Enjoy cooling foods like leafy greens, coconuts, pomegranate, avocados, mangos, or sweet juicy fruits.

· Aloe vera juice is great for reducing pitta - 1-2 tablespoons before meals

How to get better at digesting life

As whole beings, Ayurveda sees that everything we come into contact with has the potential to be food for the mind, body, or soul. Think about that...all the information, ideas, people, sights, sounds, smells, textures, and tastes as well as thoughts and emotions that you experience on a daily basis have the potential to support your health and well-being or sabotage it.

Okay, so that's a lot of stuff! And everything must be digested and assimilated just like the food you eat in order to extract the nutrients and release the waste. So when it comes down to it, your body mind is like one large digesting machine! And every day living in the modern world is like a smorgasbord on steroids. It's no wonder we're dealing with all kinds of health issues. We're doing our best to process everything but there's only so much our minds and bodies can manage.

So in order to thrive, you have to do a few key things:

- **Don't overdo it** - Moderation in all things is the Ayurvedic mantra and that's because the last thing you want to do is smother your campfire. And just like with food, it's important to ensure that you're not inadvertently "gorging" on info, ideas, sights, sounds, and the like.

- **Find your soul food** - Like the food we eat for our bodies, we need to make healthy choices for our minds as well. Empowering thoughts, information that expands our understanding of ourselves and each other, positive and compassionate messages and beliefs.

- **Tune in** - Listen and learn the signals your bodies gives when it's had enough. What do your red flags look like? How do they feel?

- **Lighten up** - Take time on a regular basis to ease the load on your mind and body. And it doesn't need to be a two week retreat in Mexico or Bali. Taking a restorative yoga class or easing up on the food and technology for one day each month can be a powerful addition to your self care routine.

- **Add warming foods and spices to your diet** - Give your digestive system a boost by eating foods that are cooked and prepared with spices that are warming like cinnamon, ginger, and pepper.

How are YOU digesting life?

How well are you doing with finding a balance between what's out there to consume and what your mind and body need?

Chapter 6

The Art of Dancing with Your world

"Life is like riding a bicycle. To keep your balance, you must keep moving." – **Albert Einstein**

How great would YOUR life be if you could spend more time "in the zone"? That sensation of effortless ease, of being more you more often, a feeling of harmony between you and your environment. Ayurveda calls it balance. I like to call it dancing with life. The goal of Ayurveda is to get you there, but it starts by embracing a single idea.

Who you are is a relationship between what's going on outside and what goes on inside.

It's no coincidence that you've heard this before within these very pages. That's because it's a VITAL point that deserves repeating. And it's the foundation for a few simple rules that will inspire and empower you to create a dynamic and supportive partnership with the foods, environments, interactions, and objects that are the building blocks of a beautiful life.

So if you're ready to let go of the struggle and step onto the dance floor, here are four simple concepts to consider:

Harmony is health - Yes, this sounds like a fairy tale. But it isn't By harmony, I mean YOU and your environment (home, work, family, friends, weather, food, basically everything around you) working in sync. That starts by acknowledging that there's a subtle and ever present give and take between your internal and external worlds. Wellness is a process of knowing when and how to pull back or lean in.

Seasons Matter - Change is the ONLY constant in life. It's also a part of who we are. Changes in your environment (weather, seasons) have a big impact on how you look, feel, and think, regardless of where you live. Seasonal changes set the tone for who we're capable of being throughout the year. Refusing to acknowledge this and make changes to accommodate seasonal influence creates mental, emotional, and physical stress, limiting what's possible in your life.

Routine Matters - Our DNA has "gifted" us with a collective understanding that "unknown = stress." These days, with the increasing number of options available to us for everything from toothpaste to careers, we're also beginning to understand that too many choices also creates mental and physical stress!

Routine can be the antidote to these insidious and ever-present stressors. Routine removes some of the unknown from your life (but not the fun!) and reduces the number of choices you're faced with in a given day. Daily and seasonal routines provide the mental and emotional underpinning for good health and real happiness. Another GREAT thing about routine is that it ensures you're doing the things that matter rather than letting them get buried underneath your busy-ness!

The key to great health is NOT JUST food and exercise.

Don't get me wrong, those things ARE important, but consider that:

- *What you believe*
- *How you think*
- *How you feel*
- *Where you live*
- *How you react*
- *Who you spend your time with*
- *How you spend your time*
- *How you feel about yourself*

are the factors that drive every decision you make around what to eat, how to move, and how to take care of yourself. These are things that we often ignore in our approach for getting healthy (because it's much easier to just make a green smoothie!).

But how much easier it would be to make healthy choices if you started by changing a few small things about your thinking, like believing that you are worthy of being amazing and healthy?

How good would it feel to know and love yourself shamelessly and to have that authentic love and inner knowing drive the choices you make to maintain your wholeness?

The only wellness advice you'll ever need...

The ancient approach to living these concepts isn't complicated (unless you choose to make it that way). All it requires is a willingness to embrace what's real and a desire to discover and step into your own natural rhythm, knowing (perhaps even before seeing) that it will support your mind and body through the challenges you'll face as you and the world around you change.

So if you're ready to start dancing, here's what to do:

Create a routine

For many people the idea of a daily routine can be SCARY! Just remember routines don't have to be inflexible or difficult to maintain. Think of a routine as a gift you give yourself every day.

Start small by choosing just a few simple things to do for yourself every day.

Don't overcomplicate it. Don't overstructure or schedule it. And remember to focus your routine around health-promoting activities, physical/emotional housekeeping, and self-care (not just ticking everything off your "to-do" list).

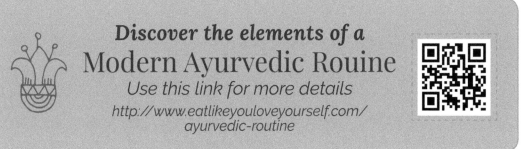

Discover the elements of a
Modern Ayurvedic Rouine
Use this link for more details
http://www.eatlikeyouloveyourself.com/
ayurvedic-routine

Observe the seasons

The best thing about the change of seasons is that you pretty much always know when it's coming. The change of seasons tends to be a transitional time for a lot of life's activities, and it's also a time that we're most vulnerable to illness and disease.

So with each new season, here's what to do:

- **Change up your food...**
  As well as eating seasonal foods, educate yourself about the qualities of the foods you eat (hot, cold, light, heavy) and be sure to make food choices that are in harmony with the qualities of the season (i.e. stay away from heavy, wet stuff in the spring, avoid too much hot, spicy stuff in the summer, etc.). It just so happens this cookbook will help you do just that!

- **Change up your clothes...**
  You would have thought it could go without saying, but you'd be surprised at how few people wear appropriate clothing for both the season and the weather on any particular day. It can make a HUGE difference on how you feel emotionally if you wear clothes that keep you suitably warm in winter and cool in summer. Trust me on this.

- **Change up your routine...**
  Again, look at the routine not as something that ties you down, but as a gift that you give yourself every day. In that way, changing it as the seasons change and new activities, weather, and other environmental factors come into play will start to feel even more like you're dancing with life rather than playing tackle football with it. For more guidance on how to change things up from season to season, check out chapter seven.

> *For more guidance on how to change things up from season to season check out chapter seven.*

Notice Everything

Yogis call it mindfulness. And it is powerful stuff. One could argue that without it, happiness, health, bliss, success, really aren't possible. And even though it's true that we operate a lot of our lives without much awareness (on "auto-pilot"), and we still manage to get things done, real awareness changes everything.

Real awareness is like turning on the lights and seeing colors for the first time. It allows for a greater efficiency and effectiveness in life. And it's a lot easier than you might think. So whenever you think about it OR just before you're about to do anything - sit down, answer the door, make a call, eat a meal, go to bed, and so on,

try asking yourself:

- **How do I feel physically, emotionally, mentally?**
  This is not a trick question just a way of focusing your awareness.
  Know before asking that answering it doesn't mean you have to do anything about it .
- **How am I behaving?**
  Does who you're "being" feel natural and authentic? Are your actions a reflection of what you truly believe?
- **What's going on around me?**
  What's happening in your environment? What's the weather? What activities are going on? What are you likely to be involved in? What people will you come into contact with? What's the pace of life like?

Then... just notice what you notice... yep, it's that simple.

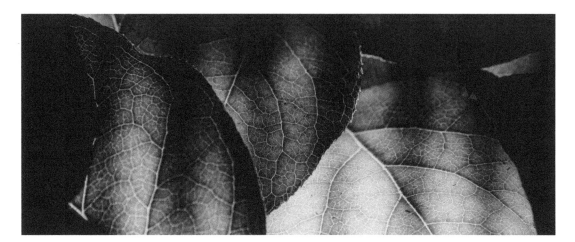

Harmonize with your environment even as it changes.

Once you're armed with an awareness of yourself and your environment, you can make easier decisions about how to create harmony in your life (that's the dance I mentioned earlier).

It can be as simple as putting on a warm coat or a rain jacket if it's cold and rainy, choosing to enjoy a cool salad over a hot and spicy chili on a warm summer day, or even making a decision to be calm and collected when dealing with a hot headed partner, friend, or colleague.

Above all it's fully embracing that life is going to "throw" stuff at you. But you have the choice to catch it, throw it back, or let it hit you in the face! My suggestion is to choose harmony, whichever option that represents.

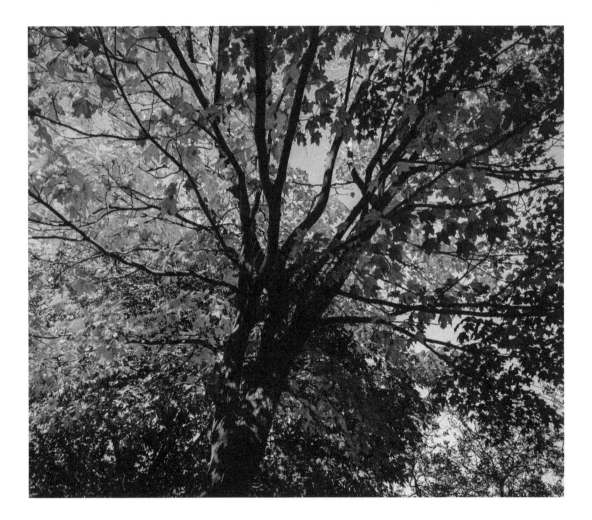

Chapter 7

The art and science of seasonal living...

"You are the sky... everything else is just the weather." – Pema Chodron

According to Ayurveda, living out of sync with the cycles of nature is one of the main causes of disease. Modern living is a story of late nights and work shifts that mess with our natural rhythms, business and leisure travel that takes us through season and time zone changes, and supermarkets that carry year-round...everything! Counteracting the damaging impacts of this way of living and harnessing the energies of each new season to fuel our dreams comes down to making simple changes to honor how you and your environment change throughout the year.

We are a part of the natural world around us and like all living things, trees, animals, flowers, etc., who we are shifts as the temperature, weather and environmental energies around us shift. And what that means is that seasons matter a lot.

Who we are changes from season to season, but the process of living has become so hectic and complex that we barely have time to notice or make simple lifestyle changes that will support who we need to be for the time and environment that we're living in. The result is inevitably imbalance (we all know what that feels like!). Avoiding this scenario, and giving yourself the opportunity for more good days, is a matter of being intentional and proactive from season to season, AND getting to know the seasons a little better.

Like everything else, each season of the year is characterized by certain qualities. These qualities will give you clues about how the seasons affect you and what you can do to stay strong, sane, and happy all year round!.

Thriving in Autumn/Early Winter

In most temperate climates, autumn to early winter is dominated by ambient conditions that are cold, dry, light, and moving (breezy, variable). These are the qualities that aggravate vata dosha, giving rise to imbalances that share these same qualities.

For that reason, autumn can be a time for both celebration and surrender. It's one of my favorite times of year, in part because it marks the beginning of the cozy season at a time when it's most welcome (at the end of a summer season of play). Creating a mind-body balance in the autumn is all about keeping a watchful eye on vata, the energy of movement, and how it moves within and around you.

Vata energy can become imbalanced during this time of year (particularly for those of predominantly vata constitution). And if that happens, your activity will start to feel out of control. Your mind may race, contributing to anxiety and insomnia. You may start skipping meals or making unhealthy nutritional choices, and your digestion may become irregular.

My balancing mantra for autumn straight through to late winter is **warming, grounding, moisturizing, routine**. It's a simple reminder of the qualities that counter the imbalancing effects of this time of year. And it can be applied to choosing to everything from your way of thinking to your yoga practice. Remember, in the pursuit of perfect healthy, everything counts. Autumn is the time of year when focus and consistency can fall to the wayside, and it's also when you need it most. So be ready to use all the tools at your disposal (exercise, self care, and food) to stay warm, juicy, and deeply connected to yourself.

Eating for balance at this time of year means choosing foods that are warming, grounding and oily or moisturizing; things like root vegetables, meats, soups and stews, curries, casseroles, warm desserts, warm salads, and warmed spiced drinks. This is the time of year when sweet, sour and salty tastes are most balancing to the mind and body, and cold, dry and light foods like salads, smoothies, crackers, popcorn, beans should be avoided.

Flourishing in Late winter/Spring

The tail end of winter is often cooler, wetter, and heavier. These conditions change only slightly as we move into spring. It's a time when we find ourselves feeling more sluggish, congested, and a little less motivated. It's also a time when we're most likely to be carrying a little extra weight resulting from the heavier, oilier foods that kept us balanced and blissful during the earlier part of the season.

This time of year is dominated by the grounding, slow, and sometimes stubborn energy of kapha. It's a heavy energy that can leave us feeling pretty stuck come spring (a not uncommon experience for many of us).

My balancing mantra for spring is **energizing, drying, stimulating, expression**. It's a clear and simple way of embracing the qualities that will help to create balance. Movement, activities and self care this time of year should focus on shaking things up and letting them go. It's a great time of year for more rigorous and expressive activities like hiking,

"*Be aware of what season you are in and give yourself the grace to be there.*"

— **Kristen Dalton**

biking, jogging, dancing, and singing. It's also a good time to take on the challenge of clearing out your mind, body, and home with a good cleanse and spring clean!

Food for this time of year should infuse lightness, dryness, and heat to shake up the complacency and melt the mucus and eliminate them from the mind and body. Easing up on the consumption of meat, eating light soups, salads and warming breakfasts. We'll also want to include more leafy greens, juices, and light drying fruits like apples, pears, berries, and persimmons as the winter gives way to spring. Doing so will leave us feeling lighter, brighter, and more clear and connected by summer.

Staying balanced through summer

Summer brings a transition from the cool heaviness of spring to a hot, light sharpness in the mind, body and environment. It's a time when we ratchet up the activity, stimulation, and intensity in our lives, increasing the potential for aggravating pitta energy. Sunburn, skin issues, heat stroke, dehydration, inflammation and short temper are just a few of the ways that overactive pitta can show up at this time of year.

Creating balance through the summer season starts with infusing **cooling, calming, moderation, and flow** into your life. Being mindful of the tendency to do too much. Taking time to slow down and tune in. Engaging in exercise and self-care activities like yoga, tai chi, walking, swimming, and volunteer work will leave you feeling connected and calm. Spend time near water or in nature, These are all simple and wonderful ways to offset the heat and intensity that can find its way into your mind and body at this time of year.

Eating for balance in summer is all about enjoying the bounty of the season -- sweet, cooling, juicy fruits like coconut, stone fruits, figs, and berries; avocados, leafy greens and bitter vegetables, salads of all kinds, juices, lighter cooler breakfasts, and simple lunches. You'll want to avoid foods that are spicy, oily, sour and salty as they can be heating and drying to the tissues and the mind.

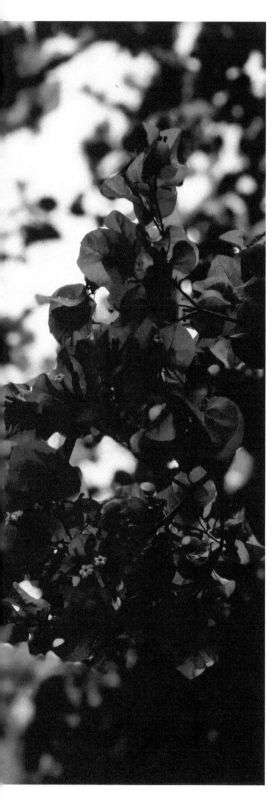

Why seasonal transitions are SO important...

Even beyond our physiology, the seasons consume our thoughts and behaviors. We look forward to the coming of summer, get nostalgic about the spring and fall, and associate winter with our favorite holidays, activities, or sporting events. But how much time do we spend thinking about the transition between the seasons?

Rarely do we close the door on one season only to open the door on the next a minute, day, or hour later. But have you ever given much thought or consideration to that period of days or weeks at the close of one season and start of the next? Ayurveda has a special name for this time of year because what happens in this "seasonal purgatory" is definitely worthy of notice.

Ritu sandhi is the Sanskrit name for the junction between the seasons. It's the four-week period that includes the last two weeks of the current season and the first two weeks of the next season. It's the timeframe for making a conscious shift from one season to the next. It's also the time of year when we're most vulnerable and susceptible to disease (think about when you most often get sick...always seems like it's that transition from one season to the next, doesn't it?).

Ayurveda associates seasonal transition with a rise in vata energy. It's an in-between place, associated with movement and change. And, not surprisingly, it can be a little destabilizing for the mind and body and leave us feeling disconnected and vulnerable.

During this time, you're likely to notice an increase in vata-type imbalance like anxiety, or dryness, constipation, fatigue, low immunity, and even low self-esteem or fear can show up during transitions.

Balance through seasonal transition

Here's a few suggestions for maintaining balance through the transitions and beyond...

The first is just to notice them and how they impact you.
- What are your mental, physical, and emotional tendencies?
- What imbalances show up for you during this time of year?

Reflect and reset

Most people wait until the beginning of each new year to reflect on the past and set goals for the year ahead. And while this is great, sometimes a more frequent and regula check-in is needed to keep us aware of what's working (and what's not, and to ensure we're sufficiently motivated and inspired to move forward.

Transition what you take into your mind and body

- **Start making the gradual shift to foods that are seasonal** for your part of the world (not always easy to know what's seasonal in this day and age when food is shipped all over the world) – use this handy dandy chart to get a sense for what's seasonal.
- **Ensure you're getting enough water.** Water consumption should stay relatively steady throughout the year (you might need a little less during the spring). This transition period is a perfect time to check in with yourself to make sure you're getting enough.
- **Be mindful of the information and entertainment you're consuming.** Realize that it makes a difference. Spring is a time for stimulation, summer is a time for cooling and calming, fall and winter are times for grounding and warming. How can the information, programs, news, and music you consume match the mood needed for the season?

Transition what you put on your body

Something most people have experience with but bears repeating is that we should dress appropriately for the season. Often we get so used to inappropriate dressing (i.e. wearing clothes that aren't warm, cool, or suitable enough for the weather) that we don't realize the impacts to our state of mind and health. I refused to wear socks for years after moving away from California just because I never had to wear them growing up (never mind the near freezing winter temperatures in Melbourne, Australia, which eventually took their toll on my poor feet before I gave in and bought some socks). Making the conscious choice to change what you wear as the seasons change is an important part of self-care and ultimately the key to happiness and well-being.

Transition what you do with your body

- **Adjusting bedtimes**. It's time to start thinking about when you wake up and go to bed and make some slight changes in consideration of the change in daylight hours. Ayurveda suggests waking up about an hour before sunrise year round! The actual time will shift slightly so make sure to adjust the time you go to bed as well to ensure that you're getting sufficient sleep.

- **Move your body right**. Make an effort to take advantage of activities (indoor and outdoor) that are appropriate for the season and be sure to take some time in nature in every season just to connect with the natural world (don't forget to wear the right clothes!!). Also consider how you might change your exercise routine to make it more suitable for the season you're moving into.

And then of course there's...

Eating in Transition...

Since transitions can be a time of variable digestion (associated with that increase in vata energy), a simple, easily digestible diet of vata calming foods is typically recommended. Warm, nourishing, and suitably spiced soups, stews and, porridges. **Kitchari** (*an ayurvedic cleansing dish of rice and dhal* - there's a recipe in this book!) has come to be our family "go to" during the change of seasons, as it's nourishing, easy to prepare, and delicious. Also use warming digestive teas and moderate portion sizes and eat meals around the same time each day.

Wondering what to eat during seasonal transitions?
Check out this video tutorial
*http://www.eatlikeyouloveyourself.com/
eating-in-transition*

Seasonal Living

	Late Winter/Spring	Summer	Fall/Early Winter
Food	Light, easily digestible, smaller portions, cleansing foods and herbal teas, warming spices, avoid heavy or fatty foods and snacks	Cooling, easily digestible, moderate portions, minimize meat consumption, best time of year for raw foods.	Warming, soothing, easily digestible meals (soups, stews), warming spices and herbal teas, avoid skipping meals or excessive snacking.
Bedtime/Sleep	Best time of the year to stay up later at night (no later than midnight)	In bed by 11pm, wake up early	In bed between 10 – 10:30pm, avoid late nights, can get up a bit later in the morning
Exercise	Active, heating exercise – yoga, running, aerobics	Yoga, walking, swimming – make sure not to get overheated with exercise	Grounding and warming exercise. Yoga, strength training. Avoid complete inactivity.
Entertainment	Stimulating music, live entertainment.	Calming, relaxing entertainment.	Grounding, warming things that make you laugh or happy.
Self Care Activities	Sunflower oil massage, declutter home, seasonal cleanse, Kapalbhati pranayama	Sunflower or coconut oil massage, connect with nature, Shitali pranayama	Sesame oil massage daily. Alternate nostril breathing. Seasonal cleansing.
Other considerations	Keep warm and dry	Minimize direct sun exposure, keep fresh, sweet smelling flowers around the home or office.	Keep warm and dry.

Chapter 8

Creating a daily rhythm that serves you...

"The secret of your success is found in your daily routine.' - John C. Maxwell

One of the most important aspects of the Ayurvedic approach to preventing disease and maintaining health and happiness, is identifying the daily steps that will deliver us to greatnes.

When you remember that who you are is a whole person in relationship with the world around you, it's easier to see that every aspect of your life contributes to your overall health and wellness. Every thought, feeling, action, and interaction plays a small or big part in your picture of well-being. Every day is an opportunity to know yourself better, and love yourself in ways that reflect that self knowledge. The key to unlocking the best of who you are is having a system of self-care that's built into your everyday.

Ayurveda defines a healthy lifestyle as one that is:

- Lived in accordance and harmony with the cycles of nature
- Is lived in accordance with one's true nature – takes into consideration your dosha
- Minimizes exposure to the effects of stress
- Includes appropriate self-care

But what does this look like from day to day?

The Daily Cycle of Energies

In chapter seven, we looked at how changes in the environment impact the doshas from season to season and how that changes the way we look, feel, and operate. We identified that each season has qualities that will increase or aggravate certain doshas, making it necessary to focus on balancing those doshas during that season.

The next thing to understand is that the energetic rhythm of the doshas is also reflected in the sun and moon cycle that governs a single day. Yes, the energies of the doshas inside and outside of you rise and fall in a single day! This highlights the power and importance of harmonizing your daily rhythm with that of the natural world, if nothing else but to avoid the stressful and exhausting experience of life feeling like a roller coaster ride!

The Ayurvedic practice of **dinacharya** – comes from a combination of two words. "dina" (day) and "archarya", which means to follow or be close to. So dinacharya is an approach to living that merges our daily cycle of activities, everything from waking up to eating to exercise, etc., with the natural cycle of the sun, moon, and doshas.

The four seasons of the day

The Ayurvedic day begins before sunrise. This is a time of day that is cool, clear, and dry. Most of us are asleep during this time, and in our sleep our minds become active and erratic. It's the time of dreams. If you spend any time in nature you'll know that the natural world begins to stir in that window of time that occurs just before sunrise, synchronizing with the prevailing energy of movement.

The beginning part of the day is very much like the spring. It feels very new, natural, and often moist and cool. And like spring, there's a heaviness in the air in the early morning that disappears as the day moves on.

Mid morning to early afternoon is the warmest part of the day, similar to summer. It's the time of the day when the sun rises to its highest point in the sky, giving us an experience of our peak temperatures inside and outside the body.

From there things start to cool down and once again become a little less predictable as we move towards the heaviness of the evening and then settle into the cooler temperatures of the latest hours of the day, a lot like the shift from fall to winter.

But at some point in the night, if you haven't managed to get to bed, you might start to feel a second wind coming on, plugging in to a whole other energy that wakes and rises hours after the sun goes down and peaks when the moon is highest in the sky before dipping into the transition that signals the start of a new day.

If this sounds or feels familiar to you, it's a confirmation that there is a natural rhythm to each day that is a part of everyone's experience. Ayurveda believes that we should live in harmony with this natural cycle of energy in order to be the most efficient, and authentically healthy and happy as possible. Dancing with life is about riding the ebbs and flows of daily living and working, using the changing energy of the day to keep you moving forward. It's a process of making lifestyle choices to offset the imbalancing influences of our internal and external worlds. So let's take a look at what that means.

Your Day ACCORDING TO THE DOSHAS

2am - 6am • Start your day during vata time...

The energy of movement intensifies during this time of day. Our brains become active in dreams and thoughts, sometimes resulting in insomnia (which always seems to happen around 3 or 4 am. Coincidence? I don't think so!). Some of my best and most creative ideas come during this time of day when my mind and body are untethered and free.

This time of day is best for: Sleeping, of course, however, Ayurveda recommends waking up during vata time, just before the sunrise, in order to take advantage of the prevailing energy of movement to get out of bed, exercise, and get the body-mind moving.

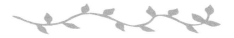

6am - 10am • Settle in during kapha time...

During this time of day there's a shift from active energy of vata to a more peaceful , heavy, and grounding kapha energy. Getting up and out of bed during this timeframe can be a challenge since you'll be working against the cold, heavy ,and dull energy of kapha (especially during kapha season – late winter and spring).

This time of day is best for: Grounding, nurturing, and routine activities, like meditation and self-care. I like to take things a little slower during kapha time and avoid scheduling anything requiring a faster pace (meetings, brainstorming, etc.) in this timeframe when the brain and body are likely to feel a little heavy and dull relative to the rest of the day. Digestive fire tends to be at its lowest during this time of day as well, so it's important to be mindful about what and how much to eat, since big heavy breakfasts can further slow digestion.

10am - 2pm • Eat and meet during pitta time...

The energy of pitta intensifies during this time, coinciding with the hottest part of the day. This is the time when our minds are most likely to be at their sharpest, most organized, and intense. Physically, our digestive fire is at its peak around this time of day.

This time of day is best for: Ayurveda highly recommends enjoying lunch during pitta time (between 11am - 1pm) and making it the biggest meal of the day! As well, I like to use this time of day for strategic planning, or any activities that require a little insight, organization, and intensity.

2pm - 6pm • Move and create during vata time...

In the late afternoon it's back to vata time, when our minds and bodies are ready to move again. This time it may be in the form of restlessness or perhaps a burst of creativity or bout of anxiety. Feeling heavy during this time may be a sign of overdoing it at lunch a little or a lot.

This time of day is best for: Anything creative or moving. Exercise, art, abstract thinking, all will be supported by the energy of vata during this time of day.

6pm – 10pm • Wind down during kapha time...

The heaviness of kapha returns in the evening. As the day cools, so too does our agni (digestive fire) and with it our ability to efficiently digest food, ideas, thoughts, and emotions. A heaviness settles into the mind, body, and environment that calls for stillness

This time of day is best for: Slow down, relax and use the heaviness of kapha energy to support activities like chilling out, meditation, and sleep. This is the time to scale back sensory input (anything that needs to be digested), including meals and snacks.

10pm – 2am • Rest and digest during pitta time...

The heat of pitta returns when the moon is at its peak. Night owls (you know who you are) often experience a "second wind" around this time, and use the fire of pitta to fuel late night work or party sessions. Resting or, even better, sleeping during this time allows us to put our pitta energy towards digestion and assimilation of the day's food and activities.

This time of day is best for: Resting and letting the body do what it does best. This is the critical time of day for regulation of digestion and other metabolic processes.

So, what does your day look like? How well do you dance to the tune of the doshas? What simple shifts could you make in your daily activities to create harmony inside and out?

The Ayurvedic Daily Cycle

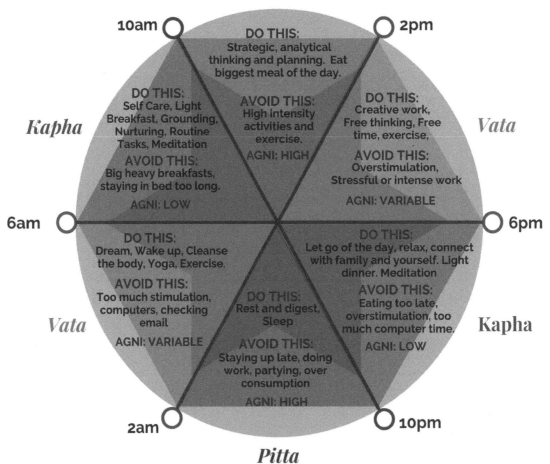

Pitta

10am — 2pm

DO THIS:
Strategic, analytical thinking and planning. Eat biggest meal of the day.

DO THIS:
Self Care, Light Breakfast, Grounding, Nurturing, Routine Tasks, Meditation

AVOID THIS:
High intensity activities and exercise.

AGNI: HIGH

DO THIS:
Creative work, Free thinking, Free time, exercise,

AVOID THIS:
Big heavy breakfasts, staying in bed too long.

AGNI: LOW

AVOID THIS:
Overstimulation, Stressful or intense work

AGNI: VARIABLE

Kapha

Vata

6am — 6pm

DO THIS:
Dream, Wake up, Cleanse the body, Yoga, Exercise.

AVOID THIS:
Too much stimulation, computers, checking email

AGNI: VARIABLE

DO THIS:
Let go of the day, relax, connect with family and yourself. Light dinner. Meditation

AVOID THIS:
Eating too late, overstimulation, too much computer time.

AGNI: LOW

DO THIS:
Rest and digest, Sleep

AVOID THIS:
Staying up late, doing work, partying, over consumption

AGNI: HIGH

Vata

Kapha

2am — 10pm

Pitta

Dinacharya: Your map for daily greatness

Have you ever noticed that we tend to treat our bodies with the same regard as our cars or other possessions (sometimes even worse)? In other words, we mostly tend to use our bodies up and take restorative action only when they break down or start giving us trouble.

We all want to be healthy, and we spend billions of dollars as a culture looking for solutions. But the real key to enduring health and happiness is taking the time to know yourself, and make your very best effort to love yourself. It's just that simple. And this is why Ayurveda recommends building acts of self-care into your every day.

Along with harmonizing the way you move and act through the day with the natural energetic rhythms, Ayurveda also recommends specific daily self-care practices to fine tune and nurture the mind and body and deepen the connection to soul.

So let's take a look at what Ayurveda recommends we do every day if we want to establish balance, and hold on to it for the long run.

But first a few more words on routine...

Routines are something that have been recognized and highly praised as valued game-changers for some of the world's most successful people. But what we don't often hear about is the fact that routines are also a highly important part of the lives of the world's happiest and healthiest people too! And that's because of a few key things:

- **Routines help to combat stress** - Routines take the guesswork out of our day. They alleviate the need to make decisions (a process that can actually be stressful on the mind and body) and they remove the uncertainty that can cause anxiety.

- **Routines make consistency possible** - Consistency is the key to having anything in our lives work. It's something that we're all consciously or subconsciously working towards, and in some cases struggling with, when it comes to making choices that are healthy for us. And routines are a vehicle for being consistent and reaping the benefits that comes with it.

So let's take a closer look at what Ayurveda suggests we do routinely every day...

Rise Early - The first moments of a day, like the first seconds of an infant's life, are minutes that can set the tone for an experience. If we allow the first attention of the day to be peaceful, grateful and infused with a sense of joy, it is more likely that our day will be pleasant.

Ayurveda recommends **Brahma Muhurta** a sanskrit word the means "The hour of God" which is a time frame corresponding to approximately one hour and thirty-six minutes before sunrise. The energy of this time of day is highly sattvic (peaceful and calming), making it great for cultivating clarity and connection to self.

Reconnect - One of my favorite teachers of Ayurveda, Dr. Vasant Lad, recommends taking time upon waking to "remember who you are". My practice is to take a few moments just before getting out of bed to ask four simple questions:

- Who am I?
- What do I want?
- What is my purpose?
- What am I grateful for?

And as I ask myself these questions, I focus on listening for the answers rather than struggling to get it right. It's a simple way of acknowledging that we change from day to day and making a practice acceptance of that.

Eliminate - *Apana* (downward) energy is active early in the morning and supports natural elimination. Regular elimination in the morning is good practice and is something that you can train your body to do if it doesn't already.

Cleanse the senses - Wash the face and ears, rinse the eyes out, and scrape the tongue first thing in the morning to clear away the stagnation and gunk (kapha) that has settled overnight. This early morning cleansing is a form of purification for the mind as well, allowing the whole of you to start new and fresh.

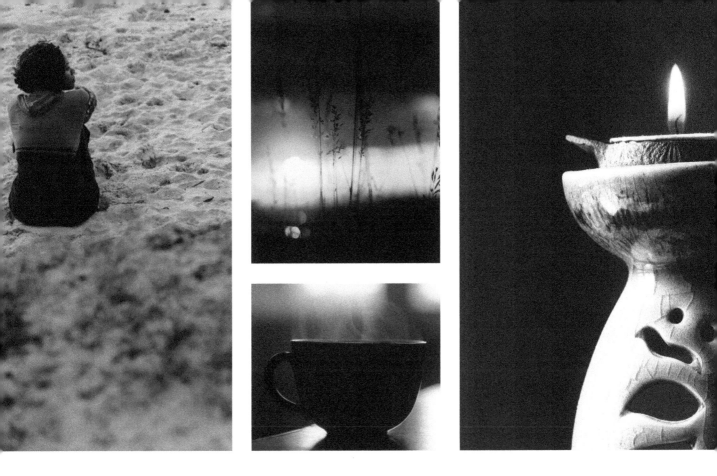

Prime the fire • Digestion can be slow or sluggish in the morning. Drinking warm water with lemon is a gentle way to wake and warm the digestive fre and stimulate peristalsis, which can also help with elimination.

Integrate • First thing in the morning, when the mind is calm, clear and unburdened, is the best time of day for yoga and meditation. So if you have a practice, it's beneficial to use this calm and energizing time of day for that.

Lubricate the body • Oil massage or *abhyanga* is a nourishing practice of self love for the mind and body. Touch is something we need as human beings. It conveys the message to every part of you that you're worthy of wellness and all that comes with it. It's also a wonderful way to lubricate the skin and joints and stave off the drying out that happens as we age.

Bath or shower • Washing the body every day is also a self-love ritual that goes beyond the actual task itself. It's recommended that one should only wash the "dirty areas" (typically armpits, genitals, feet, and neck) of the body on a daily basis and simply rinse the rest of the body so as not to dry out the skin.

Feed the fire (*but don't smother it*) • Keep breakfast somewhat light as the digestive fire tends to be low during the morning. Eating breakfast before 8am is also recommended, as well as ensuring that you get just enough nourishment to sustain you until lunchtime.

Lunch like a king • Your digestive fire is likely to be well primed by lunchtime and ready to digest the largest meal of your day. Try to consume lunch between 11am - 1pm to take advantage of this high time for metabolization. Remember not to overeat and to ensure you've had enough to sustain you until dinnertime (avoid snacking!).

Dinner light and simple • In many cultures (western and eastern alike), dinner is often the largest meal of the day, but Ayurveda recommends that you keep it light (soups, salads, light fare, moderate portions), as your digestive fire will be in the process of slowing down this time of day. Dinner before 7pm is recommended, or at least 3 hours before bedtime.

Ease into evening • Evening is a time to relax and let go of the activities of the day. It's a perfect time for reconnecting with yourself and your family, and Ayurveda recommends that you build these acts of self care into your life. Create an evening ritual to help with this. Doing so will pay you back in energy, connection, and love.

Cherish Sleep • Sleep is a vital part of healthy living. In fact, the most frequent "prescription" I give is for my clients is to get more and better sleep (it's a small thing that can have HUGE impacts in your life). Ayurveda recommends getting in bed by no later than 10:30pm, but it can vary slightly by dosha and time of year. The goal is to get the right amount of sleep for you - between 6-8 hours depending on the person. And if you have trouble getting to sleep, try oiling the feet and the top of the head before getting into bed.

The art of choosing wellness...daily

For many of us these days, our outside world can feel a little (okay a lot) chaotic! Too much information, too much to do, too little support, too little time. So many choices and voices and people to please, and what's worse is that we're running ourselves ragged trying to keep up with it all.

By refusing to turn our focus inward, we've become our own worst enemies. And we've got the fatigue, anxiety, burnout, and an extra fifteen pounds to prove it! As human beings we are programmed for survival, and in order to do that, we often compromise our well-being and enjoyment of living because under all the noise of our daily lives, we've managed to forget that self-care HAS to be a choice!

Ayurveda teaches us that thriving is available to all of us, and it starts with an understanding that in order to be our best, we must create simple systems for showing ourselves love on a daily basis.

Dinacharya is one of the most important and powerful aspects of Ayurveda, because it acknowledges that what you do every day matters more than what you do every once in a while! But it's important to understand (and appreciate) that dinacharya is a guideline. A framework for refocusing your attention on caring for yourself in ways that are the most beneficial, and more importantly... doable!

And like everything in Ayurveda, there is no "one-size-fits-all" approach to daily living. Your responsibility is to find a way to make it work for you. To use the curiosity and love that you have for yourself as your biggest ally in seeking out the foods, activities, and environments that will support you in establishing a healthy balance.

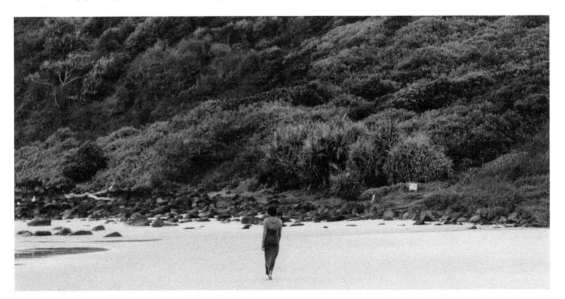

Chapter 9

The lifestyle pitfalls that
keep you from shining..

"Embrace each challenge in your life as an opportunity for self-transformation." - *Bernie Siegel*

For most of us, food is SO much more than just a nutrient delivery system; often, it's a therapist, an entertainer, and a good friend. And in a world of unlimited choices and contradictory messages about what to eat (High fat? High protein? Vegetarian? Gluten free? Organic?, etc.), our relationship with food has left us feeling powerless and confused.

So take a moment to consider your relationship with food. How did you get here?

We grow up being taught that food is both the devil and the savior. And then we seek outside of ourselves to try to understand which is which. From the earliest age we alienate ourselves from our body's intelligence and worship at the church of the wellness industry, believing that if we can master "healthy eating" we'll be redeemed.

So our quest for a healthy diet is often motivated by our deep desire to fix some part of us that's broken. We approach the process of finding the food that will feed us mind, body and soul from a critical rather than curious place and in the process set ourselves up for failure and disappointment. And in looking for that magic bullet, we avoid asking the most important question:

How can my diet serve who I am today?

The mistakes we make...

The most powerful way to answer the question of what to eat is to come from an understanding that who you are is WHOLE, not a collection of disparate and broken parts. And every time you pick up that fork, you're committing to feeding all aspects of your being in one way or another, not just your body (regardless of what shape it's in).

This is especially important when you consider that your mind makes nearly all of decisions about what you eat and your body is the physical expression of those choices. So no matter how you feel about your current state of mind or the choices you've made to date...

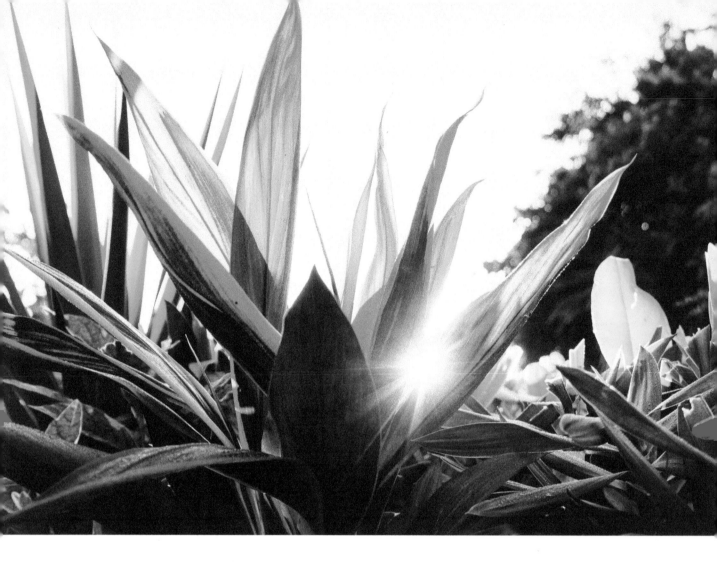

Ayurveda wants you to know that your natural state is vibrant!

And I want you to know that underneath the daily challenges that you face; fatigue, mood swings, anxiety, excess weight, foggy brain or even just a lifetime's worth of guilt and shame, **you are a graceful, energetic, calm, and balanced soul** and returning yourself to feeling alive and inspired is easier than you think. But it starts with acknowledging some of the mistakes you've made (or are still making) that are holding you back. Beginning with:

Eating someone else's diet

Ever wondered why you've tried so many different approaches to getting and staying healthy and happy, and you still haven't found the right one yet? Why you've followed all the advice and you still don't feel like you're living in the mind and body and life that's rightfully yours?

The way we see and relate to ourselves plays a vital role in how effective we can be in our efforts to shine, and so does the way we engage with advice and information from the world around us.

While some of our struggle results from a lack of commitment, our biggest challenge is in learning HOW to listen to ourselves, and others. Many of us seek out and rely on information and advice from experts in the fields of wellness to guide our actions and choices. But we listen with a view to fixing rather than understanding ourselves.

So many of us hold on to the belief that if we follow the path of our wellness mentors step by step, we can be more like them. If we "eat" their diet for living, we'll look, sound, feel, and express ourselves as they do. But we forget that where we're starting from and what we're working with is entirely different.

Taking back your power to experience yourself as healthy, happy and whole, begins with remembering that you are NOT broken. You are a unique individual with unique gifts and challenges. Finding and staying on your path requires letting go of competing and comparing.

Ayurveda wants you to embrace that you're not like anyone else.

So looking and feeling like the real YOU will happen when you ditch the diet and lifestyle that doesn't fit so that you can discover the unique foods and activities that support who you are and who you want to be.

But before we talk about how you do that, let's take a look at one of the other mistakes that's very likely standing between you and your best self. Because if you've been eating for someone other than you, chances are pretty good that you've also been...

Neglecting the fire inside

The Ayurvedic mantra is "you are what you digest" and that means everything from the news you watch on TV to the food you're eating while you watch it.

And when your digestion is compromised or broken, it looks and feels a lot like dullness, fatigue, heaviness, confusion, disconnection, cravings, fear (the opposite of confidence), and self-limiting thoughts. Any of this sound familiar? You're not alone, but here's the thing...

Your digestion gives you access to the goodness in the food and experiences you consume. It's the critical player in creating and living a soulful, balanced life. It's the fire inside that we smother with too much or the wrong kinds of food, information, interactions, and thoughts.

But the GREAT news is...

Stoking your digestive fire and keeping it burning bright is actually pretty simple with the right foods and a little awareness.

First, it's important to understand that WHAT you eat is really only the half of it.

I've seen and talked to lots of people who make healthy diet choices every day, but still struggle to feel light, bright, and fully alive. If that sounds a lot like you then it might be that far too often you're...

Dining in a minefield

When was the last time you ate a meal in a relaxed and present state? Not on the phone or watching TV, not in your car or at your desk, not in between trips to the kitchen, or in the middle of conversations. Can't remember?

Well, guess what?

All that disruption, multi-tasking, and chaos actually wreaks havoc on your digestion.

Why? Because human beings were not designed to multi-task.

What we have been brilliantly designed to do is direct our internal energy to where it's most needed. So if we're talking, thinking, driving, or running from the proverbial tiger (i.e. experiencing stress in any form), chances are pretty good that we're NOT digesting! Or at least not very well.

The bottom line is multitasking = stress = lousy digestion...and remember lousy digestion = lousy mind, body, and life.

That's three things that most people do every day and still wonder why they're struggling to look and feel healthy!

But even if you're doing all the right things and have somehow managed to escape most of the pitfalls I've outlined above, you might still have fallen prey to the one that seems to get everyone...

Living at cross purposes to nature

Ever noticed that you feel better during certain times of the day than others? Like early in the morning or maybe really late at night? As we learned in chapter eight, there's a natural cycle to the day that accounts for the mental and physical shifts we experience from dawn to dusk (and in between).

That natural rise and fall of energy through the day (similar to the one that occurs as we move through the seasons) impacts our own levels of energy, engagement, and motivation.

Attempting things like focused work when the energy around you is light and moving, trying to wake up and get out of bed in an environment that feels heavy, or digesting a big meal when the energy inside and out is slow and cold can be taxing on the mind and body and make the task feel impossible!

And that's usually the time when resistance kicks in, and then stress. The kind of stress that eventually leads to feeling overwhelmed, fatigue, and things like weight gain.

This is typically the point at which we feel disconnected, out of control, and ready to give up!

So now let's talk about what you can do about it.

But first let me just say that Ayurveda, views each one of us as a complete, whole human being capable of thriving mentally and physically regardless of our age. It also wants us to understand that who we are is the result of the choices we make every day to eat, move, and connect with the world around us and our own hearts and minds.

What that means is there is NO reason, other than those you make up yourself, that you can't look and feel radiant, be empowered and authentic in every choice you make, andconnect passionately with the world around you every day. **You just have to be willing to..**

Discover who you are
What if what you've been trying to fix isn't actually what needs fixing?

In the ebbs and flows of daily life, we often lose track of who we are and end up wanting to "fix" or change some of the best things about ourselves when the real issue is somewhere else entirely!

Knowing yourself gives you the power to know the difference between...

- YOU and your cultural conditioning,
- YOU and the person everyone wants you to be,
- YOU and the voices in your own head,
- The authentic (balanced) YOU and the imbalanced you.

Knowing who you are is your foundation, a place to call home. It's also a launch pad from which to fly. **Ready to give it a try?**

Start with these questions:

- **Who am I?** - What does the true you look and feel like? What parts of your experience of life feel balanced?
- **What stops me?** - What are the people, places, experiences, and foods that throw you off balance and make you feel less than yourself?
- **What feeds me?** - What foods, activities, and thoughts make you feel alive and inspire your greatness?

And if the answers don't come immediately:

- **Pay attention** - Notice how your mind and body react to the foods, activities, people, weather, and environments that you come into contact with on a daily basis. Identify where the stress in your life comes from and where it hides.

- **Know your dosha** - Your Ayurvedic mind-body constitution is a reflection of your true nature and will help you answer some of these questions. Discovering it is as simple as **taking a simple quiz! (like this one in the appendices!)**

And once you've done that...

Keep noticing how you interact with yourself and your environment, and above all, start accepting and loving who you are as a completely unique individual with your own special set of gifts to offer the world. Next you'll want to...

Eat for who you are right now
Food is one of our biggest allies when it comes to looking and feeling balanced and healthy!

What's important to understand is that we make really bad decisions about food and just about everything else when we're in an imbalanced state.

A diet that supports you is one that helps you re-establish mental and physical harmony moment to moment (and meal to meal) so that you can keep making choices that keep you powerfully connected to the mind, body, and life you're committed to living in!

Here's what I mean by that:

- **Feeling tired, bloated, cold, and heavy?** Choose foods that are light, warm, dry, and energizing (most smoothies don't fit this bill!). Try light soups with spices, steamed veggies with light and warming grains (millet, polenta, quinoa, buckwheat), greens sauteed in a little ghee, rice cakes, popcorn (air popped).

- **Feeling spaced out, anxious, fatigued, and distracted?** Steer clear of light and dry and go for something that's a little heavier (grounding), nourishing and soothing (root veggies, stews, baked fruit or fruit crumble, casseroles, heavier soups and chowders, rice, and pastas).

- **Feeling overheated, tense, critical, and acidic?** Reach for foods that are cooling and calming, slightly bitter, and slightly sweet (fruit salads, sorbet, anything scented with rosewater, fresh vegetable salads, coconut milk, avocados, and spices like mint, cardamom, and coriander/cilantro).

Realize that your body–mind NEEDS inputs relative to its current state (when you're cold you put on a sweater or coat, not a bathing suit and sandals, right?). So tuning into your internal state and making the choice to feed your REAL hunger is one of the most powerful things you can do for yourself, your body, and ultimately your health and happiness.

Oh, and finally...

Go with the natural flow...

Energy is something we could all use a little more of

These days most of us run our tanks all the way down to empty before even thinking about our energy levels or asking for help. We forget is that energy is all around us, and that we are defined by our relationship with that energy!

Allowing the energy of your environment to support you is one of the keys to good health and good everything. So...

What small shifts you can make in your daily routine and meal times to start using the day's energy to your advantage in order to feel lighter, brighter, more motivated and inspired, and get things done with stamina to spare?

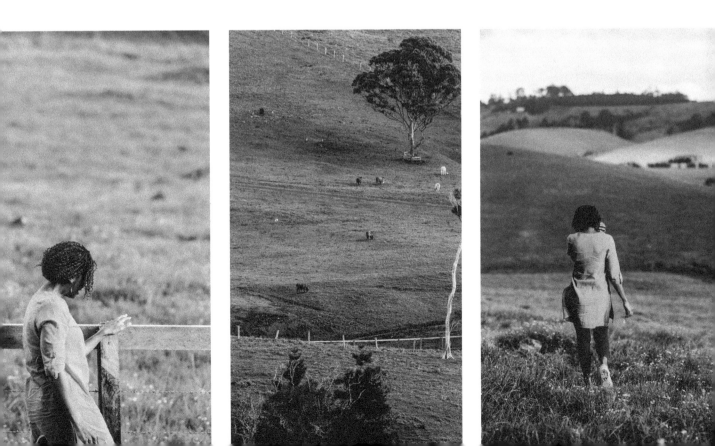

Chapter 10

How to eat like you love yourself

> *"Everything you see I owe to spaghetti."*
> **Sophia Loren**

So, what does it mean to eat like you love yourself? There are as many answers to this question as there are individuals on the planet. But regardless of how and what we choose to eat, there's no denying that our desire for food is universally driven by two fundamental human emotions: Love and Fear.

At its essence, eating is an act of love. It's a conscious or unconscious message we send to the body-mind that we want or need to soothe, nourish, protect, or grow some aspect of our being.

But more often than not, we make choices from a place of fear -- fear of not having or being enough, fear of feeling what we're feeling, fear of emptiness, fear of loving ourselves just the way we are. And it's our fears that drive what, how much, when, and why we eat.

When fear is running the show, the focus is survival, staying alive, creating comfort. Our ability to thrive becomes compromised and diminished. And our experience of life can become stagnant and dull.

Reversing this experience and reclaiming your vitality is a matter of awareness and intention, a willingness to take responsibility for your life starting with what you put into your body.

Like life, eating like you love yourself is a journey to discover the foods, environments, and routines that make your mind and body feel supported, light, strong, and energized in the moment and beyond. But more than that, it's a process of finding the courage to choose them again and again.

The rules of the road...

Eating like you love yourself isn't easy, but I'm a big fan of keeping things simple (especially the challenging things). And since figuring out what to eat is already complicated enough, I've simplified the path to eating like you love yourself down to three simple principles:

1. **Eat seasonally**
2. **Keep your fire burning**
3. **Choose balance**

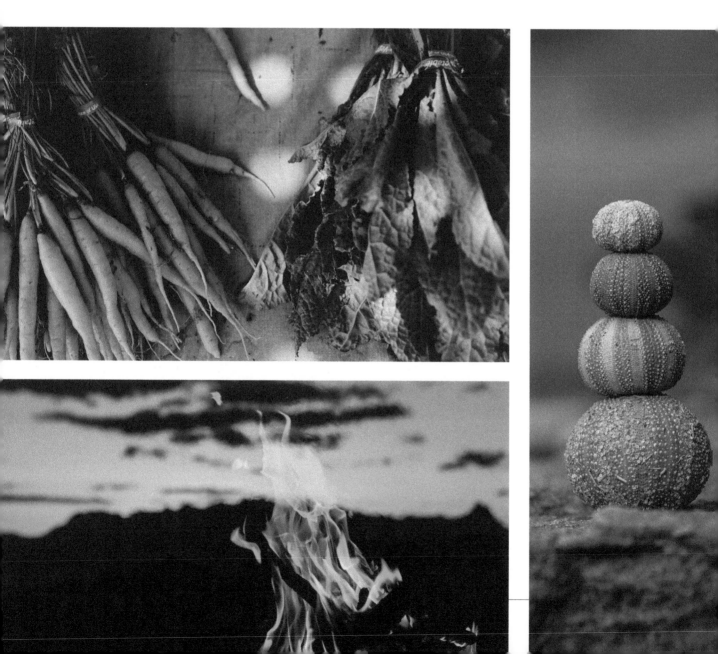

EAT SEASONALLY

When I was a kid, cherries and peaches signaled a welcome and significant shift in my life. Summer had arrived. Long warm school-free days, road trips, family picnics and Fourth of July BBQs were what we had to look forward to.

We ate watermelon, grapes, and peach cobbler until the cooler weather set in. When we'd reminisce about the good times, mourn the loss of summer heat, freedom, and trips to the beach and look forward to new beginnings as the start of school, and with it, new routines, daily schedules, and ways of eating would await us.

What's in season where you're living right now?

Most westerners have trouble answering this question these days. "Advances" in food production, farming, transportation and preservation have resulted in an almost constant abundance of foods from every corner of the planet making their way into your refrigerator almost at whim. And with these advances and growing convenience, a widening disconnect between us and the natural world around us is occurring.
Ayurveda teaches that wellness represents a state of balance or harmony between our internal and external environments. We are here to support each other. The foods that naturally grow where and when we live have the qualities that we need to create balance at that time and in those surroundings.

The foods that are in season where you live are the natural supports to imbalances that environmental factors can bring about.

Why is this important? Your medicine is all around you. It allows you to avoid illnesses and dips in immunity, energy, and clarity that have a big impact on the quality of your life. Eating the foods that are in season where you are and when you are is just another powerful step towards achieving real wellness. In other words, wellness that is unique to you.

What does this mean? Springtime produce like asparagus, peas, fresh corn, and leafy greens have light, warm, or drying qualities that offset the cool, damp heaviness that has usually set into your mind and body by the end of winter and can show up as congestion, water retention, lethargy, or even depression. As the winter blues begin to melt, these seasonal foods warm the body-mind and stimulate the processes of drying up mucus and congestion and letting go of excess weight. The same can be said about the qualities of the foods that show up in every new season. They act as a natural complement to your immune system.

What are some of the best ways to make this possible?

Eat local Make it a habit to visit your local farmer's markets regularly. I've found that farmer's markets are a great way to both connect with your local community (the ones in my area are more like a weekly social gathering) and with what you should be eating.

Educate yourself Make an effort to learn about what's seasonal in your area of the world, especially if you don't have a local farmer's market. Use this knowledge to make informed choices about what to pick at your supermarket. [LINK to guides for seasonal produce around the world]

Explore and embrace the change

Challenge yourself to step out of your usual patterns of cooking and eating, and try new recipes using seasonal foods, complementary herbs and spices, and new ways of cooking. Create a collection of treasured recipes that you and your loved ones look forward to eating with every new season.

KEEP YOUR FIRE BURNING

Ayurveda confronts traditional western thinking about what's healthy and turns it on its head. It invites us to examine the reality of our whole state of health (no matter what size we are) and embrace that true wellness is a function of not just what we consume and burn, but how well we're breaking down what we "eat"; how well

we're absorbing the nutrients from what we eat and how well we're eliminating the remaining wastes and toxins that have the potential to undermine the whole system.

Doing this in a way that leaves you feeling light, strong, clear, and centered is a sign of a mind-body digestive system that is running at its most optimal and efficient levels, which is in part the reason for the Ayurvedic adage, "Digestion is King!"

Why is this important? This is vitally important because human beings are struggling globally. We are overworked, overwhelmed and overweight, in large part due to our lack of understanding of the important part that processing all of the information, food, emotions, ideas, and stuff that we come into contact with every day plays in our overall state of wellness. And so we unconsciously seek to transform our bodies and lives by consuming more information and "healthier" but more difficult to digest foods like processed "healthy" meals, green smoothies, raw food diets, nut milks and butters, "healthy" snack foods, and vegan anything, assuming that it will fix what's broken, when what's really needed is a simple focus on keeping the fire burning. Devoting a bit of loving attention to our mental, physical and emotional capabilities for digesting our food and our lives, or what we call in the world of yoga and Ayurveda "managing your agni" (digestive fire).

What are some of the best ways to make this possible?

Know your agni Now's the time to put all of your self-inquiry to the test. What's your digestion like typically? How does it respond to the seasons and the circumstances that you most often find yourself in (stress, travel, weather, etc.)? Use this knowledge (and your new found knowledge of the agni types) to get a good feel for your digestion, allowing that understanding to be the basis for your choices.

Know your food What are the qualities of the food that you eat most often and how likely are they to kindle or smother your digestive fire? Tune in to the impacts new foods have on your digestion, especially when you're eating out or trying something new at home. The goal is to build an internal "database" of information about how your body reacts to the inputs of your daily living and use that information to make wiser choices!

Detox regularly Ayurvedic cleansing is a powerful way to renew and replenish your entire body. But most importantly it's an opportunity to revitalize your digestion. The key is building it into your life (which is why we recommend it in spring and fall).

CHOOSE BALANCE

If you've ever had a headache or fatigue or been overweight or had a bad rash, you know that when you're living with imbalance, nothing else seems to matter. Everything in your life is colored by your experience of discomfort or pain. Every choice you make is driven by some desire to feel like yourself again.

When you're living in a state of imbalance, the most important thing you can do for yourself is to move in the direction of balance. Everyday imbalances like headaches, fatigue, constipation, and even anxiety are your body-mind telling you that something is missing. It's also your signal to take inspired action to love yourself back to health. At these times, the foods you choose can be critical to your ability to recover and move beyond what's holding you back. Doing this may require a shift in the way you relate to yourself and your food.

Most people see and relate to food relative to their cultural conditioning and the messages they were exposed to as children. Food is a comfort, a nutrition delivery system, a treat for a job well done...a refuge. Our choices for food are typically driven by a few factors, namely what we've always eaten, what we can afford, what those around us eat, and what's readily available to us. But in reality, our choices are driven by how much we know and are willing to love ourselves.

Eating for balance assumes that you're willing to learn more about yourself and develop a relationship with your food that allows you to shine. Doing that in an imbalanced state requires only two things: 1. Awareness of the imbalance (what does it look and feel like); and 2. Knowing what foods can restore the balance (something you'll learn over time).

Recognizing imbalance...

An imbalance is anything that expresses itself in the form of a symptom. Ayurveda sees it as a disturbance in the delicate balance of energies in the mind and body and it can show up in myriad different ways. Choosing balance begins with recognizing imbalance.

Many of us have simply stopped seeing the body's distress signals. Our tolerance for discomfort and "dis-ease" has grown in direct proportion to the speed at which we live our lives. The result is that imbalance has quietly become a part of our everyday.

Paying attention to symptoms and tuning in to their corresponding qualities can give us the vital information we need to choose balance when we need it most.

Check out the following lists of symptoms associated with disturbances in each of the doshas (biological energies) along with some of the qualities that balance them. With this knowledge you can seek out foods, activities or even environments with the qualities you need to re-establish balance.

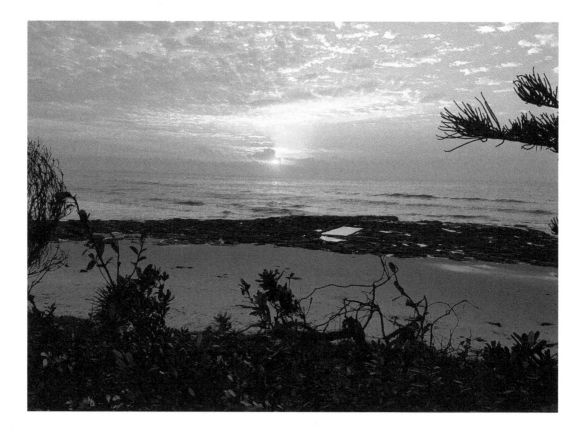

The Qualities of your imbalance

Vata Imbalance

Due to an excess of: cold, light, dry, moving, rough qualities

Symptom	Qualities in excess	Balancing Qualities
Feeling "spaced out" or ungrounded	Light, dry, moving	Heavy, moist/oily, stable
Disorganized	Moving, light	Heavy, stable
Procrastination	Light, moving, dry	Heavy, static, moist
Moody, emotionally volatile	Light, moving, rough, cold	Heavy, static, smooth, warm
Impatience	Dry, rough	Smooth, moist
Cracking or popping joints	Dry, light, rough	Moist, heavy, smooth
Muscle stiffness	Dry, rough, cold	Moist/oily, smooth, warm
Insomnia	Light, moving	Heavy, stabilizing
Dizziness	Light, dry, moving	Heavy, moist, stabilizing
Constipation	Dry, light, rough	Moist/oily, heavy, smooth
Low Energy/Fatigue	Light, dry, cold	Heavy, moist/oily, warm
Low back pain	Dry, rough, cold	Moist/oily, smooth, warm

Pitta Imbalance

Due to an excess of: hot, sharp, light, mobile, wet, flowing

Symptom	Qualities in excess	Balancing Qualities
Overly intense thinking/actions	Hot, sharp, light	Cool, dull/slow, heavy
Manipulative thinking/actions	Hot, sharp, light	Cool, dull/stable, heavy
Arrogance	Hot, sharp	Cool, Calm
Jealousy	Hot, sharp, mobile	Cool, stable, calm
Critical or judgemental	Sharp, light, mobile	Calm, heavy, stable
Anger/rage	Hot, sharp	Cool, Calm
Hot flashes	Hot, light, flowing	Cool, calm, stable, heavy
Hyperacidity	Hot, sharp, light	Cool, calm, heavy
Skin rashes/psoriasis	Hot, sharp, wet, mobile	Cool, calm, dry, stable
Ulcers	Hot, sharp, wet, light	Cool calm, dry, heavy
Inflammation	Hot, light, wet	Cool, heavy, dry
Heartburn	Hot, sharp, wet, mobile	Cool, calm, dry, stable
Diarrhea	Hot, light, mobile, wet, flowing	Cool, heavy, stable, dry

Kapha Imbalance

Due to an excess of: cold, heavy, dull, slow, wet, soft, stable, dense

Symptom	Qualities in excess	Balancing Qualities
Lethargy	Heavy, dull, slow, stable	Light, sharp, mobile, flowing
Possessiveness	Heavy, cold, dense	Light, warm, subtle
Fear of letting go	Heavy, cold, slow, dense	Light, dry, mobile, flowing
Complacency	Heavy, cold, slow	Light, warm, mobile, flowing
Depression	Heavy, slow, dull, dense	Light, mobile, sharp, flowing
Hoarding things	Heavy, slow, dense, stable	Light, mobile, flowing
Inability to express yourself	Dull, slow, dense, heavy	Sharp, subtle, moving, light
Obesity	Heavy, dull, slow, dense	Light, sharp, mobile, subtle
Colds & Flu, congestion	Cold, wet, dull, slow	Dry, warm, sharp, flowing
Yeast conditions	Heavy, wet, dull	Light, dry, sharp
Water retention, bloating	Wet, heavy dull, dense	Dry, light, sharp, flowing
Allergies	Wet, dull, dense, slow	Dry, sharp, flowing, mobile
Excess phlegm, mucus	Wet, dull, dense, slow	Dry, sharp, flowing, mobile
Heart disease	Heavy, dull, slow	Light, sharp, mobile, flowing
Intolerance to cold and damp	Cold, heavy, wet, slow	Warm, light, dry, mobile

Chapter 11

How to bring sanity into your kitchen

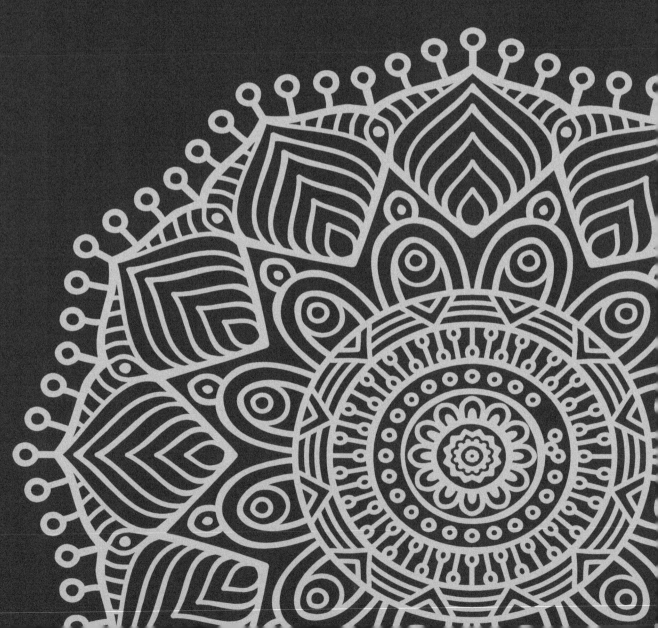

> *"Cooking is at once child's play and adult joy. And cooking done with care is an act of love."*
> **Craig Claiborne**

Why my kitchen is for dancing

These days, busy lives mean busy kitchens. And with the help of microwave ovens, endless gadgets, appliances, processed foods, and freezer meals, the focus of kitchens in many homes has changed from a physical and emotional heart of the home to its center for the convenient and efficient preparation of nutrients (sounds a little futuristic). And in that shift, we've lost the love and the soul of cooking and eating!

According to Ayurveda, the act of preparing and eating food is considered a **sadhana** (Sanskrit for sacred practice). What underlies this belief is the view that eating is as much about feeding the mind (and soul) as feeding the body. Because how we feel about the entire process of nourishing ourselves from choosing to cooking to eating will inform how we're nourished by it.

With that in mind, consider the following simple suggestions for reclaiming your kitchen from the "Sunday prep" and "microwave blitz" madness to create a sacred space where the love and the magic happens.

Eat REAL food Processed food is a necessary part of life for most people these days. Work and family schedules and commitments mean that making everything from scratch is nearly impossible. But in our era of convenience, even the healthiest minded folks among us have come to rely on processed foods to an unhealthy degree. And that's in part due to the fact that processed foods support our busy lives. They make it possible to enjoy a wide range of foods in the time and space that most of us have available (which isn't much). But the vitally important downside is that processing the food takes most of the life and nearly all of the naturally occurring nutrients out of it.

As a result, most processed foods are low in prana (life force energy) and high in nutrients like sugars, salts, and saturated fats that are best limited in order to avoid disease. Even the "healthy" processed foods like yogurt, "healthy" snack chips, and frozen "healthy" meals that are cropping up in health food outlets these days are little better than their "non-healthy" counterparts.

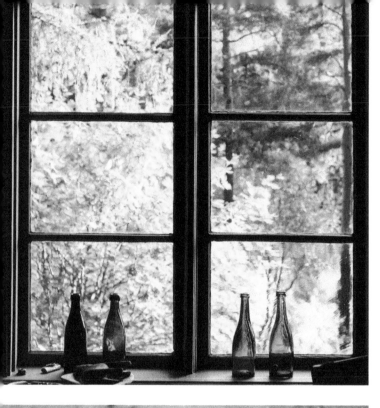
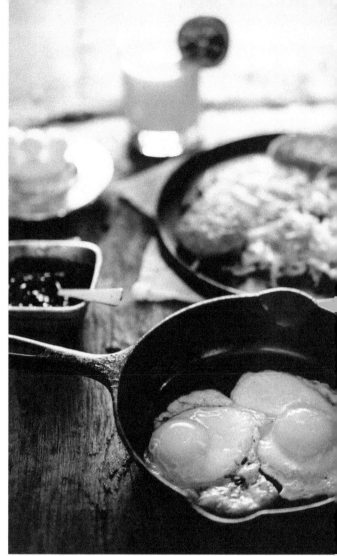
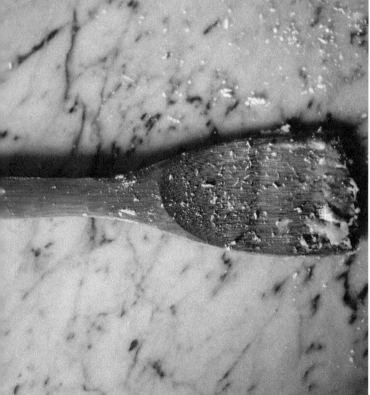
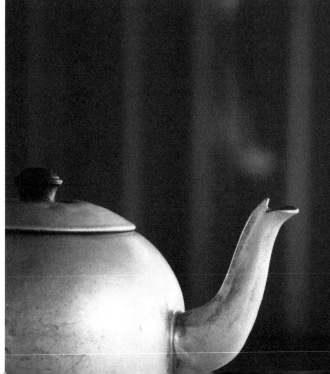
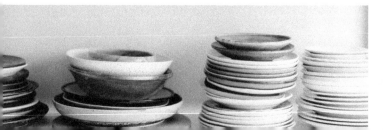

Eating real food means choosing fresh, whole, unprocessed or minimally processed wherever possible. The fewer the ingredients, the better. And while there are ongoing debates about the definition of "real food," consider that the overall goal is to consume foods that help to restore some of the natural nutrients and life force energy that we rely on to build a strong, resilient, and healthy mind and body. Most of these foods can be found at your local farmer's markets or on the outside aisles of your supermarket.

HOW TO DO IT: Do a pantry inventory and get rid of any non-essential processed foods (check the pantry list in the appendix). Make a slow and manageable transition to minimally processed sugars and grain flours. Seek out local farmer's markets for weekly fresh produce and other products. Experiment with making simple staples like yogurt, bread, nut butters, and sauces (I've included some recipes). Consider simplifying your diet to include only (or mostly) those foods that are able to be sourced fresh or made by hand. This sounds challenging, but it is SO much easier than you think! Start small with intention and give yourself space to grow into this new way of thinking and living.

Cook with love... Ever had a meal (or anything) prepared with love? Something prepared by your mother, grandmother, some family member, or friend just for you? If so then you know how it makes you feel.

Guess what? You can do that for yourself and, even better, you can do that for others. Food is a gift that we give our bodies and ourselves, the food we eat is what literally becomes our flesh and bones, so choose wisely and put all the love and goodness you can muster into the process of preparation and serving. Feed your body with love and it will return the favor.

HOW TO DO IT: Create a simple pre-cooking ritual to set an energetic intention for the food you're preparing. Whether it's for a special occasion or the everyday, taking a moment to center yourself, get present to your mental, physical, and emotional state of mind and consciously choosing the energy that you want to bring to the process of cooking, serving, and eating can take some of the stress, resentment, or hurry out of cooking. It can also benefit your digestion and set you up to enjoy every aspect of the meal prep for a change! (Check appendix for more kitchen sadhanas).

Use herbs and spices to create balance... Herbs and spices are one of our most powerful tools for regulating and strengthening the digestive fire. They provide distinct and potent qualities to help counter heaviness and congestion, ease gas and bloating, and alleviate digestion and elimination challenges. They are the foundation for Ayurvedic herbal medicine, allowing us to take advantage of the natural healing intelligence present in our backyard gardens.

Using spices to counteract some of the less attractive qualities in our food or the ones that can cause us problems, means that we can expand the quantity and variety of foods available to us in any season or environment, enhancing our ability to create balance and love life!

HOW TO DO IT: Start with educating yourself about the qualities of the herbs and spices that are readily available where you are. Get an understanding of the way that herbs work with the doshas and how they can be used to improve digestion or help to alleviate some of your most common imbalances. Buy fresh whole spices and grind them yourself for the most potent and effective result. You can also consider growing and harvesting herbs in your own backyard if you want to deepen the connection between you and the natural world. Make a spice mix for each season (make it an important part of your seasonal transition routine).

Eat in peace... How often do you eat on the run, in front of the television, reading a book, or while driving, talking, or trying to do a gazillion other things? If this is you (and let's face it, it's all of us sometimes), realize that you're compromising your digestion. Your body is a marvel of multi-tasking, but in the same way that driving and texting can be a little taxing on the brain, eating and texting (or anything else) can mess with your ability to get everything you need from your food (and create toxins to boot). So try enjoying your meals in a peaceful setting. No TV or reading, driving, OR texting. Give your body-mind the space it needs to do what it does best. Consider that your food feeds you in so many ways and by trying to do too many things while eating, you're actually missing out on the party!

HOW TO DO IT: Start with a simple question. What is it that usually stresses you out when eating? Getting up from the table to get something you forgot? The noise of the television, radio, or people speaking in another room? Ringing phone or doorbell? Consider as many things as you can and then take steps to address them before you sit down to eat. In fact, you can even create a pre-meal checklist!

Kitchen Sadhanas
Rituals for creating peace, joy and balance in the kitchen

For Cooking

- Wash your hands (mindfully)
- Keep the kitchen at a comfortable temperature.
- Clear your mind (a few deep breaths usually does the trick!)
- Give thanks (embrace a spirit of gratitude for the experience)
- Give Love (let go of resentment, anger, sadness and give love to the experience and the food).
- Listen to soothing or joyful music
- Listen to the sound of your breath

For Eating

- Turn off the TV and radio.
- Put phones on silent.
- Make sure the dining area is tidy and clear of distracting clutter.
- Get everyone to the table at the same time.
- Let anyone who's not eating know that you don't want to be disturbed during your meal.
- Make sure you've got everything you need on the table (especially if you've got kids).

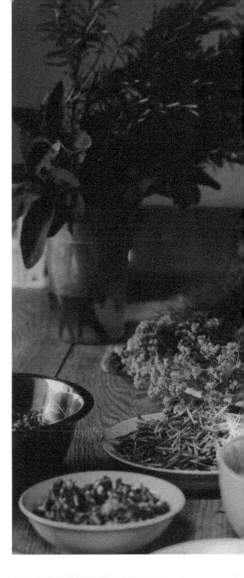

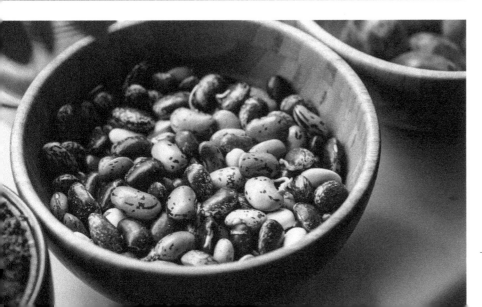

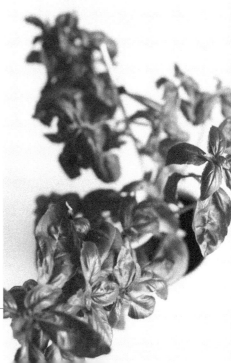

Chapter 12

Creating a food partnership to support your mind, body and soul

*"One cannot think well, love well, sleep well,
if one has not dined well."* **Virginia Woolf**

There has never been a time in the history of the human race when more options for what to eat have been as available and easily accessible to us than today.

There is SO much food available these days, so many choices of foods from all categories, and we're inventing new categories everyday to support our changing tastes and understanding of the impact our food has on our internal and external environments.

But even in the midst of all of this seeming excess, I find it necessary to ask: Are you getting enough?

And by that, I mean are you getting enough of the things that really matter in both your diet AND your life?

Our lives are packed so full these days that many of us live in a near constant state of overload. Because of that, we don't often take the time to consider what's really important, nor do we take the steps required to ensure we're getting enough of it. What results is a widening gap between daily life (the way we live it) and happiness. A gap that we fill with shiny objects, useless information, unhealthy relationships, and more and more dysfunctional food, and still end up feeling empty.

What's Your mind-body-soul food?

Because Ayurveda expands the concept of who we are from just a body with a brain to something much more, we must expand our concept of feeding ourselves to include all of our constituent "parts" if we're to live in a whole and healthy way. And so the concept of food must be expanded as well.

And if you've ever struggled with weight, fatigue, or being overwhelmed, (and let's face it, who hasn't?), it's vital to consider that more than being the result of too much food or work, that it may be a function of some part of you that's starving.

So how do YOU feed the mind, body, and soul?

FOOD FOR THE MIND

"Food" for the mind is, in a word, inspiration. It's thoughts, ideas, and emotions that incite kindness, acceptance, joy, patience, generosity, and love. In my opinion, mind food is meant to bring you closest to a state of peace, presence, compassion, and connection to your authentic beliefs.

How to find your "mind" food: You know your mind food by the way it makes you feel. Does it calm, inspire, incite, or relax? Do the ideas, thoughts, and information you consume bring you closer to you? Do they expand your worldview or challenge your beliefs about who you are? If they only tantalize and delight without truly nourishing your thinking, they might be a little closer to "mind candy" than food, and may have a similar effect on the mind as candy has on the body!

FOOD FOR THE BODY

Food for the body is a partnership. It's a give and take relationship that changes as you and the world around you change (throughout the day, month, and year!). Ayurveda recommends that food for the body be fresh, whole, pure, seasonal, and full of life-force energy (ditch anything processed, microwaved, or left over). Food for the body should be consumed with your senses in a calm and peaceful state (preferably sitting down) and in quantities intended not to overburden the digestion (about as much as you can fit into two hands cupped together).

How to choose the right "body" food: Like a great partnership, you know you've found the right food if it makes your body feel supported, light, strong, and energized, in the moment and beyond. You find your "body" food by asking questions like "Does the food I eat support who I want and need to be in the world?" and "Does it feel like a partnership that's working?", and by being willing to make changes based on your answers.

FOOD FOR THE SOUL

Food for the soul fills your heart. "Soul" food is at the center of everything. Whether you know it or not, it's what gets you out of bed in the morning and keeps you going all day. Your "soul" food reveals what you're committed to in life: laughter, quiet moments, adventure, comfort, connection. And ensuring that your soul is sufficiently fed is as vital as feeding any other part of you!

How to feed your soul: "Soul" food gives us access to parts of us that we may not know or recognize, but that feel unquestionably right. It gives us a glimpse of who we were born to be and what could be possible if we had the courage to know and love ourselves. Feeding the soul is a matter of paying attention to those experiences and connections that remind you who you really are and dare you to believe it!

Are you what you eat?

Our relationship with our food is often complicated by the view that a well-nourished body is the key to health and happiness. The result is that we are hungry minds and souls walking around in overfed bodies, seeking a sense of balance. Achieving that balance comes from expanding our view of who we are and how we can interact with ourselves and the world in order to get enough of what we really need. And THAT starts with asking a simple question...

How do you feed yourself?

Does your diet (i.e. what, when, and how you eat) leave you feeling energetic, light, satisfied, confident, guilt-free, and empowered? Would you say that it supports who you are in every possible way? If your answer is anything less than an enthusiastic, "hell yes", we've got work to do.

Why? Because eating is about SO much more than just delivering vitamins and nutrients to your body (if you've ever devoured a pizza or carton of ice cream after a victory or defeat, you know what I'm talking about). Our obsession with food has complicated our relationship with it (note to self: obsession isn't great for any relationship). Along with that, we've polarized food (and ourselves) into two buckets: "Good" and "Bad." And in doing so, we've removed the ability to see our food and how we consume it for what it really is to us: therapy, entertainment, control, camaraderie, and yes, self-medication.

So how would you characterize your relationship with food (and eating)? Guess what? It matters a lot. And if you're thinking it might be time for a change, start with awareness and these few simple practices...

Know what food is about for you... Consider that, like your spouse, partner, or closest friend, there are some things you will never know or understand about your food. What's important is that you know the basics, how you feel about it and how it makes you feel. For this you need awareness more than research. Take time to know where you stand in your relationship with food because, just like with those you love, if your diet doesn't feed and empower you, it's worth asking yourself why and making some changes in your thinking and choices.

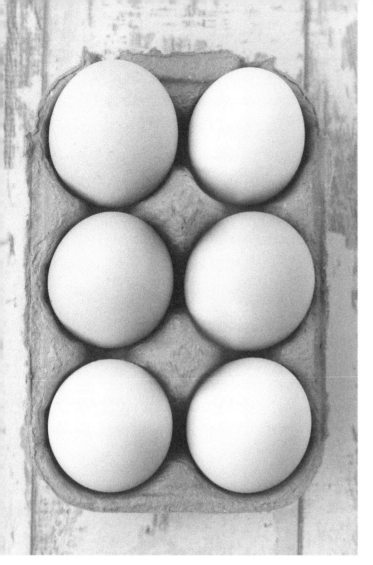

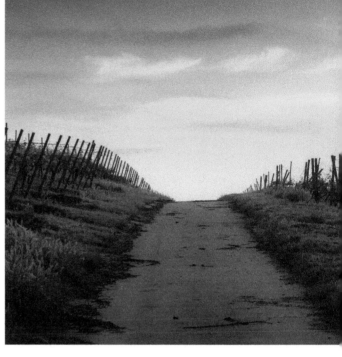

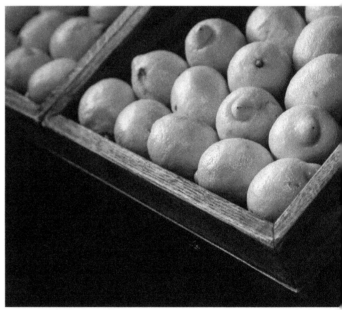

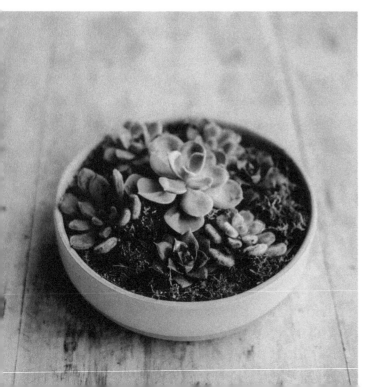

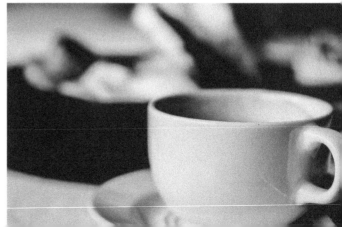

Own the process of nourishing yourself... How much do you know about what's healthy for you from moment to moment and season to season? If you're not entirely sure, don't worry, because you're not alone. There are so many voices in the health and wellness space these days that our ability or willingness to hear and trust our own has become impaired. The result is that we've stepped onto a roller coaster of health and wellness, riding the mental, physical, and emotional highs and lows from one diet to the next and from this year's junk science about what's good for us and what's not to the inevitable contradiction that will show up next year, if not sooner. Stepping off the roller coaster means committing yourself to finding out what works for you. It means tuning in to how your food makes you feel and how your thoughts, emotions, and experiences drive the choices you make about how to feed yourself. It means owning your power to thrive rather than giving it away to the wellness gurus or supplement companies. It means trusting yourself and backing yourself. It also means truly living!

Be hungry sometimes... Ayurveda says that our digestion is compromised when we eat before our last meal is digested. Most of us busy people are run by our schedules (and our emotions). When, what, and how we eat has almost nothing to do with our bodies and everything to do with our state of mind (or the time of day). Physical hunger is a novelty and a nuisance more than a gentle reminder from our bodies that it's time to eat. Allowing yourself to feel hunger does two things: it gives you the opportunity to observe how much your mind controls what and when you eat, and it actually strengthens your digestive fire. Try it!

Eat what you need until it's what you want... Bad habits are hard to break. The thing is, most of us believe that the habit we need to break is eating junk food, when the real habit we need to break is self-loathing. Your body wants and needs nourishment and love. It wants to do what it does best; it wants to feel and look strong, supple, and easeful. But the mind's natural tendency is to crave the satisfaction, comfort, escape, or even validation it thinks it can find in a diet of junk, comfort, or "health" food. Feeding our wholeness starts with a willingness to notice and transcend emotions, self-limiting beliefs, cultural conditioning, and the tendency to put ourselves last. It requires that we love ourselves enough to tune into our true physical, mental, and emotional needs in the moment, and satisfy them with the faith and understanding that self-love begets self-love.

With that in mind, here's...

Three questions to transform your relationship with your diet...

The biggest challenge for anyone who desires to learn to "listen" to their mind and body is knowing what that means and how to do it. Questions are a great way to initiate the process of tuning in and knowing what to look for. For the most part, what we consume is determined by some cross-section of what we've always consumed and what we've been led to believe is best for us to consume. But that doesn't mean it's right for us. To get to a more honest understanding about what's healthy for you in the moment, ask yourself these questions:

- *Who are you?* - What's your age, size, mental, and emotional state? What are your usual tendencies, habits, and cravings? How have they served you to date? And how do they align with who you want to be?

- *Where/when are you?* - What time of year/season are you currently experiencing? What's the energy of the environment that you're currently living or existing in, and how might the temperature, weather, people, or energy around you influence your choices?

- *What are you hungry for?* - What's your current degree of satisfaction with your mind, body, and life? What is it that you truly need (self-care, sleep, companionship, acknowledgement, food, water, or something else)?

Trust the insights and answers from these questions to guide your choices for food in the moment. And realize that like learning anything new, it will be awkward and scary to trust yourself, but given enough time and experience it will become just like riding a bike, i.e. something easy, instinctual, and fun!

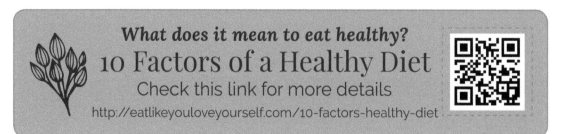

What does it mean to eat healthy?
10 Factors of a Healthy Diet
Check this link for more details
http://eatlikeyouloveyourself.com/10-factors-healthy-diet

Chapter 13

Recipes for seasonal living & eating

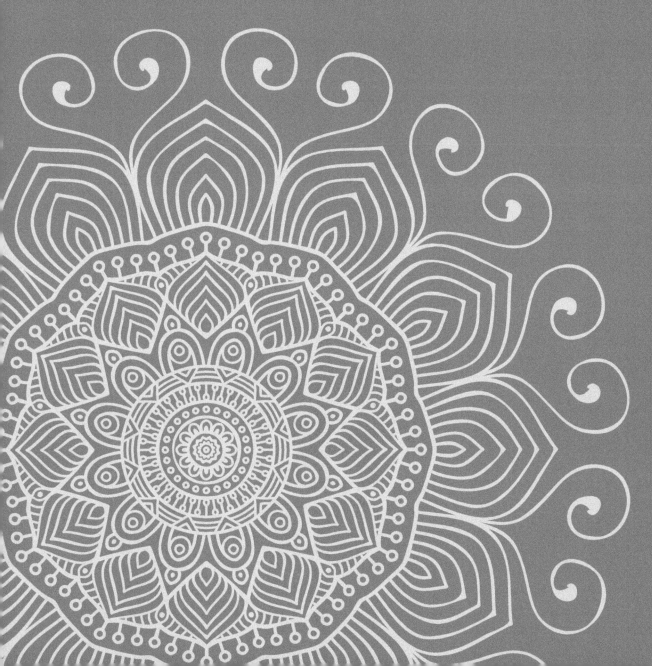

Autumn

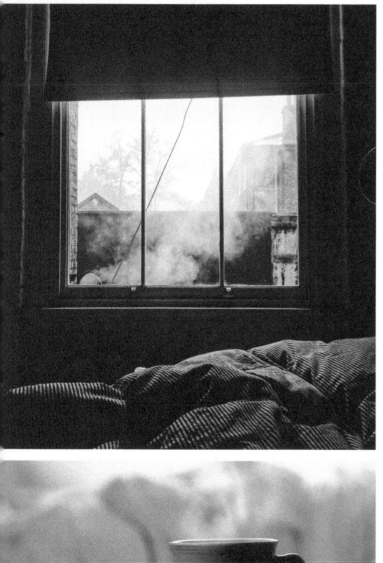

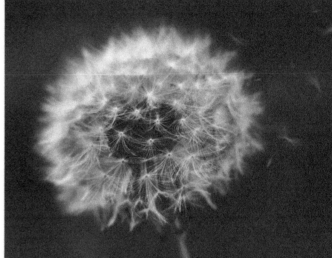

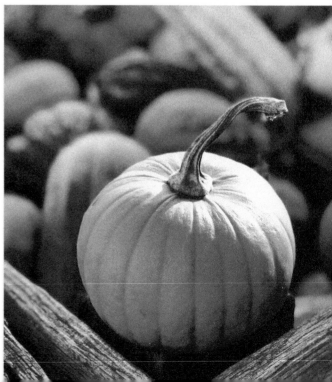

Fall is my favorite season. In fact, I sometimes wish it would last all year long (and not just for the pumpkin spiced lattes). To me it's the perfect combination of hot (pitta) and cold (vata), my two dominant energies. And of course it makes sense that it's governed by vata, since it's very much a transitional season. It's a time when the energy of movement and change swirls through the air like the cool wind, drying, distracting, stimulating, and exhausting every part of you.

Qualities of Autumn:
Cold, dry, light, moving, rough, clear

Autumn mantra for balance:
Warming, grounding, moisturizing, routine

What to watch out for:
Anxiety, fear, constipation, low back pain, dry skin, headaches, procrastination, popping joints, fatigue, impatience, impulsive spending, dizziness, feeling disconnected or untethered

Autumn Self Care Focus:

- **Stay grounded** - Grounding connects us to the present moment. It pulls us into our physical experience of right now, and in the process creates a sense of ease in the mind and stability in the body. Grounding creates calm, destroys stress, and reminds us of who we are by diverting our attention from thinking and making us feel at home in our own bodies.

- **Warm and oily** - Applying warm oil to the body is an act of love. It puts back some of what we deplete, it coats the skin in a nourishing protective layer, and, best of all in my opinion, it provides a buffer from the cold roughness of autumn. The best part about it, though, is what it does to your mind. Try it, you'll see!

- **Nourish and nurture** - Autumn is your time to regroup. Summer is fun, but exhausting. The drop in temperatures from summer to autumn can take the wind out of your sails and leave you feeling tired, overwhelmed, and depleted. Use this time of year, before winter hits, to slow down, rest. Shift from light to heavier foods and activities that will allow you to replenish your energy and spark!

- **Make the connection** - Research is showing that human connection is a powerful antidote to anxiety and depression. It's also a wonderful form of self-care for the colder months of the year, starting with autumn. Hugging reduces fear, increases confidence, and deepens your connection to yourself and others. I often "prescribe" at least two hugs a day during this season, or finding a way to deepen your connection to yourself and those around you!

A few things to add to your Autumn routine:

- **Alternate nostril breathing** - Otherwise known as "Nadi Shodhana" (channel cleansing), or balancing breath. It's a simple, powerful technique for centering mind and body, helping to stave off headaches, mental fogginess, and fatigue. It's also a great practice to settle the mind before bed, or if you can't sleep.

- **Self massage** - Make this one a priority (for the reasons I mentioned above). Put a bottle of sesame oil (you can scent it with a few drops of lavender or ylang ylang in the shower and give yourself a soothing massage right after your shower. When you dry off, leave a light coat of oil on the body. Enjoy your day!

- **Ghee... and more ghee...** I mentioned above that oiling the body is important this time of year for the health of your mind, skin, and joints. Autumn is also a good time to add healthy fats into your diet. Ghee is highly prized and recommended in Ayurveda for all its many health benefits, and is one of the most beneficial fats for balancing the effects of increased vata dosha. Taking ghee regularly (or adding a little to food this time of year) can also help to keep the digestion and elimination systems functioning at optimal levels!

- **Yoga...** Yoga is great for any time of year, but it has particularly powerful effects in the autumn. It allows you to slow down, focus your energy, feel your body, and in the process relieve tension, stress, and potentially even pain that you may be holding onto. Yoga is also a great way to remind you of your most powerful tool for reclaiming your center... the breath!

- **Cleansing…** Autumn is a time to prepare ourselves for the coming winter. It can also be a time when we're vulnerable to illness as the weather starts to become cooler and lighter. Cleansing at this time is vital to letting go of anything that isn't really serving our needs for strength, focus, and a deeper connection to what's most important to us, some of the things that we can tend to lose sight of during the long cold winters.

Eating in Autumn

Breakfast You may still be feeling the heat of the summer in the earliest parts of autumn as we ease into the cooler months. Because of that, breakfasts for us make a slow transition from light, moist, and fruity to a little heavier, warmer, and spicier by the time we make it to autumn's border with winter. Root veggies and grains are some of our favorite breakfast foods, porridge with pumpkin, rice and semolina porridge with fruit, and for something more savoury, a grounding, veggie-filled tofu scramble, with milky cups of chai - yum!

Lunch I love stewing…anything! Autumn is time for getting creative with this moisturizing, softening, yumifying method of cooking. Curries, meats, veggies, coconut milks, flavorful broths are all a possible (and welcoming) foundation for your delicious autumn creations. Lunch is the time to explore how comforting your food can get. Buddha bowls with your favorites (sauteed greens, veggies roasted with ghee and spices, braised meats, poached fish) are all great additions. Go easy on the beans and lentils as they can be a bit drying for this time of year, but feel free to go soup and stew crazy for autumn lunches!

Dinner Autumn dinners are mainly a time for us to reconnect as a family. Food tends to be simple. Leftovers from lunch, store-bought roast chicken with a few greens and some fresh bread, or a bowl of simple soup (lentil, pumpkin are the faves). As always with dinners, moderation is key, and so is ensuring that you're getting some digestive spices in there (cinnamon, ginger, cumin). The goal (especially this time of year) is to give your food time to love you (eat slow, stop before you're full), striking a beautiful balance between grounded and heavy.

Autumn tastes/qualities to favor:
sweet, sour, salty, heavy, moist, warm

Autumn spices to favor:
asafoetida, cardamom, cinnamon, fennel, cumin,
ginger, turmeric

Autumn Superfoods by Type:
These are the best foods for the season based on your constitution or imbalance.

Vata [includes vata-pitta, vata-kapha]:	Pitta [includes pitta-vata, pitta-kapha]:	Kapha [includes kapha-vata, kapha-pitta]
Dates	Watermelon	Dandelion
Figs	Apples	Watercress
Grapes	Pomegranates	Bean sprouts
Pumpkin	Avocado	Microgreens
Sweet potato	Mung beans	Asparagus
Beets	Pumpkin seeds	Dried fruit
Garlic	Acorn squash	Black & cayenne pepper
Almonds (raw, soaked, skins removed)	Coriander	Ginger (fresh, dry, tea)
Rice	Fennel	

*Get additional **autumn** info &
resources via this link!*
http://www.eatlikeyouloveyourself.com/Autumn

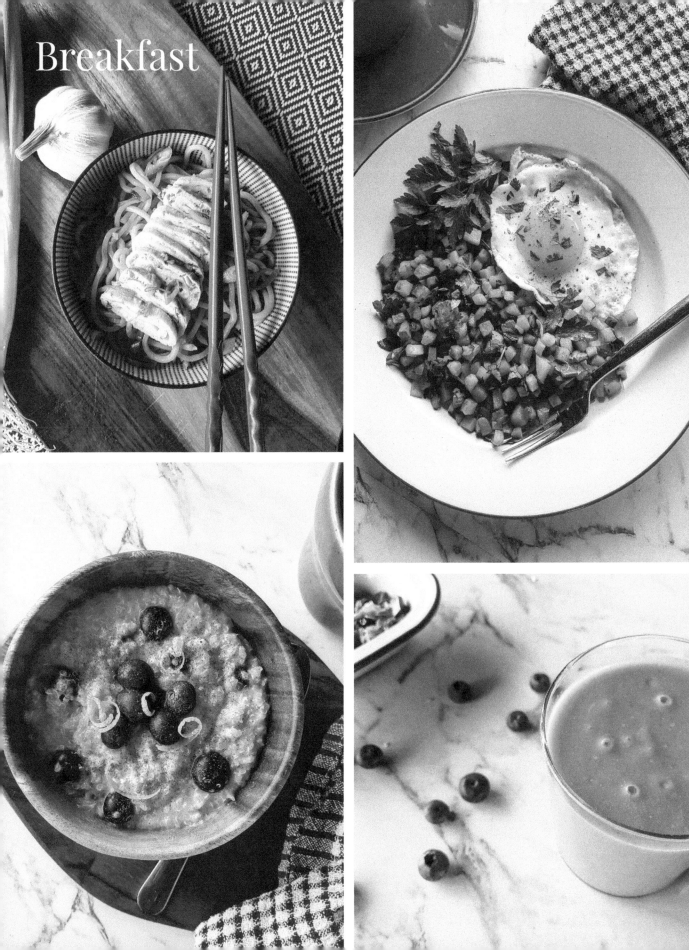

Breakfast

Egg & Sesame
Breakfast Noodles
$=V + P = K$

If you're a fan of noodles like I am, you're gonna love this simple savory breakfast. It can be eaten warm or cool, depending on your preference. The ingredients are beautifully warming and well balanced, and if you're feeling the need for just a little more lightness, the eggs can be substituted with sauteed greens. ***Serves 4; Prep + Cooking time: 20 mins.***

What's in it:

- 4 servings (cups) thin noodles (hokkien, somen, ramen, your choice), cooked and drained
- 3 eggs, lightly beaten
- 2 tablespoons soy sauce
- 2 whole green onions, sliced thin
- 1 tablespoon coconut sugar

- 2 cloves garlic, crushed
- 1 tablespoon rice vinegar
- 1 tablespoon toasted sesame oil
- 2 teaspoons olive or vegetable oil
- ¼ teaspoon of finely sliced mild red chilli (optiona)

How to make it:

- Cook the noodles as directed on the package and set aside.
- Lightly beat the eggs in a bowl and add in half the sliced green onions.
- In a frying pan on medium to high heat, add a splash of sesame oil to cover the pan. Add the eggs and swirl to create a thin layer.   Cook for about 30 seconds and then roll the eggs into a roll, and remove from the pan.
- Allow eggs to cool slightly then slice the roll into thin slices.

- Whisk all remaining ingredients (except noodles and green onions) together in a bowl. Taste the sauce and adjust ingredients as needed.
- Pour ¾ of sauce over the warm noodles and toss to coat (let it sit for a minute to allow the noodles to absorb the flavors and liquid). Add in the green onions and toss to distribute.
- Divide the noodles into bowls and top with a portion of the sliced eggs and a portion of the remaining sauce.

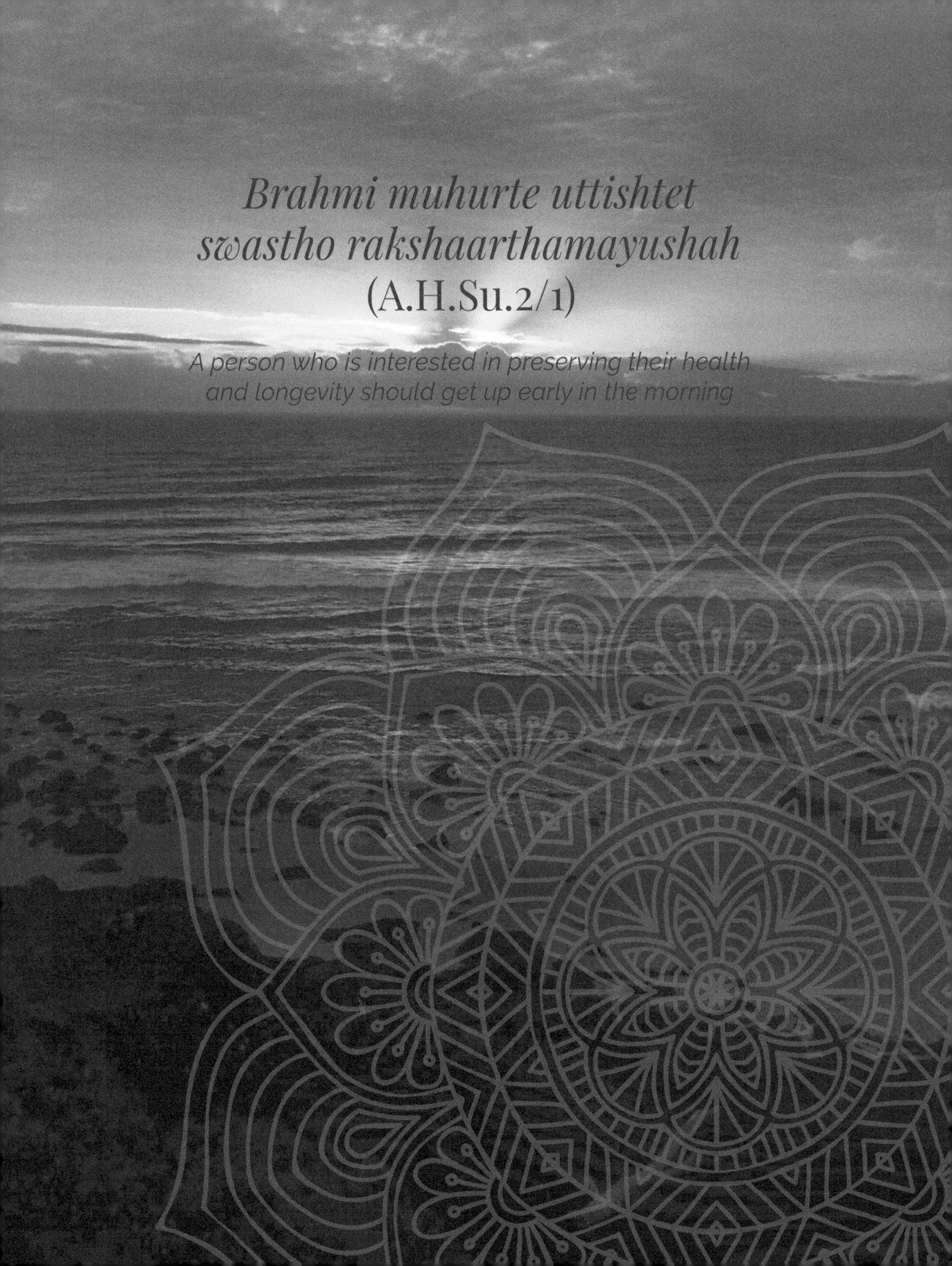

*Brahmi muhurte uttishtet
swastho rakshaarthamayushah*
(A.H.Su.2/1)

*A person who is interested in preserving their health
and longevity should get up early in the morning*

Quinoa Vanilla & Blueberry Porridge
-V -P -K

Quinoa is a very versatile grain that makes a beautiful breakfast porridge. It's a grain that balances all the doshas and it's not too hard on the digestion. I've added a few of my favorite accompaniments to this one, because what's porridge if not a vehicle for toppings! You can also throw a small handful of toasted granola or almonds onto this if you're in need of a little texture.. ***Serves 2: Prep + Cooking time: 30 mins.***

What's in it:

- 1 cup fresh water
- ½ cup quinoa
- 1 cup milk of your choice,
- I prefer almond milk
- 1 teaspoon vanilla extract

- ½ teaspoon nutmeg
- Pinch of salt
- ¼ cup blueberries (fresh or frozen).
- 1 teaspoon ghee to garnish (optional)
- Maple syrup to top (optional)

How to make it:

- Wash the quinoa very well under cold water and strain.
- In a medium size saucepan over medium to high heat, cook quinoa with water, and salt till soft.
- Add milk, vanilla, nutmeg and cook until creamy. Then finally stir through the blueberries and allow them to soften a little before taking the pan off the heat.

- If it gets too dry, just add a bit more milk or water to find your desired consistency.
- Serve in bowls and top with a drizzle of ghee and a splash of maple syrup if you're so inclined!

Root Vegetable Hash
-V -P -K

I'm not ashamed to say that my family is no stranger to hash. Being one who doesn't like to let good food go to waste, I'll sometimes find myself throwing last night's veggies with cut-up potatoes into a pan with some ghee, salt, and pepper. Throw an egg on top and voila…breakfast!

So this recipe kind of came naturally. But this time we're starting from scratch. Taking advantage of the opportunity to dive into root veggie heaven, this recipe gives you license to do just that. Use your favorites, don't hold back. Root veggies are high in fiber and vitamins A and C. They're also a great source of complex carbohydrates that can keep you satisfied until lunch and beyond! *Serves 4; Prep + Cooking time 35 mins.*

What's in it:

- 5 cups diced root vegetables - (i.e.potatoes, sweet potato,
  parsnips, carrots, celery root, beets, jerusalem artichokes, rutabaga
- 1 medium - large yellow onion diced
- 3 tablespoons ghee
- 2 teaspoons salt

- 1 teaspoon pepper
- 1 green onion, thinly sliced
- 2 tablespoons fresh parsley chopped

Optional toppings
- fried egg
- harissa sauce

How to make it:

- Add the ghee and diced onion to a large frying pan over medium to high heat. Cook until the onion is soft and nearly translucent.
- Add the remaining ingredients and lower the heat to medium.

- Slowly cook, tossing occasionally until all of the veggies are soft and cooked through. If you find the mixture getting a little dry, you can add a tablespoon of water and keep stirring.
- Serve alone or top with a fried egg or sauce.

Sweet Potato Smoothie
-V -P +K

As much as smoothies have become the health and wellness world's symbol for... health and wellness, the Ayurvedic view is that they can be hard to digest. In part because of what we put in them (a lot of sweet and heavy stuff - fruit, dairy, nuts, etc.), but also because of the fact that they are most often served cold. Here's an option for a yummy smoothie that's served at room temperature with a few warming spices to help prime the digestion. ***Serves 1; Prep + Cooking time: 10 mins.***

What's in it:

- ½ medium sweet potato, cooked and peeled
- 1 tablespoon honey ginger nut butter {Pg 283}
- 1 tablespoon chia seeds

- 1 cup unsweetened almond milk
- ½ teaspoon pure maple syrup
- ¼ teaspoon ground cinnamon
- ¼ teaspoon ground cardamom

How to make it:

Put all the ingredients into a blender and blend on high speed until smooth. Add a tablespoon or two of water if it's too thick to drink.

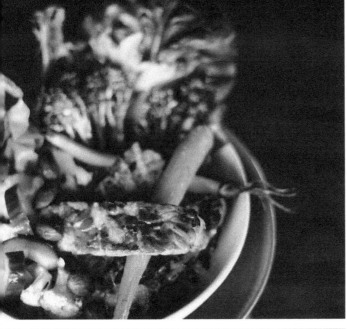

Lunch & Dinner

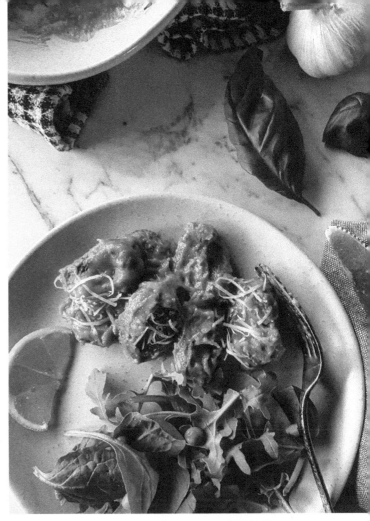

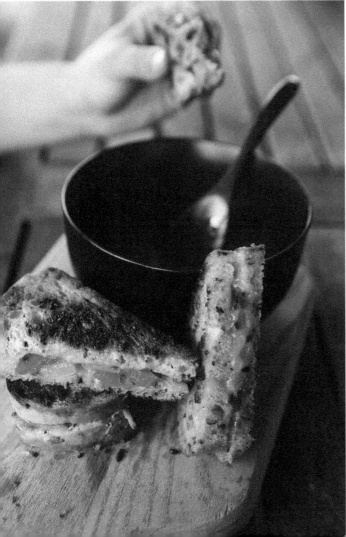

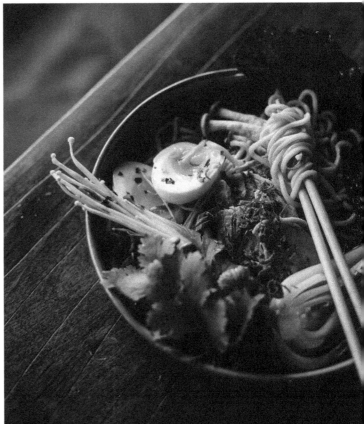

Autumn Tempeh Bowl
-V +P -K

Tempeh is a wonderful food that benefits gut and menopausal health. It's also beneficial for reducing cholesterol and increasing bone density. And my local tempeh maker tells me it's one of the world's healthiest foods.. This lovely dish is a seasonal meal in a bowl that features brown rice (or your favorite seasonal grain) as a base along with a selection of flavors representing the six tastes (including sour!!). It makes a wonderful, hearty, and simple to throw together autumn lunch. ***Serves 4; Prep + Cooking time: 40 mins.***

What's in it:

- 1 small bunch broccolini, trimmed
- 1 dozen Dutch carrots, cleaned, peeled, and tops trimmed
- 2 tablespoons ghee or olive oil
- 2 pinches salt
- 1 heaped teaspoon vata churna mixed spice (from Sauces & Basics)

- 1 block tempeh
- 1 ½ cups garden pickles [Pg 280]
- 4 cups cooked brown rice
- lemon dressing [from Sauces and Basics]
- 2 tablespoons dukkah

How to make it:

- Preheat oven to 180 C/350 F and line a baking sheet with baking paper.
- In a medium-sized bowl toss the broccolini, carrots, salt, ghee, and spice mix to coat the veggies.
- Spread vegetables on the baking sheet and bake for 15 -20 minutes or until soft.
- While the veggies are baking cut the tempeh into 1 inch (2.5cm) thick slices,

and pan fry in a little bit of ghee on medium heat until they are golden brown. Remove to a paper towel covered plate and sprinkle with a pinch of salt.

- To assemble divide the rice into four bowls, arrange the veggies, pickles and tempeh on top. Drizzle with lemon dressing and sprinkle a few pinches of dukkah over each bowl.

Golden Potato, Leek & Zucchini Fritters

-V -P -K

I'm always on the lookout for fun and interesting ways to incorporate healing spices into our diet. This simple to throw together fritter is an easy dinner or lunch option for any day of the week or weekend. It's also gluten free and a yummy way to showcase some of the season's most popular and plentiful ingredients! ***Makes about a dozen; Prep + Cooking time: 35 mins.***

What's in it:

- 3 cups raw zucchini, grated
- 3 cups raw russet potatoes, grated
- 2 cups raw leeks, trimmed, washed, and thinly sliced
- 4 tablespoons chickpea flour (all-purpose flour or gluten-free flour works also)

- 2 large eggs
- ½ cup chopped parsley
- 2 teaspoons turmeric
- 2 teaspoon salt
- 1 teaspoon ground pepper
- 3 tablespoons olive oil or ghee
- tzatziki sauce (optional) {Pg 275}

How to make it:

- Put the zucchini in a bowl and sprinkle a teaspoon of salt over the top. Set it aside until the liquid starts to release.
- In another bowl rinse the potatoes with cold water to remove some of the starch. Drain well.
- Squeeze as much water as you can out of the zucchini and add it to the potatoes along with the leeks and flour.
- Add the eggs, parsley, spices and remaining teaspoon of salt and the pepper.

- Add oil or ghee to a fry pan on medium high heat.
- Add two heaped tablespoons of the veggie mix (about ⅓ cup) in a small pile on the hot pan and flatten it out to about ½ inch thick with the back of a spoon.
- Fry for about 3-4 minutes on each side or until both sides are golden brown on the edges. Cook in batches using all the prepared mix.
- Serve warm with coconut tzatziki, chutney or on their own!

Sweet Potato, Leek & Parsnip Curry Soup
–V +P –K

Curry is the standout spice in the creamy, warming veggie soup that features the digestive spice and the subtle warming sweetness of leeks! Potato and leek soup has long been on my list of soup staples. So I thought it would be interesting to take it deeper into Ayurveda territory and switch it up a little to make it more suitable for my favorite season of the year. Sweet potatoes add a bit of stability for the mind and body. *Serves 4; Prep + Cooking time: 35 mins.*

What's in it:

- 2 ½ cups raw parsnips, peeled and diced.
- 1 medium leek (or two small ones), washed and chopped
- 2 to 3 cloves garlic, crushed
- 2 tablespoons ghee

- 1 tablespoon curry powder
- 5 cups chicken or vegetable stock
- 1 ½ cups sweet potatoes, washed, peeled, and diced
- 1 tablespoon coconut cream
- 2 pinches fine black pepper

How to make it:

- Add the ghee, parsnips, leeks, and garlic to a saucepan on medium heat. Cook gently for about 5 minutes to soften the vegetables.
- Add in the curry powder and the stock. Bring to a boil and add the sweet potatoes and coconut cream.
- Reduce heat to low and simmer until the vegetables are all tender (about 20 minutes).

- Remove the soup from the heat and using a hand blender or a regular blender, blend the soup until smooth.
- Pour out into bowls and top with a swirl of coconut yogurt.

Ramen Simplified
-V +P -K

Ramen is another one of those "blank slate" dishes that gives you the space to choose ingredients and toppings that will balance and delight you. The vata in me loves this freedom, but if you prefer a little more structure, I've provided some suggestions for how to make this a lovely autumn meal to remember. ***Serves 4; Prep + Cooking time: 35 mins.***

What's in it:

- 2 ½ teaspoons toasted sesame oil
- 1 garlic clove, crushed
- 1 teaspoon fresh ginger, finely grated
- 1 pound ground pork (optional)
- 2 cups bean sprouts, rinsed
- 2 cups chinese cabbage, shredded
- 1 green onion (scallion), thinly sliced
- 2 cups shitake mushrooms
- 1 medium carrot, washed, peeled, and julienned

- 4 cups low sodium chicken broth, dashi stock, or ginger broth
- 1 teaspoon sugar
- 2 teaspoons light soy sauce
- 4 tablespoons miso paste
- 2 packages ramen noodles

Optional toppings
- Nori sheets or strips
- Boiled Eggs
- Pickled ginger

How to make it:

- Heat 2 teaspoons of sesame oil in a medium-sized pot or wok.

- Add garlic, ginger, and pork (if you're using) and cook on medium heat until veggies are soft or pork is no longer pink.

- Add vegetables and saute for a few minutes, longer stirring to keep the vegetables moving.

- Add broth, sugar and soy sauce. Bring to a boil. Turn heat down to simmer

and add miso paste and green onion. Cook a few minutes more and add the remaining sesame oil. Remove from the heat and cover.

- Cook the noodle as directed, drain and set aside.

- Divide noodles into four separate bowls and ladle soup over the top. Top each bowl with desired toppings and enjoy!

(Kapha: Balancing in moderation and without pork)

Spinach Gnocchi with Pumpkin Pancetta Sauce

- V -P +K

This dish is an opportunity to get mindful in the kitchen as it requires you to work with your hands (no getting around it). A perfect, satisfying, and grounding dish for a cold and windy autumn or early winter's day, the pillowy gnocchi with leafy greens adds a touch of lightness to ensure you don't end up too weighed down. You'll be fed mind, body, and soul by the entire process of putting this beautiful dish together. I've added pancetta to this dish, but feel free to leave it out or substitute nutritional yeast if you'd like to make it vegetarian. ***Serves 4; Prep + Cooking time: 45 mins.***

What's in it:

Pasta
- 4 cups baby spinach
- 1 cup full-fat ricotta cheese
- (the fresher, the better)
- ¾ cups grated parmesan cheese
- 1 egg
- ¼ teaspoon grated nutmeg
- ¾ cup plain flour, plus extra to dust
- 1 pinch of salt
- 1 pinch of pepper
- 2 tablespoons unsalted butter, chopped, plus extra to grease

Sauce
- 1/2 tablespoon butter
- 2 whole fresh sage leaves
- 2 whole cloves garlic
- 3 strips pancetta or streaky bacon, chopped into small pieces
- 1 cup roasted pumpkin puree
- ½ cup milk
- ½ cup freshly grated hard cheese
- (Parmesan or Pecorino Romano)
- Salt and finely ground black pepper, to taste
- Small pinch of nutmeg

How to make it:

- Place spinach in a colander over a mixing bowl and cover with boiling water. Let it sit for a few minutes and then drain and put into cold water to stop the cooking process. Set aside to cool.

- Once the spinach has cooled, squeeze out all the water and finely chop.

- Add the chopped spinach, ricotta, parmesan, egg, nutmeg, and flour to a bowl along with a pinch of salt and black pepper.

- Mix gently with a fork to combine and then carefully with your hands to ensure the ingredients are well combined.

- Turn the dough out on a lightly floured surface and divide it into four sections. Roll each section into a long, thin sausage shape (about 1 inch in diameter).

- Using a sharp knife, cut the dough at 1 ¼ inch intervals and gently roll the dough under your index finger to form a dent and slightly flatten each piece.

- Place finished gnocchi on a baking paper lined tray, cover with cling wrap, and refrigerate for 20 - 30 minutes.

- Make the sauce while the gnocchi is chilling in the fridge.

- In a medium-sized saucepan, melt the butter over medium - low heat. Add the garlic and sage leaves and pancetta and saute for a couple of minutes. Turn up the heat slightly and cook until the pancetta is crispy on the edges.

- Add the pumpkin puree and stir constantly until the pumpkin is warmed all the way through. Add the milk bit by bit until it's fully incorporated and the mixture is smooth and creamy. Add the grated cheese and a pinch of nutmeg. Season with salt and pepper.

- Bring a large pot of water to a boil, Throw in a couple of generous pinches of salt. Remove the gnocchi from the refrigerator and gently place them into the boiling water (they are likely to sink).

- When they rise to the surface, allow them to cook for another 30 seconds and then remove them with a slotted spoon and place them into the pan of sauce. Cook the gnocchi in batches this way until they're all cooked.

- Gently toss the sauce with the gnocchi and divide onto plates. Garnish with a little fresh grated cheese and a small pinch of red pepper flakes.

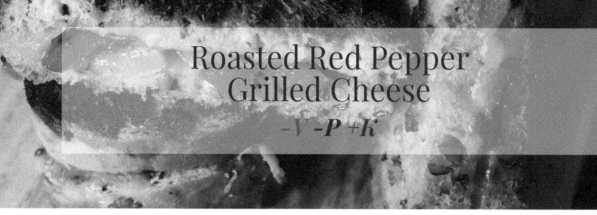

Roasted Red Pepper Grilled Cheese
-V -P +K

Growing up, grilled cheese sandwiches with Campbell's tomato soup was one of my favorite lunches. So how excited was I to discover that grilled cheese and soup are a perfect balancing meal for the autumn time, when we're looking to add more oils, heaviness, and heat to our diet and our lives. So this recipe is my more grown-up take on the sandwich I grew up eating. And it's so tasty and colorful that little kids will love it as much as big kids!
Serves 2: Prep + Cooking time: 20 mins.

What's in it:

- 4 slices whole grain, rye, or sourdough bread
- ¾ cup grated cheddar cheese
- 1 small bell pepper (red or
- yellow preferred)
- 1 tablespoon ghee

How to make it:

- On a barbecue grill, gas stove burner or oven set on broil, roast the pepper, turning it until the skin is blackened.
- Remove from heat, place into a bowl and cover to capture steam. Steam for 10 mins or until the skins are soft and pull away from the pepper. Remove the skins and cut peppers into strips.
- Spread one side of each piece of bread with a light coating of ghee and add the rest of the ghee to a warm skillet.

- Place the bread, ghee side down, into the skillet and allow to warm. Divide the cheese between the sandwiches and lay the roast pepper strips over the cheese.
- Cover with the other pieces of bread and turn the sandwiches. Cook sandwiches, flipping occasionally until cheese is melted and each side is golden brown.
- Remove, cut in half and serve. These are a perfect accompaniment to the smoky tomato soup.

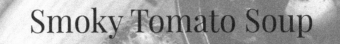

Smoky Tomato Soup
–V +P –K

This soup is so good and so simple that you'll hardly believe it! Those kinds of recipes are my favorite! Tomatoes are warming and sweet, which makes them good for balancing vata energy. In this recipe, we kick the vata balancing factor up a notch with a little smoked paprika, which also elevates the flavor of this simple soup to something definitely out of the ordinary! This makes a great lunch or quick, light, and warming autumn dinner.
Serves 4; Prep + Cooking time: 15 mins.

What's in it:

- 1 can diced organic tomatoes (or 2 cups chopped fresh tomatoes, skinned)
- 2 cans pure water
- 1 teaspoon salt

- 1 teaspoon smoked paprika
- Pinch of sugar
- Pinch of black pepper
- 1 teaspoon yogurt [optional]

How to make it:

Add all ingredients to a medium saucepan and bring to a boil, and then lower to a simmer. Adjust seasonings to your taste. Transfer soup to a blender, or use a hand blender to blend it to a smoother consistency. Serve warm, topped with a swirl of yogurt (optional).

*Kapha: Balancing (in moderation)

Harvest Vegetable Lasagne
-V -P -K

I'm convinced that this recipe was channeled to me by a higher power, or at least someone a little more tuned in than me, because it's that good,. It's a little bit of work, so it tends to be a weekend endeavor, but it delivers such a grounding, comforting, and nourishing (yep, goodbye vata) punch, that I'm sure it's probably medicine for EVERYTHING. It's chock full of all my favorite autumn veggies and can be altered to pacify the meat eaters (or those who are in need of extreme vata balancing). But our favorite way to enjoy it, is as it was conceived...a loving display of the beauty of vegetables. ***Serves about 10; Prep + Cooking time: 90-110 mins.***

What's in it:

- 3 medium to large sized eggplants (these will be used as the lasagna "noodles")
- 2 pound piece of pumpkin (any type will do), cut into thin, wide slices
- 2 cups mushrooms (prefer brown or white), stems trimmed and cut into pieces or slices
- 3-4 medium to large zucchini, washed, ends trimmed, cut into lengthwise "noodles" ¼ inch (6mm) thick

- 3 cups cooked, chopped, and drained spinach
- 2 cups ricotta cheese
- 2 cans organic diced tomatoes
- 1 medium onion finely diced
- 2 tablespoons of butter
- 1 cup freshly grated Parmesan cheese
- Pinch of nutmeg
- Salt and pepper to taste
- 3 tablespoons olive oil

How to make it:

For the lasgne

- Start by roasting the veggies. These will become the noodles and filling for your lasagna.
- Preheat the oven to 180 Celsius (350 Fahrenheit) and line two baking sheets with baking paper.

- Spread the eggplant slices out the baking sheets. Season both sides with salt and pepper and drizzle with olive oil. Bake for 30 minutes or until they've dried out some and are looking lightly browned. Remove from the oven, set aside.

- Depending on the size of your oven, you may need to roast the veggies in batches.

- Once the eggplant is done, do the same with the pumpkin and zucchini slices, roasting all with a little oil, salt and pepper until they're soft and lightly browned.

- In a medium sized bowl mix the chopped spinach and ricotta cheese with a pinch of salt, pepper and nutmeg. Stir well to combine everything. Refrigerate until your ready to use.

For the sauce:

- Add the diced onion and mushrooms to a pan on medium heat along with a splash of olive oil.

- Sautee onions until transleucent then add the two cans of tomatoes, butter, salt and pepper to taste.

- Cook sauce on low heat for 10-15mins and then set aside until needed.

- To assemble the lasagne use a 9 x 13 in baking dish (or two smaller baking dishes). Begin by placing a layer of eggplant on the bottom. Top with a bit of sauce (just a light layer), a layer of spinach ricotta and a layer of roasted veg (pumpkin, zucchini or a combination of both).

- Continue layering eggplant, ricotta, sauce and veggies until the pan is nearly full. Finish with a light layer of parmesan cheese.

- Bake for 30 - 40 minutes or until the lasagna is bubbly and the top cheese layer is browned. Remove from oven and allow to cool. Serve on its own, or with a salad and a smile!

-

Kapha: Balancing (in moderation)

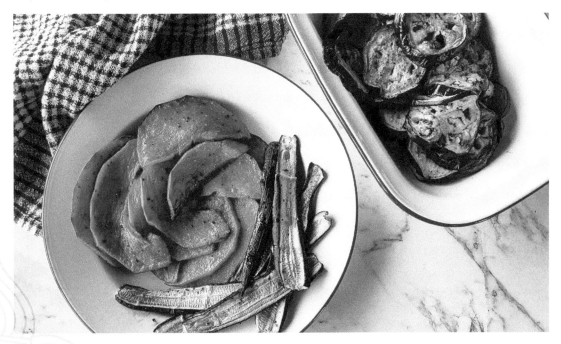

Baked Sweet Potatoes
with Spinach & Feta
-V - P - K

There's nothing better than a sweet potato, unless you count a sweet potato topped with greens and a little bit of tangy cheese. This dish is perfect for a quick lunch and can easily be packed away to take on the road if need be. It's a nutrient and flavor packed dish that will no doubt become a favorite! *Serves 4; Prep + Cooking time: 35 mins.*

What's in it:

- 2 large sweet potatoes (or four small ones), skin on, washed and patted dry
- 6 cups spinach, washed and chopped
- 1 large onion, sliced thin
- 2 teaspoons seasonal spice mix
- 1 cup crumbled feta cheese
- 4 tablespoons ghee

How to make it:

- Preheat oven to 200°C/400°F). Line a baking sheet with baking paper and place the washed sweet potatoes on the sheet.
- Cook the potatoes for 30 minutes or until fork tender all the way through.
- Make the topping while the potatoes are cooking,
- Add the ghee and onions to a medium frying pan on medium heat. Saute the onions until they soften and turn down the heat slightly. Cook the onions on medium-low heat until they begin to lightly caramelize.
- Add the chopped spinach and stir well to combine. Add the seasonal spice mix and a pinch of salt and pepper. Cook until spinach is wilted.

- Remove from heat and set aside until the potatoes are ready.
- When the potatoes are ready allow them to cool slightly. Slice each big potato in half and use a fork to fluff and loosen the potato. Divide the spinach and onion mixture into four.
- Drizzle a teaspoon of ghee (optional) and add a portion of the spinach and onion mixture over each potato half. Top with crumbled feta cheese and return to the baking tray.
- Turn the oven heat up to broil setting and cook the potatoes under the broiler for just a few minutes, until the cheese is slightly melted and lightly browned.

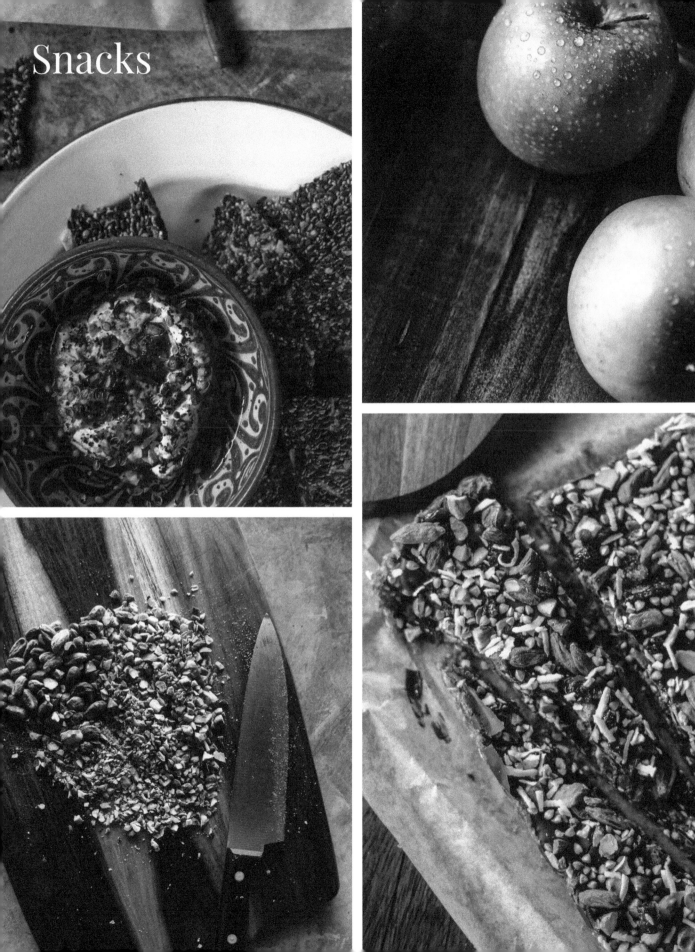

Snacks

Fruit Nut & Grain Bars
-V -P +K

Ayurveda recommends that we avoid snacking, but sometimes it can't be helped. Vatas and pittas will sometimes need a snack to calm the nerves or stave off hangriness. This lovely fruit and nut combination is just the thing. SUPER easy to make, and even easier to eat! They're pretty decadent, so practice moderation, (especially if you're a pitta). ***Makes about 15 bars or 30 squares; Prep + Cooking time: 25 mins. + fridge time.***

What's in it:

- 1 ½ cups unsalted, peeled almonds, lightly roasted
- 1 ½ cups pitted dried dates, preferably Medjool
- ¼ teaspoon salt
- 1 cup roughly chopped dark chocolate or mini chocolate chips
- 2 tablespoons dried goji berries (optional)
- 2 tablespoons toasted buckwheat groats (optional)
- 2 tablespoons cacao nibs (optional)
- 2 tablespoons chopped pistachio nuts (optional)
- 2 tablespoons shredded coconut optional)

How to make it:

- Add almonds, dates, and salt to the bowl of a food processor. Pulse until the mixture resembles coarse crumbs. Continue processing until the ingredients start to bind together.
- Add half the chocolate to the mix and pulse a few more times to combine the ingredients.
- Transfer the mixture to an 8in x 8in baking pan lined with baking paper. Press the ingredients into the pan to form a medium-sized layer.
- Melt the remaining chocolate in a small bowl suspended over a warm water bath. Spread the melted chocolate over the date and nut layer.
- Sprinkle remaining ingredients over the top of the melted chocolate and refrigerate for an hour up to overnight (if you can wait that long).
- Turn the bars out onto a cutting board and cut them into bars (or squares).
- Store in an airtight container for up to 1 week.

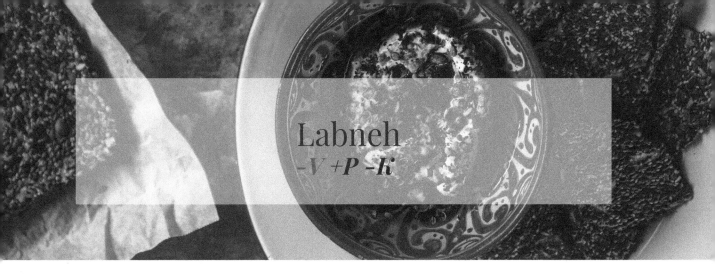

Labneh
-V +P -K

Labneh or middle eastern cheese is one of those dishes that falls into the "easy-fancy" category. It's easy to make, but it has a fanciness to it that makes it feel like a much harder recipe! It has just a handful of ingredients, which means that it can be VERY versatile. I often change up the spices that I add to it to suit the season or the purpose. Check it out.

Makes 1 ½ cups; Prep + Cooking time: 4-8 hrs. (overnight is best)

What's in it:

- 2 cups Greek yogurt (you can also use coconut yogurt for this, best if you start with a thicker consistency yogurt).
- 1 garlic clove
- 1 teaspoon black pepper
- 1 teaspoon salt
- 1 tablespoon finely chopped fresh herbs of your choosing (optional).

How to make it:

- Minimum time needed for this (for the best result) is 6-8 hours! Best to start the night before you'll need it.

- With that said, smash the garlic clove with half of the black pepper and a pinch of salt in a mortar and pestle (the idea is to create a paste). Mix the garlic pepper paste with the yogurt in a bowl along with freshly chopped herbs untilfully combined.

- Line a mesh strainer with cheesecloth or paper towel and pour the mixture into the paper towel or cheese cloth. Hang the ball of yogurt over a bowl and store in the refrigerator. Keep or dispose of the whey (liquid that drains off).

- When ready (firm texture), remove it from the cheesecloth or paper towels and store in an airtight container.

- Used it as a spread for sandwiches, stirred into salads or soups, or covered with a good quality olive oil and served as a dip with bread or biscuits.

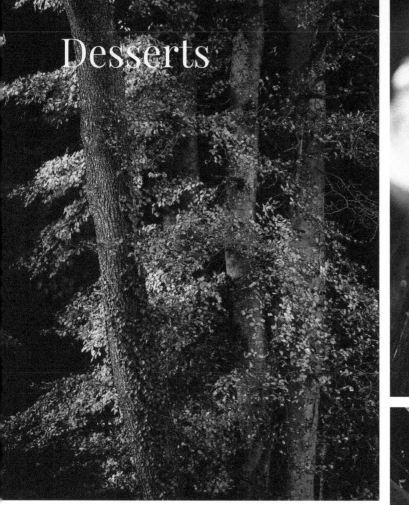

Desserts

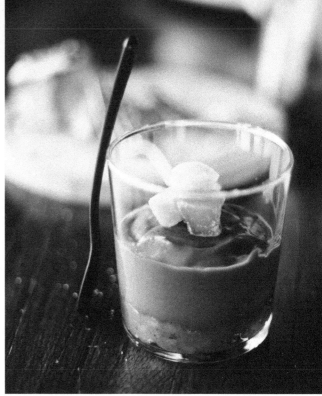

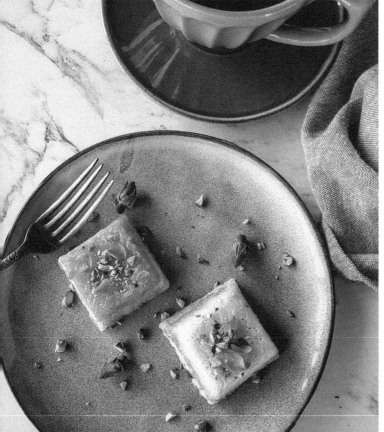

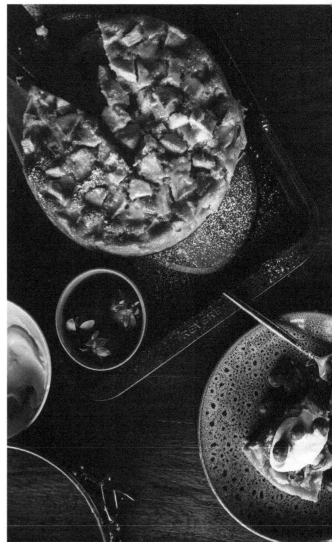

Carrot & Parsnip Halva
-V -P +K

I can still remember the day I discovered this beautiful treat. Who could forget vegetables as dessert! Since then I've done my best to introduce vegetable halva to as many people as possible. it's just one of those dishes that makes you feel happy. And then there's the surprise of cooking veggies that end up tasting like the most decadent and luscious pudding you can imagine. The best thing is that halva is sattvic, which is nourishing to the mind and body. It's also best taken in modest servings. Hope you love it as much as I do.
Serves 4-6; Prep + Cooking time: 60 mins.

What's in it:

- 2 cups coarsely grated carrots
- 2 cups coarsely grated parsnips
- 4 cups full cream milk
- 1 cup sugar or jaggery
- ½ teaspoon ground cardamom

- 1 tablespoon ghee
- 8-10 unsalted whole or chopped cashews
- 8-10 unsalted roasted almonds
- 12-15 golden raisins

How to make it:

- In a large frying pan gently roast the nuts until just lightly browned. Remove and set aside.
- Add the carrots, parsnips and ghee to the same pan and cook for 2-3 minutes or until the veggies are softened.
- Add the milk to this mixture and stir constantly as you bring the mixture to a boil. Lower the heat and continue stirring to ensure the milk doesn't burn and stick. The milk will begin to evaporate, leaving a lovely soft veggie paste.

- Once the milk has reduced by half, add the sugar and continue stirring to mix well. Continue until the milk is entirely evaporated and you're left with a loose, dough-like texture.
- Sprinkle the cardamom and half the nuts and raisins over the top and mix to incorporate them.
- Once the cooking is complete remove from heat and serve warm or room temperature, garnished with the remaining nuts and raisins.

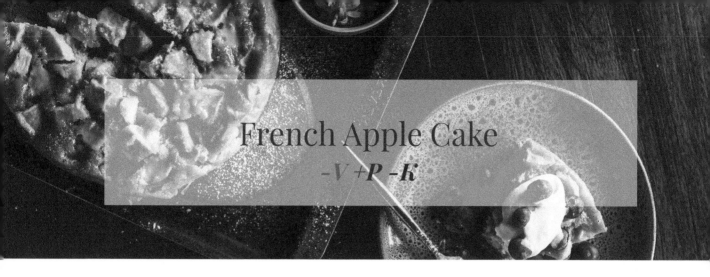

French Apple Cake
-V +P -K

This cake is perfect for drinking tea! Rich, moist, grounding, and filled to the brim with apples. It runs a close race with pumpkin anything for being the food embodiment of autumn season. It's based on an original French recipe and I've thrown in a few Ayurvedic touches (i.e. spices) in consideration of keeping your fire burning. **Serves 10; Prep + Cooking time: 90 mins.**

What's in it:

- ¾ cup all-purpose flour
- ¾ teaspoon baking powder
- Pinch of salt
- 3 large apples(I used Honeycrisp), peeled, cored, and diced in 2-inch pieces.
- 2 large eggs

- ¾ cup granulated sugar
- 1 teaspoon cinnamon
- ½ teaspoon fennel powder
- 1 teaspoon pure vanilla extract
- 6 tablespoons butter, melted and cooled to room temperature
- Icing sugar, for garnishing (optional

How to make it:

- Preheat oven to 180°C/350°F. Grease and flour an 8-inch round cake or springform pan.
- Combine flour, baking powder, spices, and salt in a small bowl and set aside.
- In a larger bowl, whisk the eggs until they're light and frothy. Add the sugar and keep going until the eggs and sugar are combined.
- Pour in the vanilla and mix until the sugar is nearly dissolved.
- Add half the dry mixture into the wet mixture and whisk to incorporate. Add half the melted butter and mix. Repeat

this with the remaining dry ingredients and butter.

- Add the chopped apples to the mix and fold gently to coat them. Pour the apple batter into the pan and bake for 55 - 65 minutes or until a toothpick inserted in the middle comes out clean.
- Remove the cake from the oven when done and allow to cool. Once cooled, run a knife around the inside edges of the pan (or release the springform) and turn the cake out on a plate. Dust with icing sugar or a pinch of cinnamon and devour!

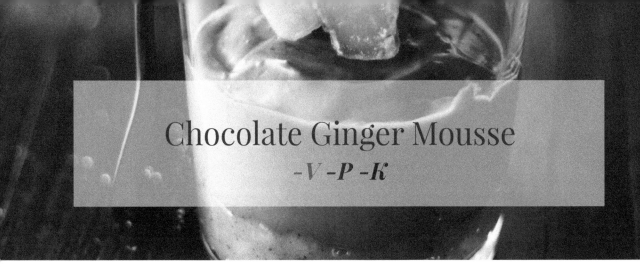

Chocolate Ginger Mousse
-V -P -K

The warming and stimulating qualities of chocolate make it a nice option for balancing the heaviness of kapha. Where we usually run into trouble with chocolate is the addition of fat and sugar, which can have the opposite effect. This recipe for a decadent (vegan) chocolate mousse uses light and creamy silken tofu and 70% dark chocolate combined with the warming and digestion-supporting qualities of a ginger surprise at the bottom for maximum impact and enjoyment! *Serves 4; Prep + Cooking time: 30 mins.*

What's in it:

- 2 cups silken tofu
- 80g/3oz 70% dark chocolate, broken up
- 3 tablespoon maple syrup (honey, or rice syrup)
- 1teaspoon vanilla extract
- Pinch of salt
- ½ cup of candied ginger
- 1 teaspoon cornstarch
- 1 cup water

How to make it:

- Place tofu inside a cheesecloth lined strainer basket to drain.

- Chop the candied ginger into fine pieces and put into a small saucepan with 1 cup of water. Cook on medium heat until the ginger has softened and begun to break apart.

- Make a slurry with the cornstarch and add to the ginger mixture. Stir until the mixture thickens. Remove from heat and allow to cool.

- Melt chocolate pieces in a bowl over a pan of lightly simmering water. Set aside to cool slightly.

- Place drained tofu in a mixing bowl and blend with a hand blender or processor until smooth and creamy.

- Add the melted chocolate, maple syrup, and vanilla and salt to the tofu.

- Mix thoroughly and check for sweetness (add additional sweetener if need be).

- Add 2 teaspoons of ginger mixture each to 4 ramekins and top each with an equal serve of the "mousse".

- Chill until firmly set. Remove from the fridge 10 minutes before eating to allow the mousse to warm to room temperature.

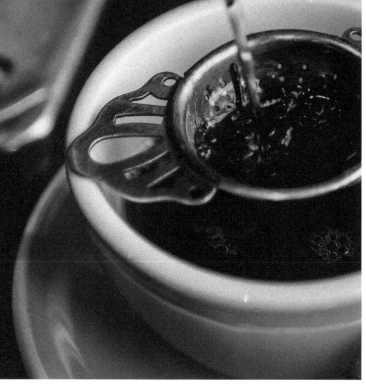

Drinks

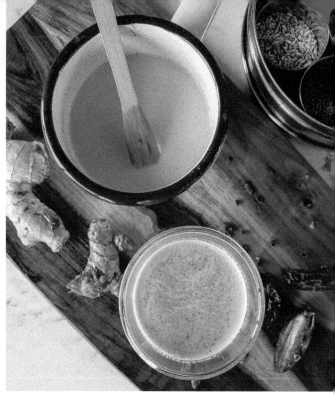

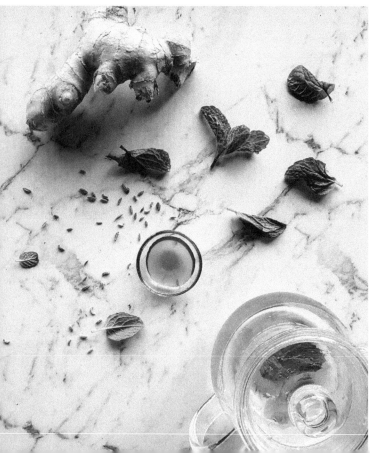

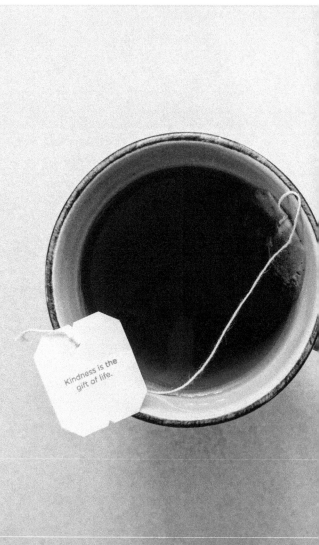

Kindness is the gift of life.

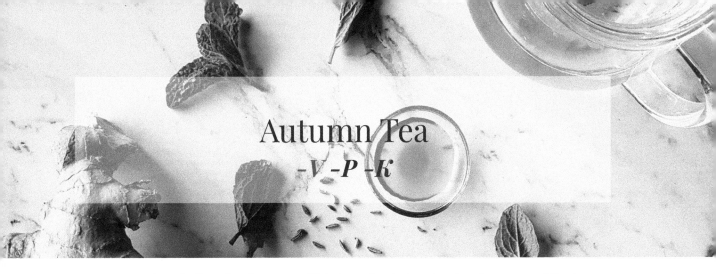

Autumn Tea
-V -P -K

Autumn can be challenging for some. This is a nice balancing tea for some of the issues that can arise in autumn season (i.e. anxiety, mental emotional or digestive upsets). It also includes a few elements for building immunity. It's a satisfying alternative to chai, is easy to make, and is beautiful to sip! *Serves 1; Prep + Cooking time: 10 mins.*

What's in it:

- 2 teaspoons fennel syrup (from Sauces and Basics)
- 1 teaspoon freshly grated ginger
- 2-3 mint leaves
- 2 cups water

How to make it:

- Place the ginger into a teapot strainer and top with boiling water.
- Allow to steep for 3-5 minutes.
- Add the mint leaves and allow to steep for a minute longer.
- Pour ginger mint tea into cups and sweeten with fennel syrup.

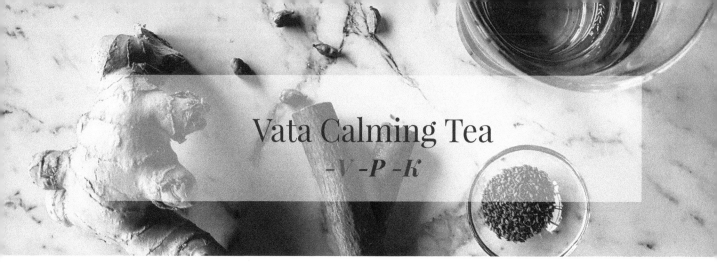

Vata Calming Tea
-V -P -K

Simple tea that includes elements to calm the mind and ground the body. I find that digestion can go a little haywire in autumn, so this soothing brew is just the thing for soothing and stimulating the system into action! **_Serves 2-3; Prep + Cooking time: 10 mins._**

What's in it:

- 1 teaspoon cardamom pods
- 1 teaspoon ajwain or caraway seeds
- 2 cinnamon sticks
- 1 teaspoon fresh ginger, grated
- 4-5 cups water

How to make it:

- Place all ingredients into a medium-sized pot and bring to a boil.
- Reduce heat and simmer for 5 minutes.
- Strain into cups and serve.
- You can sweeten with a bit of honey if you like (just wait for the tea to cool a bit before you do!).

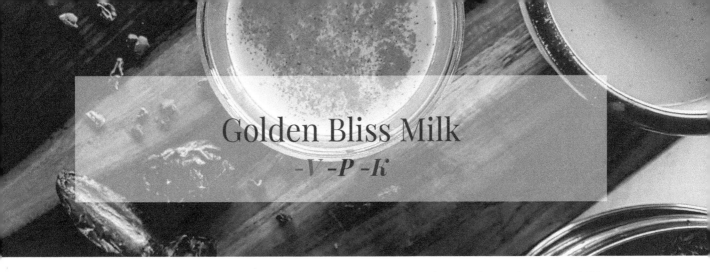

Golden Bliss Milk
-V -P -K

Golden milk is one of my favorite ways to enjoy the beauty of turmeric, so I've created this lovely warming recipe with a few additional surprises to ensure a blissful experience. This is a beautiful drink to have at breakfast time (it's warming and soothing) or when you just need a little decadence to calm you down. *Makes 2 cups; Prep + Cooking time 10 mins .*

What's in it:

- 1 (1-inch) piece turmeric, thinly sliced, or 1/2 teaspoon dried turmeric
- 1 (1/2-inch) piece ginger, thinly sliced
- 1 cup unsweetened coconut or almond milk
- 1 cup water
- 4 cardamom pods (slightly crushed to open pods)

- 2 teaspoons cacao nibs
- ¼ teaspoon nutmeg
- 1 (3-inch) cinnamon stick
- 1 tablespoon virgin coconut oil
- ¼ teaspoon whole black peppercorns
- ¼ teaspoon of molasses or coconut syrup for serving (optional)
- ground cinnamon (for serving)

How to make it:

- Add all but the last two ingredients to a small saucepan on medium heat.
- Whisk as you bring the mixture a low boil. Reduce heat and simmer for about 8-10 minutes (or until the flavors have combined).

- Strain the liquid through a fine mesh tea strainer into cups and season with ground cinnamon and molasses.

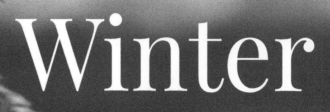

Winter

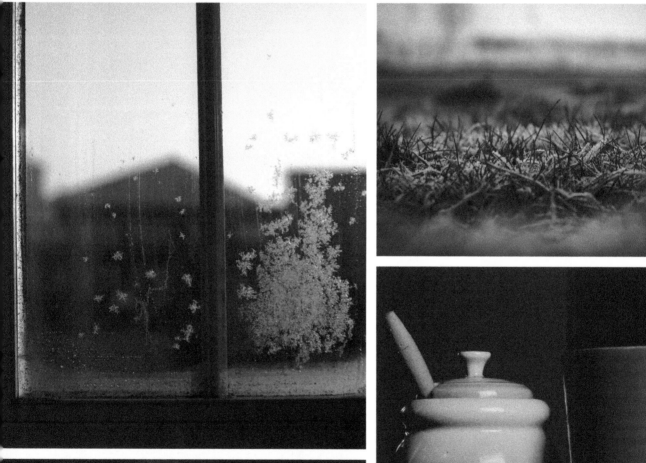

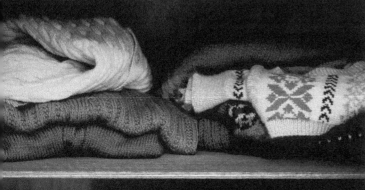

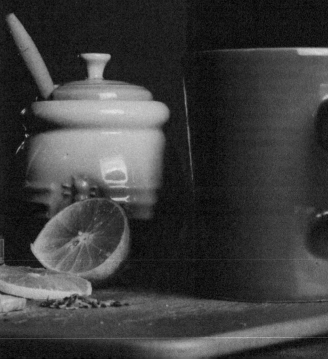

Winter season can be a little two-faced sometimes: cold, dry, and light in the beginning, often morphing into colder, wet, and heavy by the end. It's a time of year to stay tuned in to what's going on in your mind and body and allow your inner wisdom to guide your choices for maintaining balance and bliss.

Qualities of winter...

Early Winter: *Cold, light, dry, variable*
Late Winter: *Cool, heavy, damp, dull*

Winter mantra for balance:

Early: *Warming, grounding, moisturizing, routine*
Late: *Enegizing, stimulating, drying, expression*

What to watch out for:

Anxiety, fear, constipation, aches and pains, insomnia, mood swings, cold hands and feet, depression, lethargy, water retention

Winter Self Care Focus:

- **Sleep** - Great time to get your sleep schedules on track. Ensure that you're getting enough, but not too much sleep. Waking up a little later in the winter is okay.

- **Hydrate** - Hydrating during this time of year is critical, as cooler temperatures can tend to dry out the body and mind! Ensure that you're getting sufficient water every day.

- **Oil** - Oiling the body via daily self massage practice will keep the muscles, joints and skin supple and toned. Self massage is a powerful practice for showing yourself love during one of the more difficult seasons of the year. Oil pulling with sesame oil is good to add to your winter routine.

- **Connect** - Tune in to what feeds you. Early winter is a great time for introspection and turning inward. Later in winter you'll want to ensure that you are getting sufficient connection with friends and family to feed your mind and soul.

- **Stay warm, but not hot** - Do what you can to maintain a comfortable body temperature. It will do wonders for the mind and body this time of year.

A few things to add to your winter routine:

- **Spice water...** Our digestion can typically be strongest in winter, but it might still need a little boost. Sipping warm water througout the day is a great suppor for wintertime digestive health! **You can find the recipe for my favorite winter drink here!**

- **Oil massage...** Winter is a great time to treat yourself to a professional massage (or a series of them). A gentle and oily focus can soothe the nerves in early winter. While more rigoruous massage late in the season can be the stimulating boost your body needs.

- **Laughter...** Laughter is a powerful medicine, and one of the best ways to keep the winter blues at bay! Create a "laugh list" of comedy movies, books, and even live experiences to ensure you have a steady supply!

- **Nasya oil...** Keep the sinuses clear, moist and happy by adding nasya into your daily routine. A preventative mesaure for colds, flus and springtime allergies, and a great way to keep your "gateway to consciousness" happy and healthy!

- **Chyawanprash...** This Ayurvedic rejuvenative jam. is great all year round, but particularly supportive through the winter season. Find a brand you like and take 1-3 tsp daily. To strengthen mind and body against the winter cold.

- **Nadi Shodhana...** Otherwise known as alternate nostril breathing, this balancing breathing practice is a simple, powerful way to cleanse the mind, body and channels! It's especially good for early winter.

Eating in Winter

Breakfast In winter are warm, oily, soft, and easily digestible. I like to keep the portion sizes more modest than in the autumn (just a natural reaction to how I feel) and porridges are pretty much the star of the show! Oats, buckwheat, semolina, polenta. They can be dressed up with stewed fruit and a few nuts (sometimes even a dollop of coconut yogurt for that warming sour quality).

Lunch Soups, curries, and warm sandwiches or warming Buddha bowls are a perfect winter lunch. You can mix and match the flavors and ingredients creating a variety that takes advantage of produce available this time of year. Stews with grains are a great lunch for winter as well. Tune in to your digestion. This is the time of year when heavier foods will be most nourishing to your mind and body. If you can digest them, it's a good time to dive in.

Dinner I like to keep winter dinners pretty light. We do a lot of soup in the wintertime. Creamy soups, soups with root veggies, and a little bit of meat or lentils is a satisfying meal, and yet still feels light this time of year. Stay tuned in to portion sizes (especially as you make the shift from larger to lighter dinners), and if possible, eat before the sun goes down and use your evening to wind down, take care of yourself, and connect with those you love.

Winter tastes/qualities to favor:
sweet, sour, salty, heavy, oily, and moistening

Winter spices to favor:
Ginger, cinnamon, cardamom, asafoetida, fennel,
basil, turmeric, cumin

Wintertime Superfoods by Type:

These are the best foods for the season based on your constitution or imbalance.

Vata [includes vata-pitta, vata-kapha]:	*Pitta* [includes pitta-vata, pitta-kapha]:	*Kapha* [includes kapha-vata, kapha-pitta]
Nuts and seeds	Kale	Mung beans
Olive oil	Beets	Brussels sprouts
Ghee	Artichoke	Pumpkin seeds
Avocados	Apples	Grapefruit
Meat & fish	Coconut Oil	Ginger tea
Ashwagandha	Chamomile	Turmeric
Licorice & cinnamon tea	Licorice & cinnamon tea	
	Brahmi	

*Get additional **winter** info & resources via this link!*

http://www.eatlikeyouloveyourself.com/Winter

Breakfast

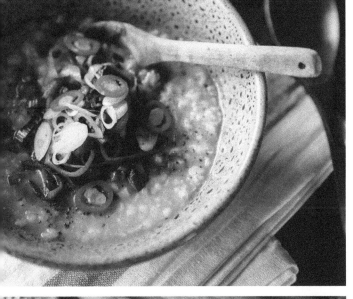
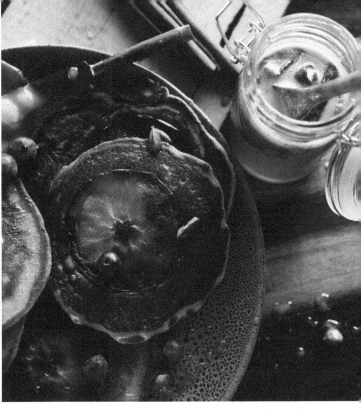
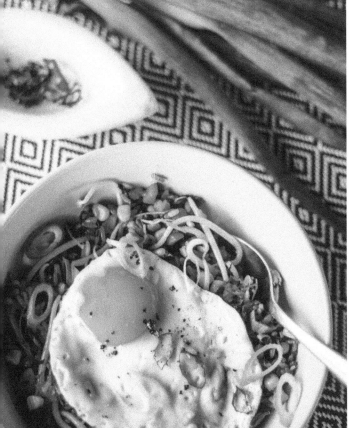
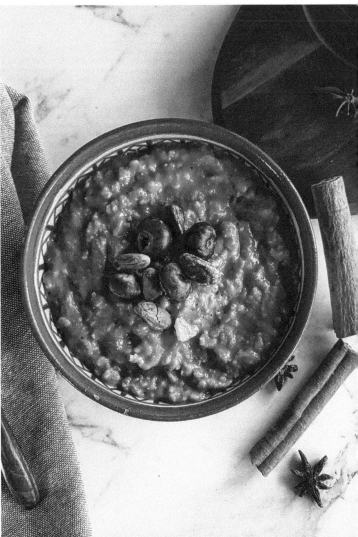

Spiced Apple Cinnamon Pancakes
-V -P =K

Pancakes are are perennial favorite in our house, and if you're a fan like I am, know that there's a version of pancakes that could be considered good for just about every season, depending on what you put in them. This one is basically simple, classic pancakes with a little bit extra. I've added some fruit into the mix to make them more interesting and definitely moreish! ***Makes about a dozen; Prep + Cooking time 35 mins***

What's in it:

- 1 cup flour
- 2 teaspoons baking powder
- ½ teaspoon salt
- 2 tablespoons sugar
- 1 large egg, lightly beaten
- 1 cup milk

- 2 tablespoons melted unsalted butter
- 2 tsps ghee
- ¼ teaspoon cardamom
- ¼ teaspoon cinnamon
- 1 medium apple

How to make it:

- Cut apple in half and core. Slice each half into large, thin slices. Sprinkle with lemon juice and set aside.
- Add flour, baking powder, salt, cinnamon, cardamom, and sugar to a large bowl and whisk together to mix.
- In a separate bowl, mix together the egg, milk, and butter. Add the wet ingredients to the dry and stir just to combine ingredients. Don't worry if there are lumps in the batter.
- Heat a large skillet or griddle on the stove to medium heat.

- Add a teaspoon of ghee to hot pan. Place two apple slices into the pan and cook until slightly tender. Top cooked apples with 2-3 tablespoons of batter.
- Flip the pancakes when the batter bubbles and resist pressing them down! Cook until golden brown on the bottom. Repeat for all apples and batter.
- Keep pancakes warm in the oven until you're done with everything.
- Serve these on their own or with a drizzle of honey or maple syrup.

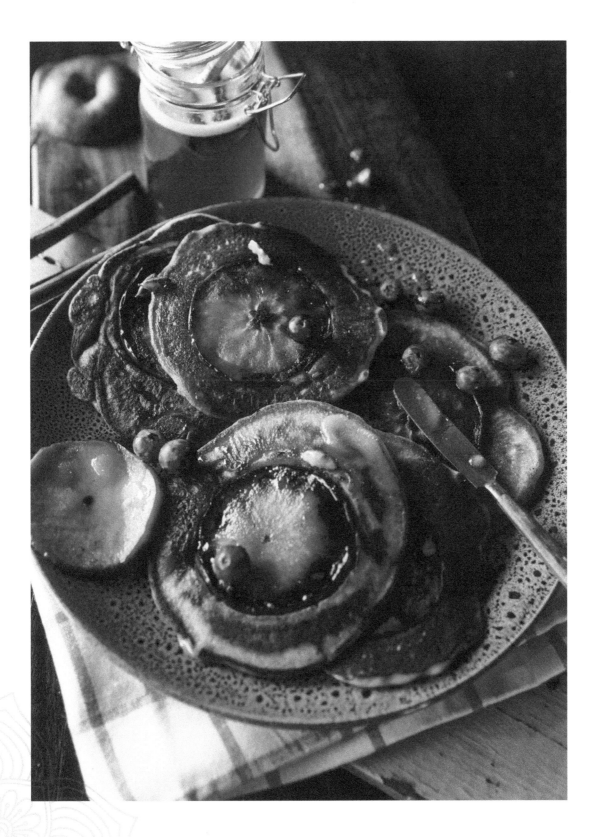

Chai Tea Oats
-P -K

If you're a fan of chai (which I definitely am) and a fan of oatmeal, this recipe will revolutionize your breakfast and blow your mind at the same time! Not only does it allow you to have your tea and breakfast combined, you'll get all the digestion-stimulating goodness of the warming spice hit of chai masala PLUS the mind-body stimulating effects of the black tea. It's also really yummy. *Makes 3 servings; Prep + Cooking time: 20 mins*

What's in it:

- 1 ½ cups traditional rolled oats
- 2 ½ to 3 cups of chai tea (why not use the Warm Winter Chai recipe - Pg 199)
- ¼ teaspoon salt

Optional toppings:

- Cooked fruit (apples are great)
- Homemade granola
- Coconut flakes
- Honey
- Homemade yogurt

How to make it:

- Add tea, salt, and oats to a large pot over medium to high heat. Heat slowly, stirring often until the oats have expanded to the texture you desire (I like chewier oats for vata season and runnier oats for kapha season).

- If you like a little sweetness, you can add a little bit of molasses or maple syrup.
- Transfer portions to bowls and top with toppings of your choice (or none at all).

Quick Nasi Goreng
-V +P -K

Ayurveda says that the life force energy we feel comes largely from the energy in our food. Which means eating fresh food as much as possible and avoiding leftovers and processed foods. I do my best to finish any leftover food within twenty-four hours of when it was first prepared, so this dish is one of my breakfast (or lunch) "go to dishes". You can use leftover rice (or make a small batch of fresh if you've got a rice cooker), along with fresh or left over veggies. And approach it as a way of breathing new life into food that might otherwise be wasted. *Makes 2 servings; Prep + Cooking time: 35 mins*

What's in it:

- 1 small brown onion, finely diced
- 2 cups of cooked jasmine rice, best to cook the day before
- ½ cup vegetables of your choice (great to use leftover veggies), chopped into small to medium sized pieces

- 1 tablespoon toasted sesame oil
- 2 teaspoons soy sauce
- 1 teaspoon sesame seeds (optional)
- 1 tablespoon scallions (green onions) finely sliced
- 2 eggs

How to make it:

- Add the sesame oil and onion to a frying pan on a medium heat setting, and stir until softened and slightly browned.
- Add the chopped veggies and stir just to warm through.
- Add the rice to the pan with the veggies, along with the soy sauce, sesame seeds and half the sliced scallions.
- Toss the rice and veggies to warm and combine well. Remove from heat and cover to keep warm.

- In another frying pan, heat a teaspoon of sesame oil to medium high heat.
- Fry the eggs in the pan to your desired degree of doneness.
- Divide the rice and place into bowls, topped with a fried egg.

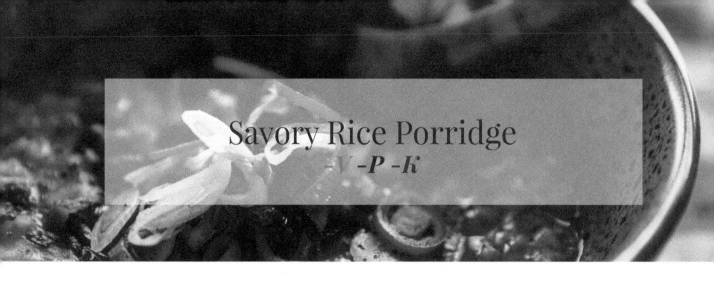

Savory Rice Porridge
-V -P -K

Nothing's simpler than porridge. What I love the most is how versatile it can be. This one's a take on congee (Chinese rice porridge), and meant to be served warm with savory toppings. This is a great dish for a light fast or as part of a cleanse regimen. It's also lovely when you're feeling a bit tired and heavy and need something that's satisfying and nourishing that won't weigh you down. My favorite way to "dress" it up is by adding a few tablespoons of cooked green mung beans, and some crunchy fried shallot to it! *Serves 2-3; Prep + Cooking time: 30 mins.*

What's in it:

- 1/2 cup uncooked brown basmati or jasmine rice
- ½ tsp himalayan pink salt (or smoked salt)
- ¼ tsp black pepper
- 1 inch sized piece of fresh ginger peeled and finely chopped.
- 4 cups water, plus more as needed

Optional extras

- ¼ cup cooked green mung beans
- 1 tablespoon thinly sliced green onions
- 1 tablespoon crunchy fried shallots
- ¼ cup cooked chicken (optional)
- Red pepper flakes to taste (optional)

How to make it:

- Add the rice, water, salt and ginger to a large pot. Bring to a boil and reduce to simmer.
- Cook uncovered for 60 - 90 minutes, stirring occasionally and adding more water as necessary to maintain the soupy texture.
- Porridge is ready when the rice is fully cooked and begins to fall apart. If you like a little less texture, you can continue to cook until the texture is more like a smooth soup.
- Serve warm with added optional ingredients, stirred through.

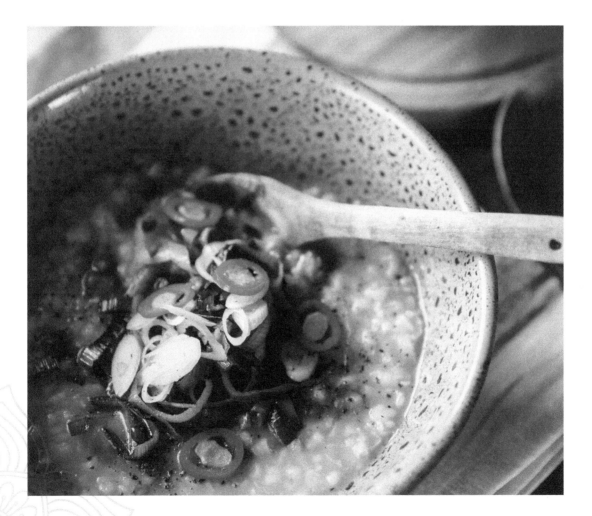

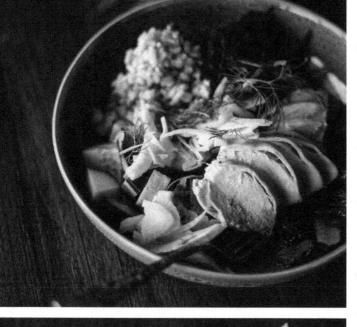

Lunch & Dinner

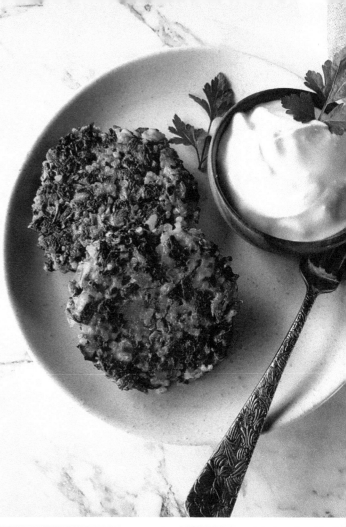

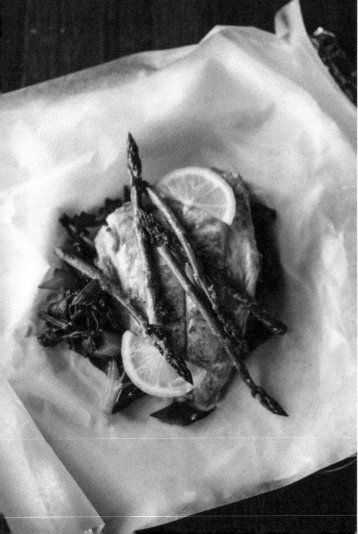

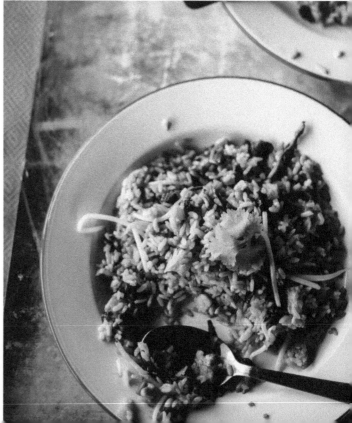

Fish In Parchment Paper
-P -K

If you've ever thought that cooking fish was hard, you'll definitely want to give this a go. This nearly foolproof method of cooking fish is a great way to ensure the fish stays moist and flavorful. It's also super easy to cook and clean up! A great weeknight meal to ensure that you're getting all of your veggies (and tastes) in! ***Serves 1; Prep + Cooking time: 25 mins.***

Cooking time will depend on the type of fish and the size/thickness of the piece you choose. You'll know the fish is cooked when the center is no longer opaque. This is a really versatile dish that is a great simple meal for winter or even spring. I would go with freshwater fish in spring accompanied by seasonal greens!

If cooking for more than one, make a separate parcel for each piece.

What's in it:

- 170g (one good sized piece) skinless snapper (or any local fish available)
- 1 handful of spinach or chard
- 1 clove garlic, chopped finely
- 1 tablespoon olive oil
- ½ lemon, sliced
- salt and pepper to taste

How to make it:

- Preheat the oven to 180°C/355 °F
- Start with a piece of aluminum foil and parchment/baking paper that are the same size. Place the parchment on top of the foil layer and the spinach on top of the parchment.
- Lay the fish on top of the spinach and sprinkle with salt, pepper, garlic, and lemon juice.
- Bring the outside edges of the foil/ parchment together and fold the top edge down about an inch. Make another inch fold, and then fold the sides in (like a wrapping a gift). The foil should ensure that the package stays closed.
- Bake in a hot oven for 5-6 minutes or until center of fish is no longer opaque.
- To serve, open the parcel on a plate and enjoy all the flavours that were trapped inside.

Winter Chicken & Fennel Bowl
-V -P -K

This simple seasonal bowl is a great lunch option for in home or on the go! The ingredients are mildly heating without being too heavy and the addition of cumin and fennel help to pump up the flavor and the digestion balancing qualities. In my opinion, we just don't eat enough fennel! It's a beautiful seasonal veggie that adds some serious depth and support for balancing the mind and body this season. ***Serves 4; Prep + Cooking time: 35 mins.***

What's in it:

- 3 chicken breasts
- 1 large fennel bulb sliced into thin strips
- 1 bunch silverbeet, washed and torn into large strips
- 2 teaspoons salt
- 1 tablespoon vegetable oil (sunflower or olive is best)
- 3 garlic cloves, sliced

- 2 tablespoons ground cumin
- 1 tablespoon ground fennel seeds

Fresh ingredients for garnish

- 1 large grated beetroot
- 1 cucumber, sliced
- 2 cups of cooked farro, brown rice, or couscous

How to make it:

- Mix the cumin, fennel, garlic slices, salt, and oil in a bowl.
- Line a baking dish with a sheet of baking paper and spread the fennel, silverbeet leaves and chicken breast, then sprinkle with spice and oil mix.

- Cover the tray and bake for 20 minutes on 180°C/355°F
- Remove the tray from the oven and let the mix rest for 10 minutes.
- Slice the chicken and assemble all ingredients in bowls using grains as a base.

Pitta: Balancing - in moderation

Kapha: Balancing (less chicken, more greens)

Kale & Carrot Fried Rice
-V -P +K

This one has become a staple in our house, because who doesn't love fried rice? This one's got heaps of fresh veggies, a little egg for protein, and a lot less oil than your Chinese restaurant or takeout variety! My kids love it, so there's a good amount of dancing in the kitchen when this is being made. This makes a great lunch, served with a light soup, or an easy light dinner served on its own. ***Serves 4; Prep + Cooking time: 45 mins.***

What's in it:

- 4-5 stalks Tuscan kale, washed, spines removed, chopped into small sized pieces
- 2 medium carrots, peeled and diced
- 2 cups mushrooms, diced
- 3 scallion stalks (green onions), finely sliced

- 3 eggs
- 2 cups medium grain rice, cooked
- 1 tablespoon soy sauce
- 1 tablespoon oyster sauce
- 1 tablespoon toasted sesame oil
- Bean sprouts (optional)

Pitta: Balancing (substitute tamari for soy sauce, eat only in moderation)

How to make it:

- Lightly beat the eggs in a bowl, adding in a small handful of the sliced scallions.
- Add one teaspoon of sesame oil to a hot pan over medium heat, and scramble the eggs until they are on the drier side. Break the eggs into smallish pieces. Remove from heat and set aside.
- Add a teaspoon of sesame oil to a large, heavy-bottomed pan or wok.
- Over medium heat, cook the carrots and mushrooms together until most of their water has been released and evaporated (you don't want them to be wet and mushy, more like dry without being crispy).

- Add the kale to the mushroom and carrots and cook until wilted. Add the eggs to the pan and combine.
- Add the warm rice to the pan, along with the soy sauce, oyster sauce, and 2 teaspoons of sesame oil.
- Combine all ingredients until completely mixed and coated with the sauces.
- Add bean sprouts at the end and toss through.
- Serve immediately to the hungry mob of folks eagerly awaiting their lunch. Or dinner.

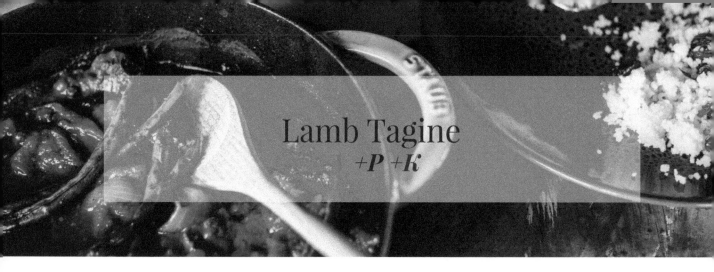

Lamb Tagine
+P +K

Whenever I hear the word tagine, I just melt. It's the thought of the gorgeous mix of all of my favorite spices (including cinnamon) in a hearty, nourishing stew! This dish reminds me of travelling (ate a lot of it in Morocco), and has a heaviness that is great for grounding (something that travellers really need). It can be made with chicken or just vegetables (I prefer root veggies), and the spice mix alone is enough to make your digestion smile. Don't be frightened by the long list of ingredients. This one is pretty easy and can be put in a slow cooker if you want the house to smell like heaven when you get home from work!! *Serves 4-5; Prep + Cooking time 3 hrs.*

What's in it:

- 1 tablespoon olive oil
- 1 ½ pounds lamb leg or shoulder diced into small, stew-sized pieces
- 1 ½ teaspoons salt
- ½ teaspoon freshly ground black pepper
- 1 large yellow onion cut into small slices/wedges
- 4 cloves garlic
- 1 ½ cups veggie stock (you can use beef stock for slightly richer flavor)
- ½ cup golden raisins
- 2 medium sized carrots, peeled and cut into medium-sized chunks
- 100g green beans, washed with ends trimmed

- 1 can organic chickpeas, drained and rinsed (you can also use ½ cup of chickpeas that have been washed soaked overnight)
- 1 400g can organic diced tomatoes
- 1 ¼ teaspoons ground cumin
- 1 ½ teaspoons ground cinnamon
- 1 teaspoon ground coriander
- 1 teaspoon smoked paprika (you can also use sweet paprika if you prefer)
- ¾ teaspoon ground turmeric
- ½ teaspoon ground ginger
- Small bunch of fresh coriander leaves (cilantro)

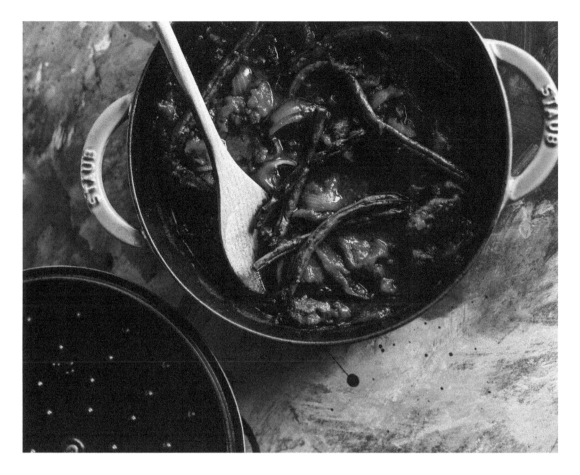

How to make it:

- Preheat oven to 150°C/355°F. Season lamb pieces with salt and pepper.

- Heat a Dutch oven or a large ovenproof skillet with a lid over medium-high heat. Add oil to the pan and cook lamb pieces for 5 minutes, until nicely browned. Transfer lamb to a plate and set aside.

- Add onion and garlic to pan and sauté 4 minutes, stirring occasionally, until softened. Add spices: cumin, coriander, paprika, turmeric, ginger, and 1 teaspoon salt. Cook, stirring constantly, for 1 minute. Add broth and scrape the pan to loosen browned bits.

- Throw the lamb pieces back into the pan along with tinned tomatoes and bring to a simmer.

- Stir in chickpeas, cover, and place into heated oven covered with lid.

- Cook covered, for 1 ½ hours. Add the carrots and cook for an additional 45 minutes to 1 hour. Add green beans and cook for an additional 20 minutes or until the lamb falls apart and the green beans are tender.

- Remove from oven and serve with couscous or on its own, topped with chopped coriander leaves (cilantro) for garnish.

Pork &Ginger Dumpling
-P +K

Ayurveda says that cooking is an opportunity to bring us closer to ourselves by bringing us closer to those elements that become who we are. I feel this most powerfully when making things like dumplings. Dishes that require just you and the food, no tools (really), but things like this take time which is why we rarely do them. Consider this dish your chance to dive in. Super simple, incredibly flavorful and a beautifully versatile and nourishing dish for any time of year (depending on the fillings and style of cooking). Give it a go!

Makes 2-3 dozen; Prep + Cooking time: 90 mins.

What's in it:

- 1 pk egg wonton dumpling skins

Filling
- 300g ground pork
- 1 tablespoon finely grated ginger
- 2 cloves garlic, grated
- 1 shallot (Asian shallot)
- 1 tablespoon sesame oil
- 1 tablespoon soy sauce

- ½ teaspoon salt
- 2 whole eggs

Dipping sauce
- ½ cup soy sauce
- 2 teaspoons sesame oil
- 2 teaspoons rice wine vinegar
- 1/2 of one red chilli, chopped
- 1 clove finely chopped garlic

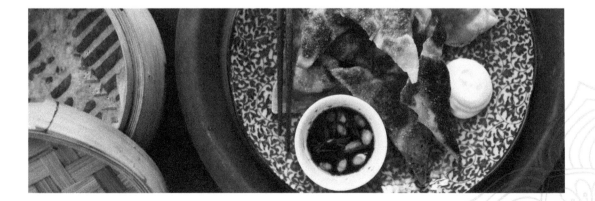

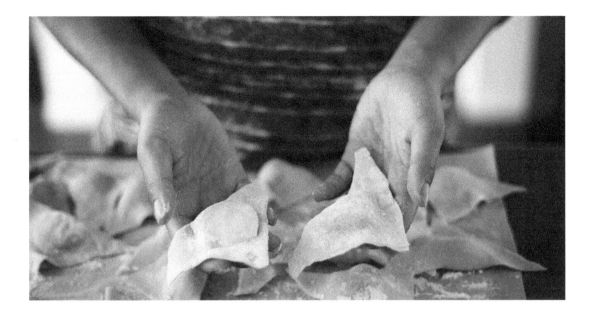

How to make it:

You can make the dipping sauce first or put it together, while the dumplings are steaming (if you choose to steam them).

- To make it, combine all the dipping sauce ingredients together and mix well. Set aside or refrigerate.

- Put all the filling ingredients into a bowl and combine well using your hands. Be careful not to over mix the filling, using your hands first and then pinching the filling through with fingers. Set aside.

- To make the dumplings, first let go of any issues you've got with perfection! Then lay out the dumpling skin and put 2 teaspoonfuls of pork mixture in the center of the wrapper. Brush edges with water. Fold over to enclose filling. Pinch edges together. Place on a tray lined with non-stick baking paper. Repeat with remaining wrappers and pork mixture.

- Now to cook them! Here's where you've got some options.

- To steam the dumplings, place them in a bamboo steamer on a piece of oiled baking paper on top of a 1/2 full pot of boiling water. Cook about 2 minutes.

- To pan fry the dumplings, add 1 teaspoon of toasted sesame oil to medium hot frying pan or skillet. Carefully place the dumplings into the pan and fry for up to a minute on each side or until golden. Add a couple of tablespoons of water to the hot pan and cover to finish steaming the dumplings.

- Serve dumplings with dipping sauce and enjoy!

Pitta; Balancing (steamed in moderation)

Roasted Veggies & Grains Salad
–V –P +K

The title for this one is a little vague in that I haven't specified the "veggies." We typically use roasted pumpkin or sweet potato for this dish, but you could also go with roasted carrots or beets in a pinch. This is a substantial enough salad to enjoy as a lunch or dinner in the winter or spring. *Serves 4-6: Prep + Cooking time: 60 mins*

What's in it:

- 1 cup couscous (can substitute quinoa
- for a gluten-free option)
- ¾ cup water (or vegetable stock)
- 1 ½ cups butternut pumpkin, cut
- into medium-sized chunks
- ½ cup crumbled feta cheese
- 3 cups baby spinach
- 2 cups mixed salad leaves
- (baby romaine, arugula, etc.)
- 2 cups sunflower or pea sprouts
- ¼ cup pine nuts

- ¼ cup dried cranberries -
- chopped into small pieces
- salt and pepper to taste

- **Salad Dressing**
- 2 tablespoons olive oil
- ¼ cup orange juice
- 1 teaspoon lemon juice
- ½ teaspoon salt

How to make it:

- Preheat oven to 200°C/400°F. Line a baking sheet with baking paper.

- Toss pumpkin pieces in a bowl with 1 teaspoon of olive oil, salt, and pepper. Spread pieces on a baking tray and roast for 30 minutes or until fork tender and browned on the edges.

- Remove roasted pumpkin from oven and allow it to cool to room temperature [this job can be done up to a couple of hours ahead of salad assembly time].

- While the pumpkin is roasting, bring water/veggie stock to boil in a saucepan. Add the couscous and chopped cranberries, stir, cover, and turn off heat and let stand covered for 5 minutes or until water has been completely absorbed. Fluff with a fork and allow to sit uncovered to cool slightly.

- In a big salad bowl, add spinach, salad leaves, and sprouts, and set aside.

- Toast the pine nuts in a fry pan on medium to low heat until they are lightly brown. Watch closely as they can easily burn if you turn your attention away from them for what seems like an instant! Set toasted nuts aside to cool slightly.

- For the dressing, put all ingredients into a small jar and shake to mix. You can season with salt and pepper to taste.

- When all ingredients are cooked and cooled to room temperature (or slightly warmer), throw the pumpkin, couscous, feta cheese, and pinenuts in with the salad leaves. Drizzle some of the dressing over the top and toss to coat everything.

- Serve and enjoy!!

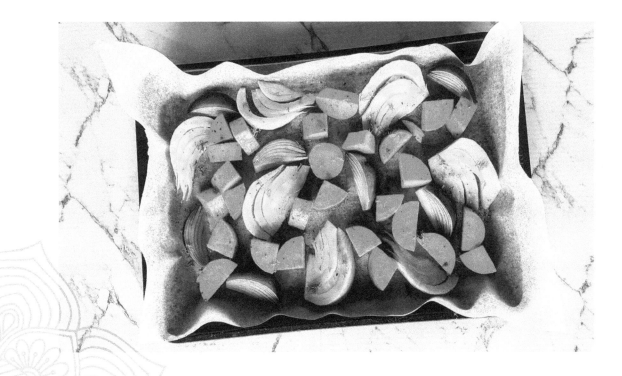

Winter Grain & Veggie Cakes
-P -K

My family loves these. What I like most about them is the versatility. You basically combine grains that work for the season (check the references, but for winter I use quinoa, amaranth, or couscous) with seasonal veggies and a little bit of fat and salt (i.e. cheese) for glue (and happiness). These make a terrific light dinner or a great lunch coupled with a bowl of soup! I dare you to use your imagination and come up with a combo that will thrill you and your family and friends!! *Makes 1-2 dozen; Prep + Cooking time: 90 mins.*

What's in it:

- 1 ½ cups cooked quinoa, amaranth, or even couscous
- ½ cup finely chopped onion
- 2 garlic cloves, finely chopped
- 5 ounces (140g) chopped baby spinach
- 1 cup diced pumpkin pieces
- 2 large eggs, beaten
- 2 ounces (55g) crumbled feta cheese
- ¼ teaspoon grated lemon zest
- ¼ cup bread crumbs
- Coarse salt and freshly ground black pepper
- 1 tablespoon extra-virgin olive oil or ghee

For dipping sauce
- ½ cup plain yogurt
- 2 tablespoons finely chopped scallions (green onion)
- 2 teaspoons freshly squeezed lemon juice
- 3 tablespoons finely chopped fresh parsley
- ½ teaspoon ground cumin
- ½ teaspoon ground coriander seeds

How to make it:

- Make the sauce by mixing together the yogurt, scallions, lemon juice, 2 teaspoons of parsley, and spices in a small bowl. Add salt and pepper to taste. Cover and refrigerate for at least an hour to allow the flavors to combine. Serve sauce at room temperature.

- To make the veggie cakes, heat the olive oil in a large skillet over medium heat. Add the onion and garlic and cook until softened, about 4 minutes. Add the pumpkin and cook for about 4-5 minutes or until slightly softened, then add the spinach and cook until wilted. Transfer the vegetable mixture to a medium sized bowl and allow to cool slightly.

- To the veggies bowl add the quinoa, feta, the remaining parsley, lemon zest, and ¼ teaspoon black pepper and mix well. Mix in the bread crumbs and let the mixture sit for a few minutes to allow the bread crumbs to absorb some of the moisture.

- Heat a skillet and add 1 tablespoon of oil or ghee.

- Form patties about 2 1/2 inches in diameter and 1/2 inch thick. Place the patties in skillet in batches if necessary. Cook the patties until they're browned on the outside, 4 to 5 minutes per side, and then flip.

- Serve warm with yogurt sauce.

*Kapha: Balancing (in moderation)

Snacks

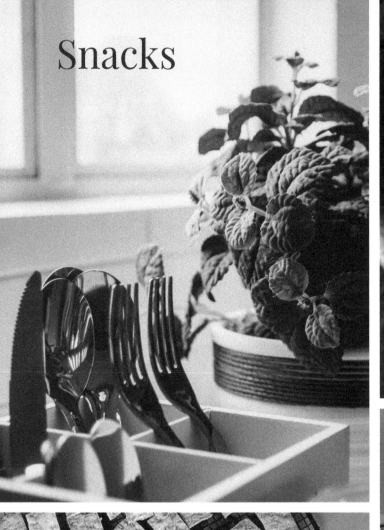
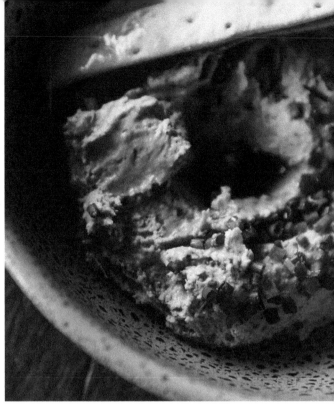
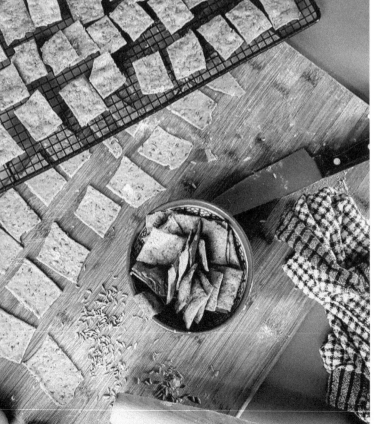
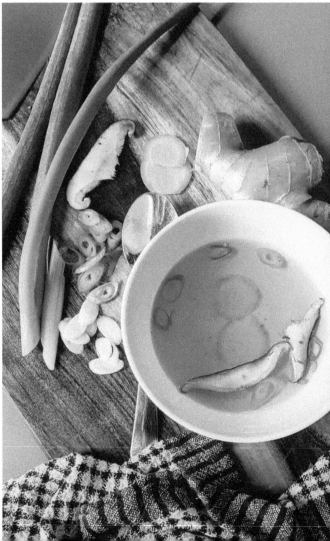

Fennel Seed & Turmeric Crackers
-P -K

I'm a cracker-a-holic, which can be an issue for my vata (crackers are dry and rough, just like vata). So I always have them with something warm and oily). I've incorporated some warming spices into the recipe to help with digesting. Those qualities make them a great option for winter (to have with soup or a warm spread for a light dinner). If you've never made your own crackers, you've definitely got to try them. ***Makes around 60 crackers; Perp + Cooking time: 40 mins.***

What's in it:

- 1 ¼ cups all purpose flour (whole wheat, spelt, gluten free will all work).
- 4 teaspoons fennel seeds
- 2 teaspoons ground turmeric
- 2 teaspoons sea salt
- ½ teaspoon baking powder

- ¼ teaspoon freshly ground black pepper
- ½ cup water
- ¼ teaspoon apple cider vinegar
- 2 tablespoons olive oil

How to make it:

- Whisk dry ingredients together in a large bowl.
- Combine water, vinegar, and oil in another bowl and pour into dry ingredients. Knead the mixture into a soft, smooth dough
- Shape the dough into a ball, cover with plastic wrap, and refrigerate for at least 30 minutes.
- Then preheat oven to 220°C/425°F. Line a baking sheet with parchment paper and set aside.
- Remove refrigerated dough and divide into pieces and roll into balls.

- Roll out each ball on a lightly floured surface to about ⅛ inch (3-4mm) thickness.
- Using a sharp knife, slice the dough into cracker sizes and shapes.
- Transfer to lined baking sheet, and bake for approximately 10 minutes, or until firm and edges are beginning to brown.
- Repeat with remaining dough balls or refrigerate/freeze dough for later use.
- Let crackers cool completely before serving. Store in an airtight container for up to a week.

Vata: Aggravating (have them with something oily or not at all)
Kapha: Balancing (in moderation)

Ginger Broth

+V -P -K

Super simple and delicious, this light broth can make a nice savory snack when the weather is cold or a light lunch or dinner just about any time of year. It's made with ingredients that will give your digestion a boost and is stimulating and fragrant enough to make you feel truly alive! ***Serves 4-5; Prep + Cooking time: 15 mins.***

What's in it:

- 4 cups vegetable or chicken stock
- 1 teaspoon soy sauce
- 1 tablespoon thinly sliced scallions (green onion)
- 3 slices fresh ginger root (thin to medium thickness)

Optional additional items

- handful fresh spinach leaves
- drizzle of toasted sesame oil (for a more Asian flavor)
- 2 thinly sliced mushrooms
- ¼ cup medium to firm tofu chunks

How to make it:

- Add stock, soy sauce and ginger slices to a medium-sized saucepan and bring to a boil. Reduce heat to simmer and add scallions.

- Enjoy this as a simple broth or add in your choice of optional extras to make it slightly more substantial.

Pitta: Balancing (use tamari instead of soy sauce)

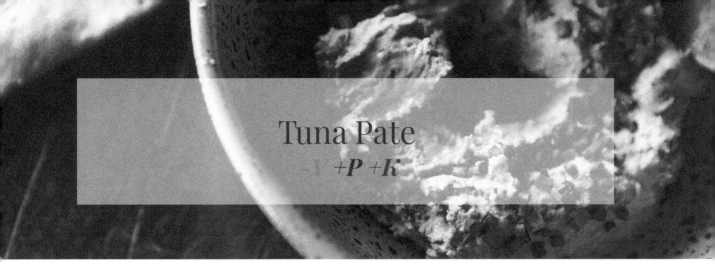

Tuna Pate
–V +P +K

Winter dinners in our home can sometimes look more like snacks than the traditional heavier dinnertime fare. If you're in need of a snack or perhaps a light meal, this lovely dish fits the bill. It's got quite a few warm and heavy elements, along with a bit of unctuousness that can help to keep winter vata at bay. ***Serves 4-6; Prep + Cooking time: 25 mins.***

What's in it:

- 1 tablespoon olive oil
- 2 shallots (60g), finely chopped
- 2 garlic cloves, finely chopped
- 4 anchovy fillets, rinsed, drained, and chopped
- ¼ bunch dill, finely chopped

- 425g can tuna in olive oil, drained
- 250g cream cheese
- 1 tablespoon lemon juice
- salt and freshly ground
- black pepper, to taste

How to make it:

- Warm the oil in a pan on medium heat and saute the shallots until they are soft.
- Add the garlic and anchovies and cook until the anchovies have softened (a couple of minutes should do it!). Remove from the heat and set aside.
- Blend, process, or mix dill, tuna, and shallot mixture, cream cheese, lemon juice, and pepper until smooth or the desired consistency (sometimes a little chunkier is nice!). Season with salt as needed.
- Transfer the pate to a serving bowl and chill to set.
- Remove from the refrigerator before eating and allow to warm slightly to just under room temperature. Serve with fresh bread, pita bread, or crackers

Desserts

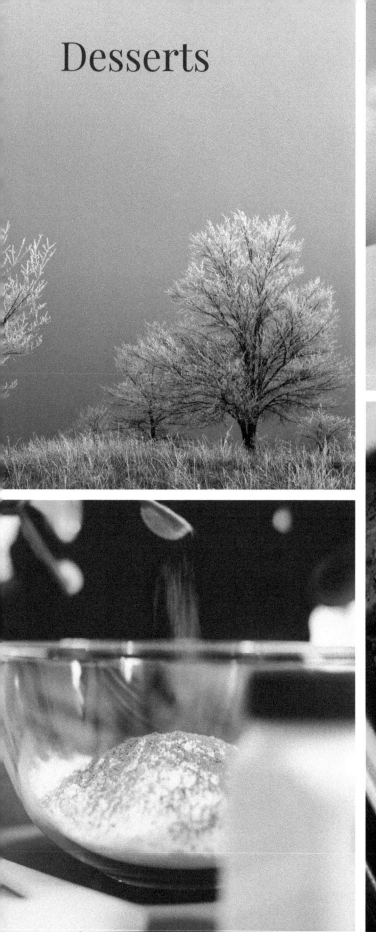
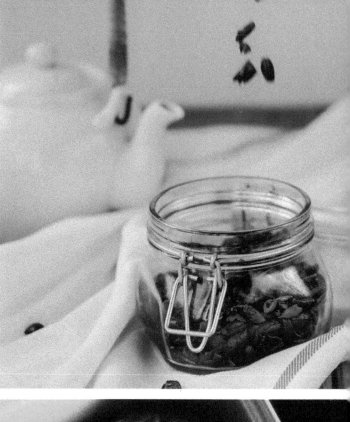
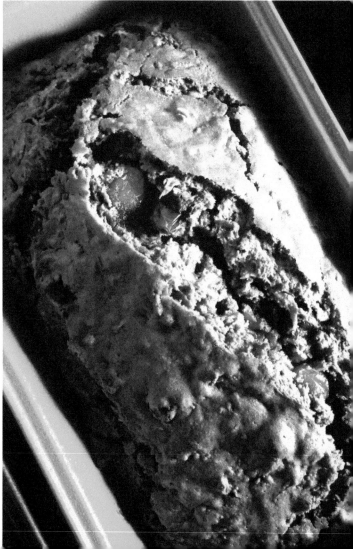

Cranberry Zucchini Bread
-P -K

The unique combination of sweet, sour, bitter and astringent is actually perfect for early autumn when both vata and pitta energies can become imbalance. It takes me back to my days living in NYC where the super hot summers would give way to cool, breezy autumn days. And a cranberry-zucchini muffin with a cup of chai could make everything right with the world. Use fresh cranberries if you can find them! ***Makes 2 loaves; Prep + Cooking time: 90 mins.***

What's in it:

- 3 to 4 cups grated fresh zucchini
- (700 to 900 ml) - usually about 3 small to medium zucchinis
- 3 cups (390 g) whole wheat flour
- 2 teaspoons baking soda
- 2 teaspoons cinnamon
- ½ teaspoon ground ginger
- ¼ teaspoon ground nutmeg

- 1 ⅓ cup (270 g) raw cane sugar, Sucanat
- 2 eggs, lightly beaten
- 2 teaspoons vanilla extract
- ½ teaspoon salt
- ¾ cup (170g) butter, melted
- 1 -2 cups (120 - 240 g) fresh or frozen whole cranberries

How to make it:

- Preheat oven to 175°C/350°F. Grease and flour two 5 by 9 inch loaf pans.
- Place the zucchini in a tea towel or paper towels inside of a colander or strainer to drain.
- In a bowl whisk together the flour, baking soda, cinnamon, ginger, and nutmeg.
- In a large bowl, whisk together the sugar, eggs, vanilla extract, and salt, until the sugar has mostly dissolved
- Stir in zucchini and melted butter. Add the cranberries to the mixture.

*Kapha: Balancing (in moderation)

- Add dry ingredients to the wet ingredients a third at a time, stirring to fully incorporate, while being careful not to crush too many of the cranberries.
- Divide the batter equally between the loaf pans. Bake for 50 minutes or until a toothpick or skewer inserted into the center comes out clean.
- Cool in pans for 10 minutes. Turn out onto wire racks to cool thoroughly.
- Serve warm with butter or a light drizzle of ghee!

Drinks

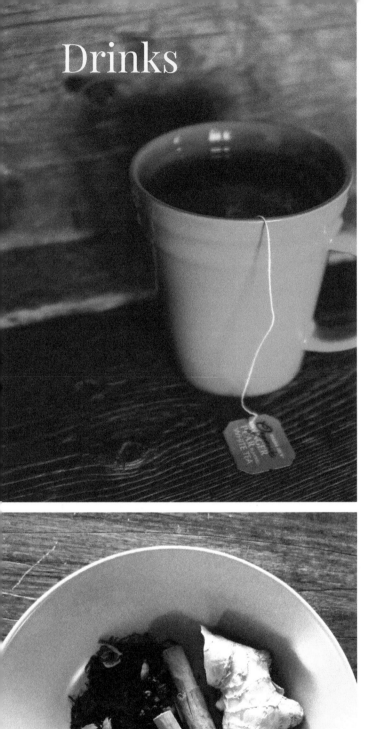
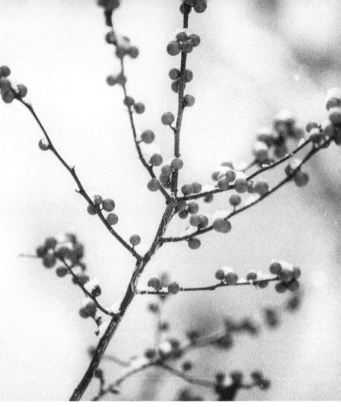
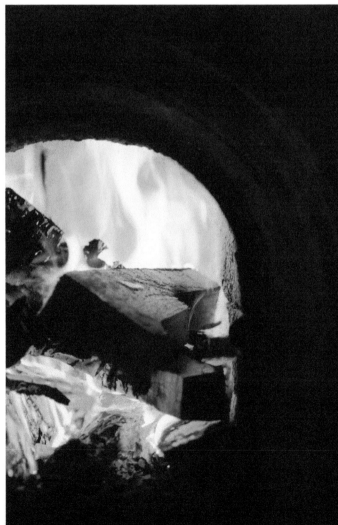

Warming Winter Chai
-*P* +*K*

Tea is one of my favorite things to drink throughout the year, but on cold wintry days it feels more like medicine! Winter is a great time to spice up your tea, providing a double benefit of warming you from the inside out AND applying healing properties to soothe your potential imbalances. Black tea is quite stimulating and can help to wake up sleepy digestion and moods this time of year. Warming spices help to keep winter digestion happy and healthy. But, while keeping the mind and body warm is important this time of year, too much heat can cause drying effects that can aggravate vata.

That's why I'm a big fan of milk teas in winter or using demulcent (soothing) spices like cinnamon or licorice to stave off the drying or irritating effect that too much heat (or cold) can have on the mind and body. Here's my favorite winter chai recipe. ***Serves 2; Prep + Cooking time: 10 mins***

What's in it:

- 4 tablespoons black tea - I typically use assam
- 1 one inch piece fresh ginger root
- 6 cardamom pods - crushed to open the pods
- 2 star anise
- 1 cinnamon stick
- 1 teaspoon cacao nibs (optional - for the chocolate lovers)
- 3 ½ cups pure filtered water
- 2 ½ cups milk of your choosing (this can be any kind of milk or nut milk)

How to make it:

- Add the water and spices to a sturdy -bottomed saucepan and bring to a boil.
- Add the black tea and allow to continue at a low boil for 3-5 minutes.
- Stir in the milk and lower the heat to simmer for 1-2 minutes.
- Strain the warm tea into cups. Top with a pinch of cinnamon or Magic Dust.

Spring

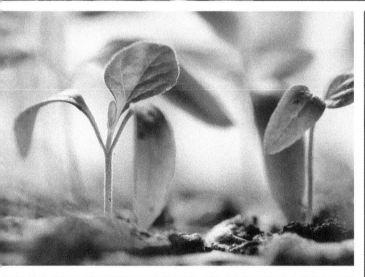

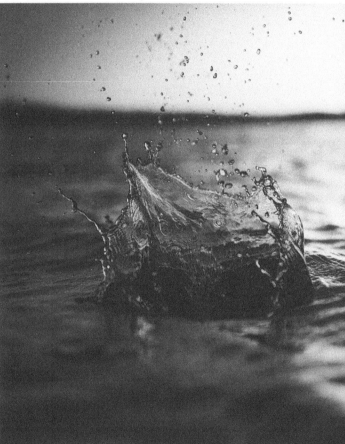

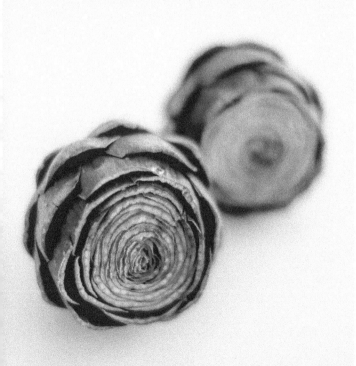

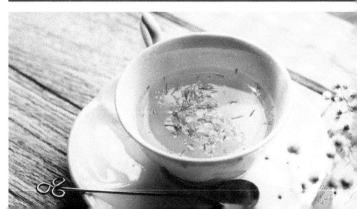

Ayurveda calls spring the king of seasons, and we all know why. Spring is a fresh start, a chance for renewal, a long awaited parole from winter's incarceration. It's the official season for cleaning up your act and clearing away anything that's standing between you and your best you (even though technically you can do that any time of year!). It's also our signal to shed the layers of winter before they get too heavy and walk towards the light by balancing kapha dosha.

Qualities of spring:
Cold, damp, heavy, sluggish, slow, dull

Springtime mantra for balance:
Warming, drying, stimulating, expression

What to watch out for:
Weight gain, depression, congestion, lethargy, complacency, attachment, diabetes, colds and flu, allergies.

Spring Self Care Focus:

- **Lighten up** - Spring is a time to counter the heaviness of the end of the winter season by lightening up! Turn up the light in your food (go with light and easy meals -- you may even have been drawn to them), your activities (get outside, move, invite a feeling of freedom into your mind and body), and even your clothes (great time for light and bright colors to reflect or create a sense of lightness and clarity in your attitude).

- **Clear out** - We've all heard of spring cleaning! It's a powerful way to signal to the world (and yourself) that you're creating a capacity for new things to come into your life. Clearing the clutter in your life (things, ideas, relationships, beliefs), has a profound effect on the mind! It's a great way to lift your spirits and inspire your greatness (seriously!).

- **Express yourself** - Having taken the time and space for inward reflection over the winter season, spring is a time to let yourself go! It's a great time to connect with nature and the people you love, to feel and speak your truth, and be a sounding board for the people in your life. Holding back our feelings, desires, and emotions is a recipe for congestion, dullness, and depression. So express yourself unapologetically this season in order to thrive!

- **Warm and dry -** If you find yourself feeling a little cold and wet, don't worry, it's just the season. Balance that heaviness by staying and eating warm and dry. Popcorn is a favorite springtime snack, while you're wrapped in a light shawl with a cup of ginger tea! Whatever you need to feel comfortably warm and dry this season...just do it!

A few things to add to your spring routine:

- **Kapalabhati breathing...** is an energizing and clarifying breathing technique (pranayama) that is great for spring mornings to clear the channels, awaken the mind and body, and warm you from the inside out.

- **Dry brushing...** Clear away dead skin and dullness with this invigorating practice of dry massage. You can use a soft brush (made specifically for this task) or a raw silk glove (garshan). Great practice for mornings before showering.

- **Time with friends...** Spring is usually the time when we're feeling stuck. At the tail end of winter, we find ourselves needing activities and inputs that remind us of who we are and what's important to us. I love organizing coffee or lunch dates with friends around late winter and spring. It's a chance to express yourself and be inspired. It's also great for shaking off the winter blues!

- **Nasya oil...**Nasal care can be critically important during the cold, flu, and allergy season. Keeping the nasal passages oiled creates an optimal environment for the nose to do its work of keeping out nasties. Oiling also soothes irritated nasal passages and keeps skin on and around the nose moist and supple.

- **Cleansing...**Spring is one of the key times of year for cleansing and detoxification which are an important part of the Ayurvedic approach to health and happiness. Ayurveda offers lots of options for detoxing, but the simplest form of Ayurvedic cleansing can be done at home in just a few steps and with a little bit of guidance (check out chapter fourteen for more details).

Eating in Spring

Breakfast Spring breakfasts are the beginning of moving toward lighter foods/ meals first thing in the morning. If it's cold outside, I might have a bowl of warm, soupy oats with fruit. Or, if I'm going really light, a nice mug of Yogi Breakfast. For a more substantial springtime breakfast, I like eggs with spring veggies like fresh peas, asparagus, fresh corn and beans or hearty greens (like kale). I've noticed that my tastes change like clockwork, desiring the shift to these lighter options as the season shifts from winter to spring. I'll usually start adding a bit of honey into my warm lemon water around this time of year too!

Lunch The challenging thing about spring lunch is striking a healthy balance between heavy and light! You want lunch to be your biggest meal, but you want your choices to be on the dry side, a little spicy with a warming element. Soup, or toasted sandwich, light pizzas, and even salads with grilled veggies or seafood. Spring is a great time to bring out the leafy greens! And you can get creative with them. Beans or lentils cooked with greens over rice or light grain (like buckwheat or millet), simple two or three ingredient salad with a splash of oil all make an easy and delicious springtime lunch.

Dinner Spring dinners are pretty easy in our house! We're all fans of fresh spring rolls and often set them up "roll your own" style. Usually one or two is enough to satisfy and settle us into our evening routine. Our other pretty common go to for spring dinners is soup! Asian style soups with corn and asparagus or maybe an egg thrown in are a great way to make the most of springtime farmer's market superstars!

Spring tastes/qualities to favor:
bitter, pungent, astringent, easy to digest, and warm

Spring spices to favor:
coriander, cardamom, asafoetida, fennel,
mint, turmeric (late summer)

Spring Superfoods by Type:

These are the best foods for the season based on
your constitution or imbalance.

Vata [includes vata-pitta, vata-kapha]:	*Pitta* [includes pitta-vata, pitta-kapha]:	*Kapha* [includes kapha-vata, kapha-pitta]
Apples (cooked)	Asparagus	Dandelion
Beets	Apples	Watercress
Corn	Blueberries	Bean sprouts
Carrots	Cabbage	Microgreens
Garlic	Dandelion	Asparagus
Eggs	Spearmint	Dried fruit
Amaranth		
Asafoetida		

*Get additional **spring** info &
resources via this link!*

http://www.eatlikeyouloveyourself.com/Spring

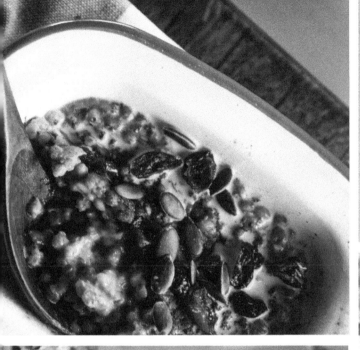

Breakfast

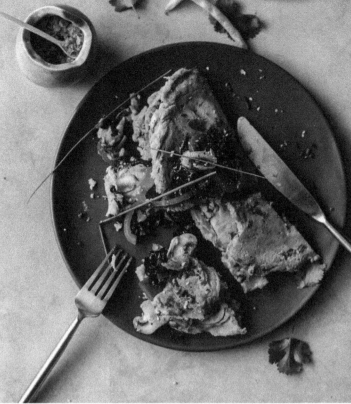

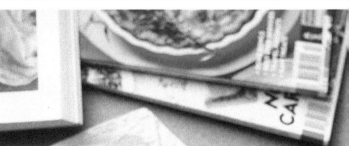

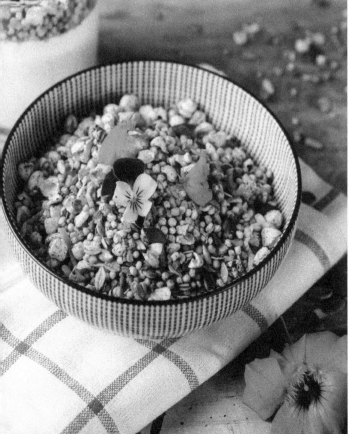

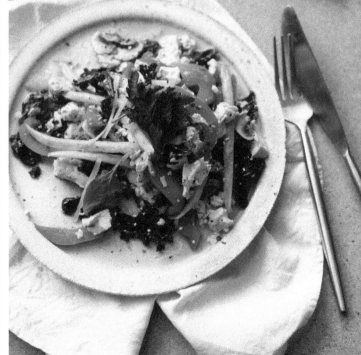

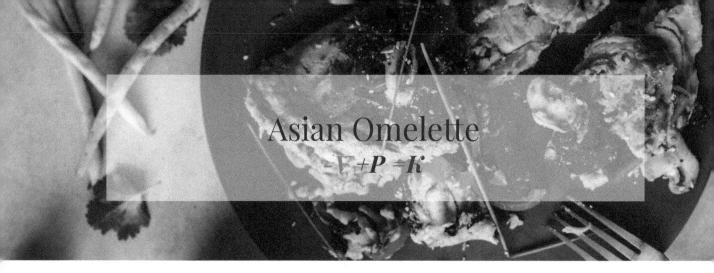

Asian Omelette
~V +P ~K

Omelettes are one of the simplest meals around. They're also a great way, outside of salads to incorporate veggies into your diet. And since they're cooked, they make a perfect meal for springtime. I've pushed outside of the traditional mushroom or cheese with this one to introduce some of my favorite asian flavors, which are a perfect complement to spring! *Serves 2; Prep + Cooking time: 25 mins.*

What's in it:

- ½ cup bean sprouts
- 1 green onion, thinly sliced
- ½ cup of red bell pepper thinly sliced
- 1 long red chili, thinly sliced
- ½ inch piece ginger, finely grated
- 1 garlic clove, crushed

- 2 tablespoons oyster sauce
- ¼ teaspoon fish sauce
- 4 eggs
- 2 teaspoons toasted sesame oil
- Finely ground black pepper to taste

How to make it:

- Beat eggs with fish sauce, a pinch of green onions, and 1 tablespoon of cold water. Season with pepper.
- In a small bowl, combine garlic, oyster sauce and ginger with 1 tablespoon of warm water.
- Add one teaspoon of sesame oil to a pan on medium high heat. Quickly saute the bell pepper along with a pinch of green onion, just to warm them. Remove and set aside.

- Turn up the heat on the pan and add additional sesame oil plus ½ of the egg mixture and swirl to coat the pan. Cook for 30 seconds until set and remove from the pan.
- Top one half of the egg "pancake" with half of the cooked peppers and half of the bean sprouts. Fold over the empty half and drizzle with the sauce.
- Repeat for the other half of the egg mixture.

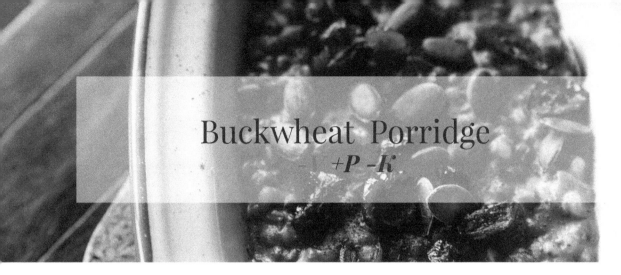

Buckwheat Porridge
+P -K

If you've started to get used to the usual porridge grains, I definitely encourage you to step out of the box and explore making porridge from the grains that are suited to the season, like this lovely spring option. Buckwheat is one of the only "grains" with a warming energy and that's because technically it's a seed. It has sweet, pungent and astringent qualities that can help to reduce water retention, dry up mucus and congestion, and warm you from the inside out. This hearty porridge is a nice way to start the day! *Serves 2-3; Prep + Cooking time: 35 - 45 mins.*

What's in it:

- 1 ¼ cup buckwheat groats
- 1 teaspoon of ground cinnamon
- 1-2 teaspoon of ground ginger
- ¼ teaspoon ground nutmeg
- 1 cup fresh filtered water
- 2 cups soy milk (or your favourite milk of any kind)

- A pinch of salt
- 1 teaspoon ghee (optional)

Optional toppings
- Stewed fruit (try the roasted rhubarb)
- Dried fruit
- Toasted buckwheat for a bit of crunch)
- Spiced seeds

How to make it:

- Soak the buckwheat groats overnight.
- Drain and rinse soaked buckwheat, and place into a medium sized saucepan along with the filtered water and spices.
- Bring to a boil and then reduce heat and cover.
- As the porridge begins to absorb the water, add half of the milk and stir. Allow it to simmer, checking and stirring occasionally. As the liquid absorbs add more milk and keep the porridge simmering until it's thickened to your desired texture.

- Cooking can take anywhere from 20 - 40 minutes, but is well worth it for a porridge that is beautifully textured and more easily digestible. Add liquid through the cooking process as needed to achieve the desired texture.
- When you've achieved the right texture, add a teaspoon of ghee (if using) and sweetener of your choosing (I use a bit of molasses, make sure to cool it before adding honey) stir through the porridge.

Nut Free Turmeric Granola
-P -K

I LOVE granola! But I've found that commercial granola has far too much sugar and is a little heavy on oil to make it a good spring option. This gorgeous recipe combines light grains with warming spices and just a touch of sweetness to make this a great springtime pick for a light breakfast. ***Makes about 9 cups; Prep + Cooking time: 35 mins.***

What's in it:

- 4 ½ cups puffed quinoa
- 2 cups puffed buckwheat
- 1 ¼ cup rolled oats
- ¼ cup shredded coconut
- ½ cup Pepitas
- ⅓ cup sunflower seeds

For the flavour syrup

- ⅓ cup maple syrup

- ¼ cup coconut oil or ghee
- 1½ tablespoons ground turmeric powder
- ½ teaspoon ground cinnamon
- ½ teaspoon cardamom
- ¼ teaspoon allspice
- pinch of salt
- pinch of black pepper
- 1 teaspoon vanilla extra

How to make it:

- Line a baking sheet with baking paper and preheat oven to 160 Celsius [325 Fahrenheit].
- In a medium sized bowl, combine the seeds and grains and mix together.
- In a small saucepan, combine all of the flavour syrup ingredients and mix until the coconut oil has fully melted. Pour the syrup mixture over the seeds and grains and mix well to coat everything.
- Spread mixture out on the lined tray in a single layer. Bake for 25 minutes, stirring every 5-8 minutes to ensure an even toast. Remove from the oven, and allow to cool before transferring it to an airtight container.

Vata: Balancing (in moderation with warm milk)
Pitta: Balancing (in moderation - omit black pepper)

Spiced Up Tofu Scramble
-P -K

This dish is a tridoshic (and vegan) substitute for scrambled eggs. The beauty of it is that you can adjust it by adding in veggies and spices that are good for your dosha (since you're starting with a balanced base). I'm a big fan of tofu in the spring time (if you haven't already guessed), but this one is also good for summer (just go easy on the heating ingredients). Feel free to enjoy this dish as is or try your hand at "dressing" it up a bit with your favorite seasonal veggies! ***Serves 1; Prep + Cooking time: 25 mins***

What's in it:

- 1 tablespoon ghee (or vegetable oil)
- 1 cup firm tofu, crumbled
- ¼ cup fresh coriander (cilantro) leaves, coarsely chopped
- 2 tablespoons onion, minced
- 2 tablespoons bell pepper (capsicum), minced

- 1 tablespoon fresh ginger, minced
- ⅛ teaspoon finely minced fresh or ground turmeric root
- ⅛ teaspoon ground cumin
- ½ teaspoon salt

How to make it:

- Add ghee/oil to a frying pan on medium heat. Saute onions and ginger until the onions are soft and translucent.
- Add coriander, peppers, turmeric, salt and cumin, and continue cooking until veggies are soft.

- Add the crumbled tofu plus a little fresh black pepper to taste.
- Cook on medium heat until the tofu is warmed through and maybe a little brown on the edges. If it the mixture goes a little dry, you can add a tablespoon of water.

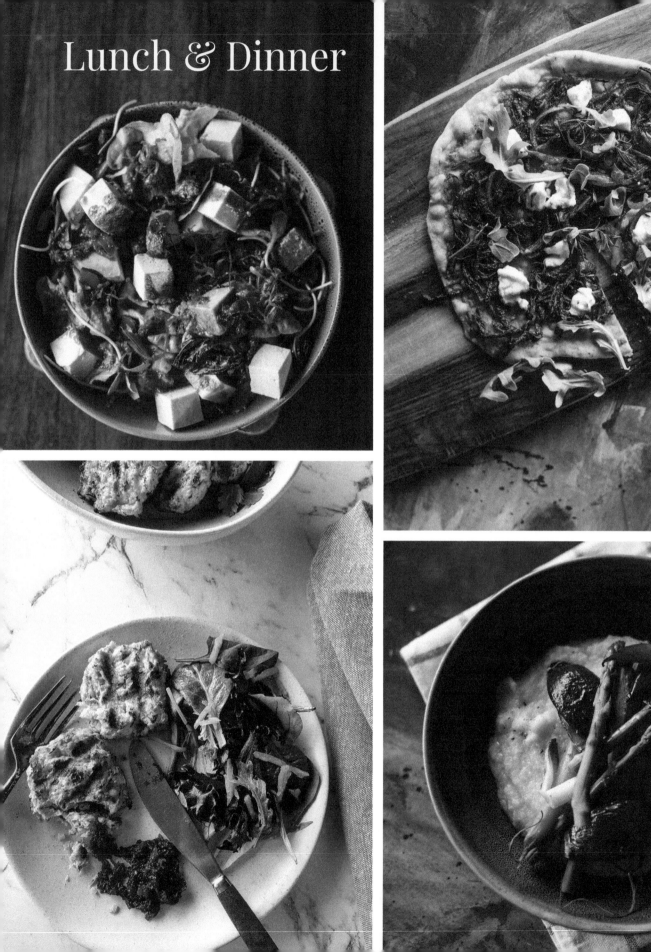

Lunch & Dinner

Asian Scented Asparagus Soup
-V -P -K

A fresh, bright soup with clean, warming Asian flavors. Asparagus is a beautiful springtime veggie that is incredibly versatile. It's got bitter and astringent qualities that make it great for cleansing. The Asian spices in this simple dish give it an aromatic kick to enliven the senses! Soup is a great springtime lunch or dinner option as it's light and warming and easy to make! ***Serves 4; Prep + Cooking time: 30 mins.***

What's in it:

- 1 large onion, finely chopped
- 1 tablespoon ghee or canola oil
- 3 pounds asparagus, washed
- with ends trimmed
- ½ teaspoon black pepper
- 1 cup lite coconut milk

- 4 to 5 cups vegetable broth
- 3 tablespoons finely minced lemongrass
- 3 tablespoons finely chopped ginger
- ½ teaspoon fresh lemon juice
- Pinch of red pepper flakes (optional)

How to make it:

- Cut asparagus into ½ inch pieces.
- In a large heavy pot, cook onion with ghee on moderately low heat until softened (about 8 - 10 minutes). Add in the chopped ginger and lemongrass, and cook until the vegetables are soft.
- Turn up the heat slightly to medium and add in the asparagus pieces, salt and pepper and cook, stirring frequently for about 5 minutes.

- Add the broth and coconut milk, and lower heat. Simmer covered until asparagus is quite tender.
- Puree soup in batches in a blender or with a stick blender until smooth. If the soup is too thick, add a bit more broth to bring it to the consistency that you're looking for and cook for another 5 minutes. Just before serving add lemon juice and stir through.
- Can be served with fresh cilantro leaves as garnish!

Pitta: Balancing (omit red pepper flakes)

Caramelized Onion Flatbread

+P =K

This springy flatbread features one of my favorite warming veggies -- onions!! I've also thrown in a little leafy green bitterness, to balance out the richness of the onions and goat's cheese! All atop a nice digestible sourdough crust or you can go with your favorite gluten free crust! *Makes 2 pizzas; Prep + Cooking time: 60 mins.*

What's in it:

Base:
Simple flat bread {Pg 289}

Topping

- 4 medium sized red onions (you can also use yellow or brown)
- 2 tablespoons of oil (I use ghee or a combination of olive oil and ghee)
- ½ cup of goat cheese
- 2 handfuls of rocket leaves
- 2 tablespoons of spring pesto sauce {Pg 229}

How to make it:

- To caramelize the onions, slice them into thin slices and separate all layers.
- Add onions and oil to a medium sized pan on medium heat. Stir gently to coat the onions in the oil.
- Allow the onions to cook slowly, checking and stirring every 5-10 minutes. The caramelization process should kick in after about 20 minutes. Cook the onions for up to 35 minutes (they should be brown but still whole, rather than broken down into a jammy texture). Remove from heat and set aside.
- Preheat the oven to 200°C/400°F Line a large baking or pizza sheet with baking paper or place a pizza stone into the oven.
- Place prepared flatbread on a piece of baking paper.
- Top each base with 1 tablespoon of spring pesto sauce and spread it to cover the entire base (it will be a very thin layer, use your hands if you need to to spread the sauce).
- Top the bread with the caramelized onions and small pieces of goat's cheese.
- Bake in heated oven for up to 10 minutes, crust should be cooked and lightly browned on the edges. Goat cheese should be lightly brown on top.
- Remove from the oven and allow to cool slightly. Scatter a handful of rocket leaves over the flatbread and serve.

Clear Soup With Chicken & Veggies
–V –P –K

Tender chicken is accompanied by spring vegetables in this gorgeous dish that looks more difficult than it is. This is a very simple weekday meal It's also perfect for when you need something slightly more substantial than soup. Great mid winter to early spring when digestion can be slightly stronger, and there's a need for meals that are a nice balance of light and nourishing. *Serves 4-6; Prep + Cooking: 75 mins.*

What's in it:

- 1 organic 3-pound/1.5 kg chicken
- 4cups vegetable stock
- 4 cups water
- 1 bay leaf
- 1 sprig thyme
- 1 sprig rosemary
- Salt and pepper

- 4 cloves garlic peeled
- 2 leeks cleaned, trimmed and thickly sliced
- 4 medium onions, peeled
- 1 small bunch of carrots, peeled with the leafy tops removed
- 2 celery stalks, cut into finger lengths

How to make it:

- In a pot large enough to hold the chicken with room to spare (a good sized dutch oven works really well for this purpose), place the chicken, breast side down (tie the feet together with string beforehand), and cover with the stock and water.
- Bring to a low boil, and allow to cook for about 30 minutes, occasionally skimming off the foam that rises, until the foaming stops.
- Add the thyme, rosemary, bay leaf, salt,

garlic and leeks. Cover and simmer for 15 minutes.

- Turn the chicken breast side up and add the onions, celery and carrots to the pot. Cook until the juices in the chicken breast run clear and the veggies are fork tender.
- Remove from heat and pull pieces of the chicken away from the bone (should be this tender).
- Serve chicken and vegetables in bowls topped with a generous ladle of soup

*Pitta and Kapha: Balancing (in moderation)

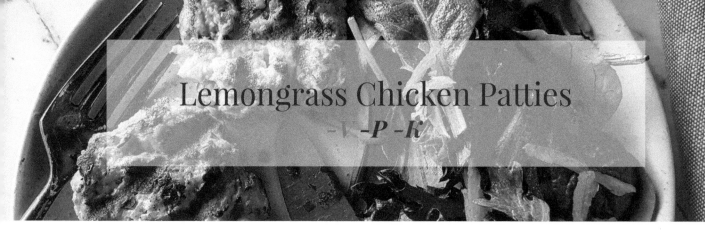

Lemongrass Chicken Patties
-V -P -K

Super simple spring meal that can be thrown together quickly (yay!). It features one of our favorite warming Asian spices, lemongrass, combined with a bit of ginger to give it some depth and an exotic flare. These can be accompanied with rice and some braised or steamed Asian greens for a hearty lunch or enjoyed on their own with a chili dipping sauce and simple salad for a light dinner. *Serves 4-5; Prep + Cooking time: 30 mins.*

What's in it:

- 3 chicken breasts
- 1 red onion diced
- 3 tablespoons soy sauce
- 1 stick of lemongrass finely chopped
- ½ bunch of coriander chopped

- 1 tablespoon vegetable oil (toasted sesame, canola, or sunflower)
- 1 whole egg
- 1 pinch salt

How to make it:

- In a blender or food processor, blend chicken breasts into a smooth paste.
- Transfer chicken paste to a medium sized bowl and add onion, soy, lemongrass, coriander, salt and mix to combined well .
- Add the egg and 1 tablespoon of vegetable oil to the bowl and mix to combine. Use fingertips to gently

- knead the mixture being careful not to overwork the meat.
- Scoop out chicken mix into small balls and roll into patties.
- Cook patties on a medium hot grill for a few minutes each side. Remove and serve.

Garlic Polenta With Roasted Spring Vegetables
-P -K

Polenta or cornmeal has light, dry and slightly warming qualities that make it a terrific option for spring! And if you're a lover of porridge, this savory veggie topped meal will be an absolute delight! Feel free to use whatever seasonal veggies you can find for this one.
Serves 4; Prep + Cooking time: 45 mins

What's in it:

- 2 medium size red onions cut into quarters
- 12 asparagus spears, washed and trimmed
- Small bunch of fresh baby carrots
- (with tops trimmed)
- 3 handfuls of green beans,
- washed and trimmed
- 1 garlic clove, thinly sliced
- 3 garlic cloves (leave the papery skin on)

- 2 tablespoons of oil or ghee
- 1 ½ teaspoons salt
- 1 ½ teaspoons finely ground black pepper
- Juice of half a lemon

For the polenta

- 4 cups water
- 1 teaspoon salt
- 1 cup polenta or yellow cornmeal
- ¼ grated parmesan cheese (optional)

How to make it:

- Preheat oven to 180°C/375°F. Line a baking sheet with baking paper. Spread all vegetables including all garlic on the baking sheet. Drizzle with oil/ghee and salt and pepper to taste.
- Roast the vegetables for 30 - 35 mins or until tender and browned on the edges, turning once or twice during the cooking to ensure even browning. Remove and set aside.
- Let the garlic cloves cool and remove the skins (squeeze out the garlic pulp). Set aside

- Cook the polenta by bringing the water to a brisk boil over medium-high heat. Add the salt and whisk the polenta into the water, pouring in a steady stream.
- Whisk until the polenta thickens, add the garlic paste and continue cooking until you get a porridge like consistency.
- Stir in the cheese and add salt and pepper to taste and divide the polenta into bowls topped with roasted vegetables and a squeeze of lemon juice.

Lentil Shepherd's Pie
-V -P -K

A different take on a classic, this vegetarian version is no less flavorful or rich. We've just left out the heaviness of the meat and replaced it with the dry, light and slightly astringent qualities of lentils. Lentils are great for kapha, but they can sometimes be a little challenging to digest, so I've slowed the cooking time on this one to give the lentils time to break down a little. The dish is topped with yummy cauliflower mash! *Serves 4; Prep + Cooking time: 90 mins.*

What's in it:

- 2 medium sized carrots, peeled and diced
- 2 sticks celery, diced
- 1 lb (500g) cremini mushrooms, brushed and sliced
- 2 tablespoons ghee (or butter)
- 1 small yellow onion, diced
- ½ cup dry white wine
- 1 ½ cups uncooked lentils, rinsed and soaked (best is brown or green lentils)
- 4 cups vegetable broth (plus more for cooking)
- 2 teaspoons fresh thyme leaves, chopped
- ½ cup of whole milk

- 2 cups of sliced kale leaves
- salt and pepper to taste

For the garlic rosemary cauliflower mash layer:

- 2 lbs (32oz/907g) potatoes - Yukon Gold or Russet - washed peeled and chopped into medium sized pieces.
- ¼ cup whole milk
- 2 tablespoons ghee
- ¾ teaspoons salt
- 4 cloves garlic crushed
- 2 tablespoons fresh rosemary, finely chopped.

How to make it:

- Preheat the oven to 200 Celsius [400° Fahrenheit].

- Place the chopped potatoes in a large pot and cover with water and a large pinch of salt. Bring water to the boil and lower heat to simmer. Allow potatoes to simmer for about 10- 15 minutes or until they are tender.

- Drain the potatoes and return them to the pot. Add milk, ghee, garlic and rosemary, and mash (or use a hand blender) to the desired level of smoothness.

- While the potatoes are cooking, add a couple tablespoons of ghee to a large frying pan. Add carrots, onions and celery and saute until slightly soft and fragrant (up to about 10 minutes). Add the mushrooms to the mixture and cook until softened and most of the liquid has dried up.

- Add the white wine to the mix and scrape the bottom of the pan to get all of the caramelized bits off the bottom. Stir for 3-5 minutes as the alcohol burns off and then add the lentils, thyme broth and kale.

- Simmer for 30 - 40 mins to allow the lentils to absorb the liquid (add more broth as necessary). Once lentils have softened, add milk, 2-3 tablespoons of the mashed potatoes, and a generous pinch of salt and pepper.

- Pour the mixture into an ovenproof dish and top with a nice layer of mashed potato.

- Place it on a baking sheet and bake for 20-30 minutes or until the top is slightly crisp and golden brown.

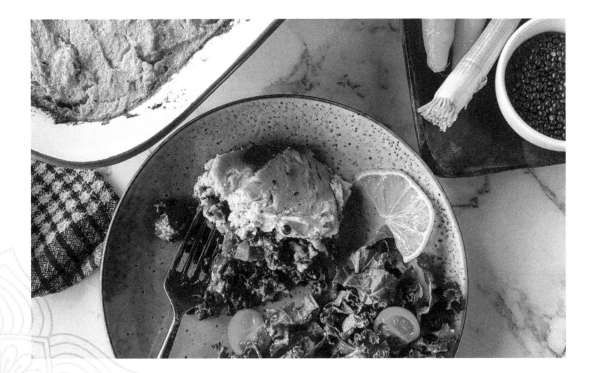

Sheet Pan Spicy Tofu & Beans
-V -P -K

Quick meals are a godsend to the soul. This one is as simple as they come and tasty too! It satisfies veggies and protein requirement with just enough flavor and umph to make it quite likely a mainstay in your household. The flavors of this one, bitter, spicy, dry and a little sweet are a perfect answer to the wet, cold or muggy heaviness of spring. ***Serves 3-4; Prep + Cooking time: 40 mins.***

What's in it:

- 400g Firm tofu, torn into bite sized chunks
- 200g (a few generous handfuls) green beans, washed and trimmed
- 1 tablespoon of olive oil or ghee
- Juice of one lemon
- 1 teaspoon smoked paprika
- 1 teaspoon cumin powder
- 1 teaspoon coriander powder
- small handful coriander leaves (cilantro)
- 1 teaspoon salt
- Black pepper to taste

How to make it:

- Line a baking sheet with baking paper and set aside.
- Place the tofu pieces in a large mixing bowl with spices, oil/ghee and lemon juice. Stir or mix with your hands to coat everything and allow to sit covered for up to 1 hour.
- Preheat oven to 180°C./350°F
- Using tongs or a fork, remove all the tofu pieces from the bowl and place them on the baking sheet, leaving the residue of lemon juice and spices behind.
- Bake the tofu for about 35 mins or until it starts to bubble and slightly brown.
- Add the green beans to the marinade bowl and mix to coat them with the juice and spices.
- Remove the tofu tray from the oven and add the green beans and any remaining juice and spice mix to the tray. Put the tray (tofu + beans) back into the oven and bake for a further 15-20 mins or until the beans are fork tender (they may look a little dry, that's okay, they'll taste amazing!).

*Pitta: Balancing (in moderation, leave out black pepper)

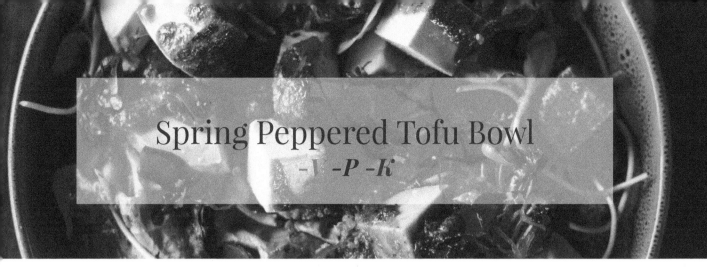

Spring Peppered Tofu Bowl
-V -P -K

A clean, crisp and light meal in a bowl with warming flavors and heating and drying qualities to remove heaviness from the mind and body! Tofu is generally balancing for all doshas and is sattvic in nature. It's light astringency makes it a good option for springtime.
Serves 2; Prep + Cooking time: 30 mins + Marinade time.

What's in it:

For the tofu marinade
- 1 cup (250g) firm tofu cut into cubes
- 1 tablespoon ground coriander
- 1 tablespoon ground black pepper
- ½ teaspoon rock salt
- 1 tablespoon of sunflower oil

For the salad
- ½ cup shredded red cabbage
- 2-3 handfuls of mixed lettuce leaves
- 1 cup sunflower sprouts

For the dressing
- ½ bunch dill
- 1 tablespoon olive oil
- teaspoon salt

How to make it:

- In a medium sized bowl, mix the tofu cubes with the coriander, pepper, salt and oil, to coat all tofu pieces. Refrigerate a minimum of 4 hrs or (even better) overnight.
- Pre-heat oven to 180°C./350°F and line a baking sheet with baking paper.
- Spread out the marinated tofu pieces evenly and bake for 15-20 mins until the surfaces are dry and slightly crispy. Remove and set aside to cool.

- To make the salad dressing, blend together the dill, olive oil and salt in a blender or with a hand blender until smooth.
- Add lettuce leaves to all elements in a bowl, stir in dressing toss to coat. Serve in a bowl.
- **Note**: for a little more substantial meal, you can add a base of cooked buckwheat or amaranth.

Snacks

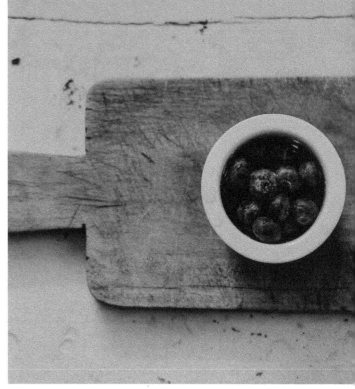

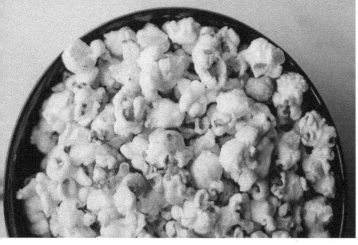

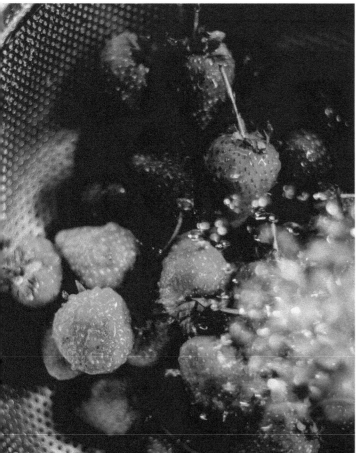

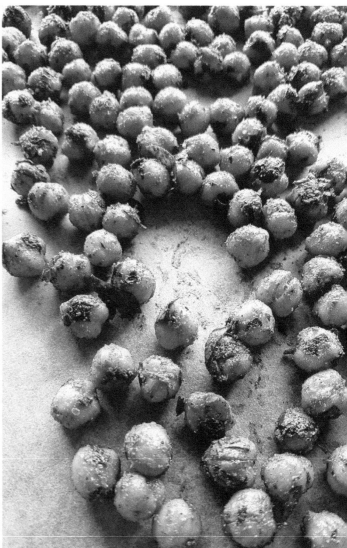

Crunchy Roasted Chickpeas
-P-K

A light dry and crunchy snack that's so easy to make with the perfect qualities for creating balance in spring. All beans are slightly astringent, and adding a bit of spice to these gives them a touch of warmth. These are a simple and healthier substitute for chips or processed snacks and a great way to sneak some balancing spring spices into your diet! *Makes 3 cups; Prep + Cooking time: 30 mins*

What's in it:

- 3½ cups cooked chickpeas from dried - or 2 15oz cans chickpeas
- 2 tablespoons olive oil
- 1/2 to 3/4 teaspoon salt
- 1 tablespoon finely chopped parsley
- 2 to 4 teaspoons spring spice mix churna [Pg 287]

How to make it:

- Preheat oven to 200C/400F, and line a baking sheet with baking paper.
- Spread the chickpeas out on a paper towel and pat dry.
- Add cooked chickpeas to a bowl with olive oil, spice mix and a small pinch of salt and pepper. Toss to coat.
- Spread the chickpeas evenly across the baking sheet and bake for 20 - minutes.
- Remove from oven and allow to cool before eating.
- Store in an airtight container for up to three days.

Savory Spiced Popcorn
+V -P -K

Popcorn is one of my favorite snacks. It's naturally warm, light and dry, so I've added a stimulating kick to it with spices like curry powder, paprika, and black pepper to turn the spring season balancing power up a notch. These warming spices will awaken your mind, body and spirit, and set you free! This snack is incredibly moreish, so remember moderation in all things! ***Serves 2; Prep + Cooking time: 15 mins.***

What's in it:

- 1/3 cup popcorn kernels
- 2 teaspoons ghee

Spice options:

Smoky spiced Popcorn

- 1 teaspoon smoked paprika
- ½ teaspoon pink salt
- ½ teaspoon ground black pepper

Curry Popcorn

- 1 teaspoons curry powder
- ½ teaspoons salt
- ¼ teaspoon fresh ground black pepper
- ½ teaspoon ground turmeric
- 1 pinch cayenne pepper

How to make it:

- Mix together your prefered spices in a small bowl and set aside. Prepare popcorn.

Stove Top Method:

- Put popcorn kernels and ghee in a heavy bottomed pot on medium heat. Cover tightly and listen for the sound of popping.
- Once the popping starts, shuffle the pot over the heat to keep the popcorn from sticking to the bottom. Once the popping stops, remove the popcorn immediately into a bowl and sprinkle spice mix through, tossing to coat.

Air Popper Method:

- Pop popcorn per popper instructions. Top with melted ghee (optional) and sprinkle spices through, tossing to coat. Enjoy!

Dessert

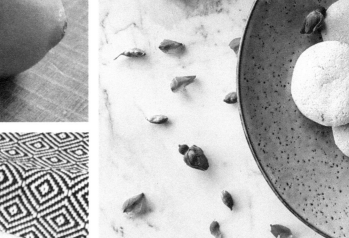

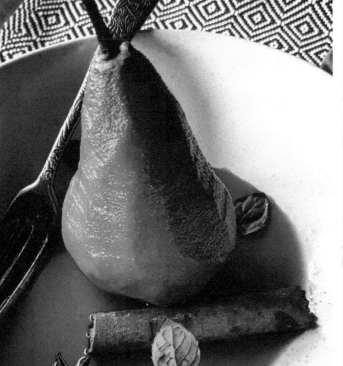

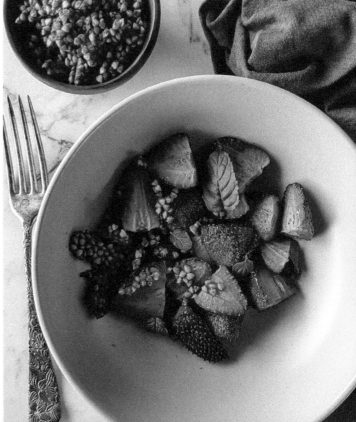

Cardamom Roasted Strawberries with Buckwheat Crunch

-P -K

The beauty of simplicity. I love the way spices and a little cooking can change your whole experience of something you've always known. This dish will transform the way you think about (and eat) strawberries. Roasting softens and intensifies the beautiful sweetness and unmistakable flavor of this favorite seasonal fruit. The buckwheat adds a bit of lightness, warmth and texture to the experience. Dessert couldn't be simpler, or more delicious. Try it, you'll see! **Serves 2; Prep + Cooking time: 30 mins.**

What's in it:

Strawberries:

- 500g (1 pound) fresh strawberries, washed and sliced
- 1 teaspoon vanilla
- ½ teaspoon cardamom
- ⅛ teaspoon finely ground black pepper
- 1 teaspoon lemon juice
- 1 teaspoon maple syrup
- 1 teaspoon water

Buckwheat crunch:

- ½ cup raw buckwheat groats
- 1 tablespoon "Magic Dust" Spice mix {Pg 284}
- 1 teaspoon coconut oil (melted)

How to make it:

Buckwheat Crunch

- Put the buckwheat groats in a bowl and cover with water. Cover the bowl and soak the groats overnight.

- When ready, drain and rinse the buckwheat and pat it dry with a paper towel.

- Preheat the oven to 140C/200F and line a baking sheet with baking paper.

- Spread the buckwheat out evenly over the tray and sprinkle with spices and coconut oil. Use your hands to mix and coat the buckwheat with oil and spices.

- Bake until the buckwheat is dry and crunchy (about 40 - 50 minutes). Allow it to cook and store in an airtight container to use as needed.

To make the strawberries:

- Preheat oven to 180C/350F and line a baking sheet with baking paper.

- Add cut strawberries to a bowl along with the spices, lemon juice, maple syrup and vanilla. Toss to coat. Spread the strawberries evenly over the baking sheet.

- Bake until the strawberries are soft and slightly juicy. Remove, allow to cool slightly and divide into bowls. Top with a teaspoon or two of the crunchy buckwheat and a drizzle of honey if you must!

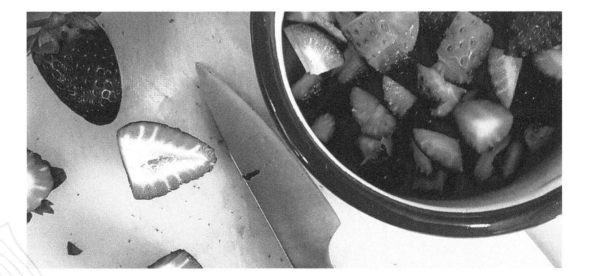

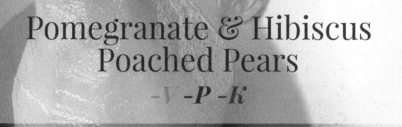

Pomegranate & Hibiscus Poached Pears
-V -P -K

Spring is the time when fresh fruit starts to become more of an option, but I still really love this recipe for cooking pears that is simple, but beautiful. Pears have a slightly astringent taste, which makes them nice for spring. I'm adding pomegranate and hibiscus to this recipe along with a few warming spices to make this a more balancing option for this time of year. These can be served warm or cooled down depending on the kind of spring you're having! *Serves 4; Prep + Cooking time: 90 mins.*

What's in it:

- 4 pears just ripe, peeled with stems attached
- Peel of ½ lemon, cut into thin strips (make sure to get the peel only, not the white pith)
- Juice of 1 lemon
- 2 cups pomegranate juice

- 1 cup water
- ¼ cup of dried hibiscus flowers
- 1 teaspoon vanilla extract
- 3 cinnamon sticks
- 2 whole star anise
- 2 small slices of fresh ginger

How to make it:

- Prepare the pears for poaching by cutting a thin slice off the bottom to make them more level.
- In a medium sized pot on medium heat, add all the ingredients (except the pears) and stir to combine. Add the pears (it's okay if they end up on their sides). Cover the pot and bring to a gentle boil.
- Reduce the heat and simmer uncovered for about an hour or until the pears are

tender and a rich red color. Baste the pears during cooking to ensure that the juice mix covers them.
- Carefully remove the pears and set them aside.
- Boil the syrup until reduced and thickened (about 5-10 minutes).
- Serve cooled pears on a plate with a drizzle of the pomegranate syrup.

Rosewater & Rice Flour Cookies

-V -P =K

These light and luscious cookies are inspired by a Persian recipe. They're gluten free, melt in your mouth and good for the mind (sattvic). Rose is balancing for all the doshas, but has a cooling energy. It's considered something of an aphrodisiac and is beneficial to the heart and nerves. It's also known to lift the spirits! *Makes a dozen cookies: Prep + Cooking time: 45 mins + overnight*

What's in it:

- 3 tablespoons ghee
- ⅔ cup unsweetened applesauce
- 2 eggs, lightly beaten
- 2 tablespoons rosewater

- 2 ¼ cups rice flour
- ¼ teaspoon baking powder
- ¾ teaspoon ground cardamom
- Pinch of salt

How to make it:

- In a medium sized bowl, mix together ghee and sugar until creamy (sugar has dissolved). Add the eggs and mix to combine before adding the rose water. Set aside.

- In a separate bowl whisk together flour, baking powder and cardamom. Add dry ingredients into the wet ingredients and stir to combine. This should form a firm dough. Refrigerate the dough overnight (or for a minimum of 4 hours).

For baking

- Line a cookie sheet with baking paper and set aside. Preheat the oven to 180°C/350F.

- Remove dough from the refrigerator and scoop out walnut sized spoonfuls. Roll into balls and place onto cookie sheet. Flatten with your hands. Space cookies about 1 inch apart.

- Bake cookies for 15 - 20 minutes or until firm and slightly cracked on top. Remove from the oven and allow to cool slightly before transferring them to a cooling rack.

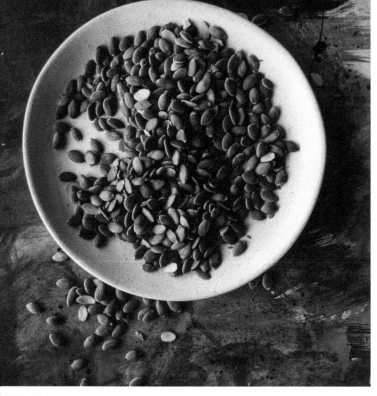

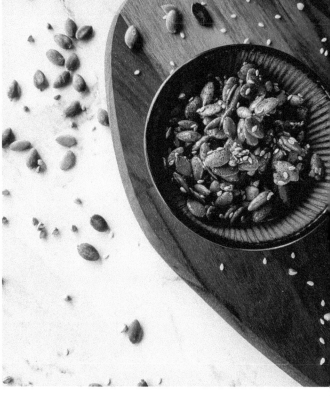

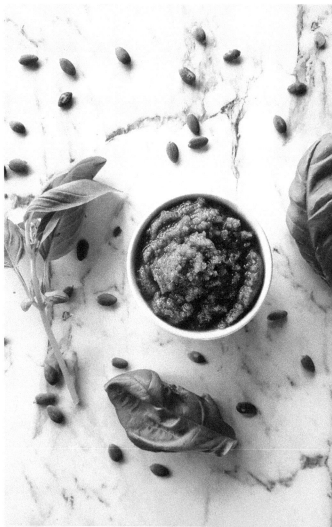

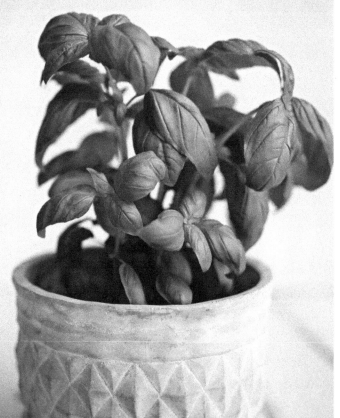

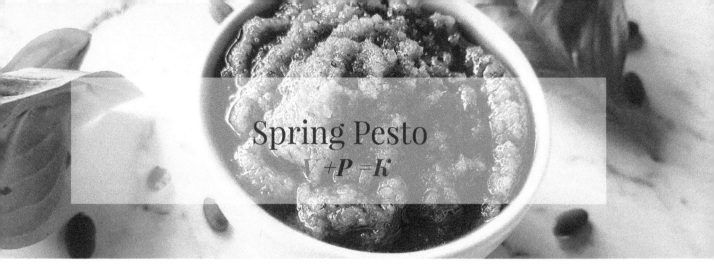

Spring Pesto

$V + P = K$

Basil is warming and great for spring time, so I've lightened up this sometimes heavy sauce with a few extra spices and a change of nuts and oil. Pumpkin seeds are drier and lighter than the traditional pine nuts, which also contributes to making this one more spring-worthy. Enjoy this one as a sauce for pasta dishes or topping for just about anything! *Makes about 1 ½ cups; Prep + Cooking time: 10 mins.*

What's in it:

- ½ cup pumpkin seeds (shelled, roasted)
- 2 cloves garlic
- ¾ cup basil leaves
- ¾ cup fresh parsley leaves
- 2 tablespoons fresh lemon juice
- 2 tablespoons olive oil
- ⅓ cup ghee
- Pinch of red pepper flakes (option

How to make it:

- In a frying pan on medium heat, lightly toast the pumpkins seeds, tossing for a few minutes. Remove before they go brown and allow them to cool

- Add the pumpkin seeds, parmesan, garlic, and red pepper flakes in a blender or food processor and pulse until the seeds are nearly ground.

- Add parsley, lemon juice, basil, olive oil and ghee, and blend until combined. If the sauce is too thick, add an additional tablespoon of olive oil.

- Serve immediately or refrigerate up to 2 days.

Kapha: Balancing (in moderation)

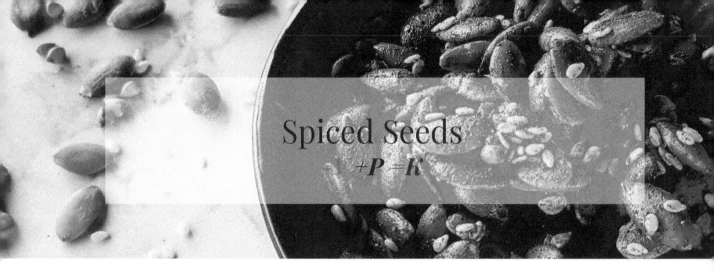

Spiced Seeds
+P =K

This is a simple way to add a little texture and warming energy to spring dishes. This simple combination of seeds and spices is a great addition to springtime porridges, stewed fruits and even yogurt. Seeds are warming and can be a little challenging to digest, so I've roasted them to make them slightly lighter, and spiced them up with some digestive spices to help move them through the system. The only challenge now is to consume them in moderation! *Makes about 1½ cups; Prep + Cooking time: 15 mins.*

What's in it:

- 1 ¼ cups raw, shelled pumpkin seeds
- 1 tablespoon sesame seeds
- 1 tablespoon buckwheat groats
- 1tablespoon pure maple syrup
- 1 teaspoon ground cinnamon
- ⅛ teaspoon salt
- pinch of cayenne [optional]

How to make it:

- Line a large baking sheet with baking paper and preheat oven to 180°C/350°F.
- Add all ingredients to a medium sized bowl and toss together to coat and combine.
- Spread the seeds in an even layer on the baking sheet. Roast in oven for 10 minutes, tossing once halfway through.
- Let cool completely and store in an airtight container.

Drinks

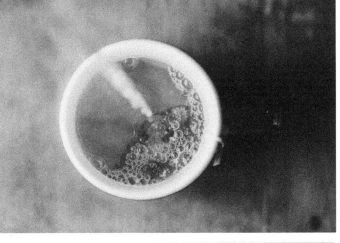

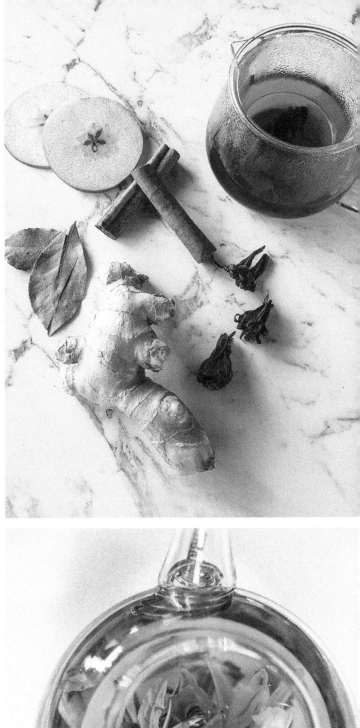

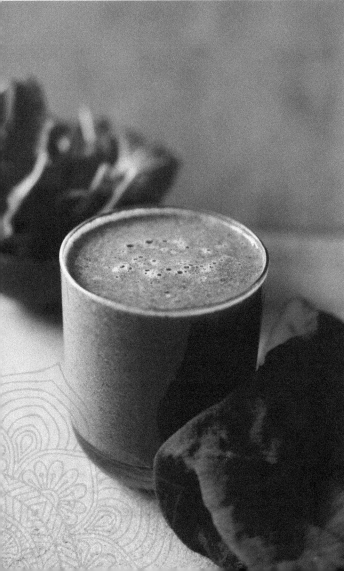

Springtime Tea
-V -P -K

Springtime teas are warming, stimulating and clarifying and although spring can be one of the best times of the year for teas with a bit of caffeine (like black and green teas), I wanted to introduce you some caffeine free options that give you a sense for the balancing power of herbs and spices. Here are a few of my springtime favorites that are both tantalizing and easy to make. *Serves 2; Prep + Cooking time: 10 mins.*

What's in it:

Hibiscus-Bay Tea
- 1 tablespoon dried hibiscus flowers
- 1 medium sized cinnamon stick
- 1 bay leaf

Ginger Apple Tea
- 1 tablespoon coarsely
- grated/chopped ginger
- 2 tablespoons coarsely chopped apple (your choice of apple)
- 1 small cinnamon stick

How to make it:

- Add the ingredients to the strainer of a teapot and cover with 3 cups of boiling water OR
- Bring 3 cups of water to a boil in a saucepan and add the tea ingredients.

- Steep tea for 5 minutes. Strain into two cups and enjoy.

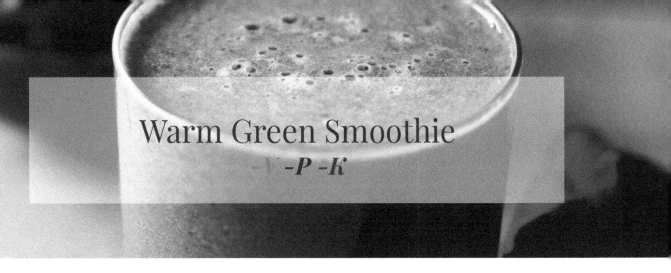

Warm Green Smoothie
-V -P -K

This is not your typical smoothie! The cold, heavy, and often rough qualities of smoothies mean that in the Ayurvedic world they are often seen as less than healthy as they can be challenging to the digestion and promote heaviness and congestion. This smoothie turns the typical smoothie on its head. We use fruit and leafy greens with astringent qualities to dry up congestion, and warming spices to counteract the wet heaviness of spring. And then we warm it! The experience of this yummy warm concoction may just change your smoothie game for good. *Serves 2; Prep + Cooking time: 20 mins.*

What's in it:

- 1 medium gala, honeycrisp or pink lady, apple, quartered, stem and seeds removed
- 1 small Bosc or Taylor Gold pear, quartered, stem and seeds removed

- ¼ teaspoon cinnamon (or to taste)
- ½ teaspoon grated fresh ginger
- ⅛ teaspoon nutmeg
- 3 large handfuls baby spinach

How to make it:

- Place apple, pear, and spices in a medium sized saucepan. Add 3 tablespoons of water, cover, and cook until fruit is fork tender.
- Pour the contents into a blender.
- Add spinach, blend on low for 20 seconds, then high for another 20 seconds or until completely blended.

- This smoothie can be enjoyed on its own or used as a base for a warm smoothie bowl.

Summer

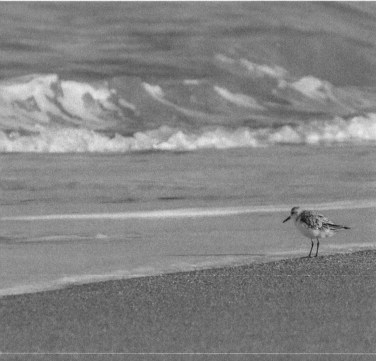

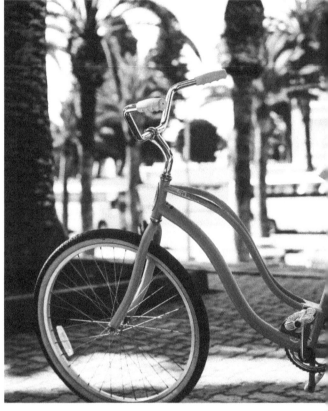

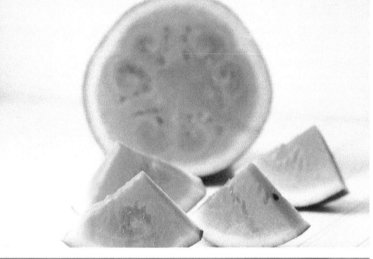

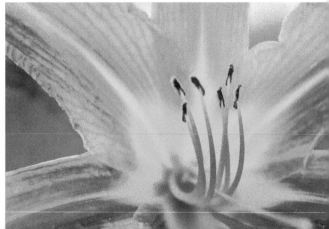

Summer is one of the busiest times of the year and life can get pretty intense. If we're not careful, we can start to feel the heat inside and out. One of the keys to staying balanced during this time of year is tuning in to your own tendency to push yourself or overdo it. Pause and take a closer look at how the intensity on the outside is impacting your internal weather, and then ask yourself what you can do to create calm.

Qualities of summer:
Hot, sharp, intense, light, mobile, oily

Summer Mantra for Wellness:
Cooling, *Calming, Moderation, Flow*

What to watch out for:
Inflammation, skin issues, anger, aggravation, impatience, diarrhea, reflux, digestive upsets

Summer Self-Care Focus

- **Sleep** - Summer can be a time when we're tempted to stay up late into the night. Getting the right amount of sleep is critical during this time of year to offset the challenging effects of the environment. Get to sleep no later than 11pm and get up early!

- **Hydrate** - Hydration in summer is important for keeping the body cool and replacing the water and electrolytes that are depleted as we engage in outdoor life and pursuits.

- **Cool** - hang out in cool spots like the pool, the beach, or the movies. Use the cooling power of the breath (sheetali pranayama, and chandra bhedana, "left nostril breathing") as your own internal A/C, weave steadiness and release into your yoga practice with forward bends, gentle twists, and easeful standing poses.

- **Reflect** - Balance the mental and physical intensity of the season by resolving to find as many ways as possible to keep your cool, which can actually be as simple as just thinking… I'm cool!

A few things to add to your summer routine:

- **Don't forget to meditate...** Summer can be a busy time when you feel so good that you forget to do some of the things you need to do to feel so good. Meditation is an important mental housekeeping exercise all year long, but it can be especially helpful to keep your summer mind calm, cool, and collected. So don't let it slip this time of year!

- **Agua frescas...** All day long. Cooling doesn't have to mean icy, which can mess with your digestion. Going with drinks that have cooling qualities is the best way to save your digestion while boosting your hydration!

- **Coconut oil on feet and scalp...** before bed to calm and ground, counteract insomnia, and to prevent hair fall.

- **Selfless Service...** Give selflessly in the summer through volunteer work or projects to infuse a cooling humility, grounding, and gratitude into your thinking and being. It's also a great way to connect, which is good for overall wellness.

- **Skin care...** Practice sun safety by wearing a hat and sunglasses when outdoors. Use all natural skin protection products. Maintain awareness of the impacts of the sun and keep the skin cool, clean and hydrated.

Eating in Summer

Breakfasts are light, sweet, and juicy. Fruit salads are a great summer breakfast, but if you're in need of something more substantial you can stick with porridge (chia porridge or puddings with fruit are good for this time of year. I love cooked fruit cooled to room temp), and lightly steamed cooling summer fruits. This is one of the best times of the year for smoothies, but be mindful of portion sizes AND the state of your digestion before you dive in (would a juice be better?). Also be careful of raw foods if your digestion can be sluggish or variable and include a few warming spices like ginger and fennel to keep the fire burning.

Lunch Grain salads and veggie soups are typically my go-to lunch for summer. Open-faced sandwiches are a gorgeous and easy lunch option too! Chock full of fresh veggies and salad. I like using hummus in summer instead of mayo, paired with a sweet mango chutney. Grain and veggie bowls are a great way to mix greens, grains, and veggies and even a little stewed fruit if you want to get creative. If we're having meat, we'll have it at lunchtime. Freshwater fish on the grill and in salads is a summer staple. Soup is an easy workday lunch with bread and a lovely summer spread (hummus, beetroot spread).

Dinner We often skip dinner in the summer if we're feeling more than satisfied from lunch and are hankering to hold on to the light, clear feeling in the mind and body. Light broths with noodles and veggies, simple veggie salads, fresh spring rolls, or even a few bites of chia pudding with fruit are great options for a light, clean summer dinner. Stay tuned into your body (i.e. digestion) during this time of the year. And definitely follow any instincts to go light (or even skip a meal.

Summer tastes/qualities to favor:
sweet, cool, and moistening

Summer spices to favor:
coriander, cardamom, asafoetida, fennel,
mint, turmeric (late summer)

Summer Superfoods by Type:

These are the best foods for the season based on your constitution or imbalance.

Vata *(includes vata-pitta, vata-kapha):*	Pitta *(includes pitta-vata, pitta-kapha):*	Kapha *(includes kapha-vata, kapha-pitta)*
Beets	Asparagus	Dried fruit
Sweet potatoes	Apples	Bell peppers
Papaya	Blueberries	Corn
Avocados	Pineapple	Swiss chard
Mangoes	Coconut Oil	Bean sprouts
Figs	Dandelion tea (greens)	Dandelion tea
Freshwater fish	Tofu	Hibiscus tea

*Get additional **summer** info &*
resources via this link!
http://www.eatlikeyouloveyourself.com/Summer

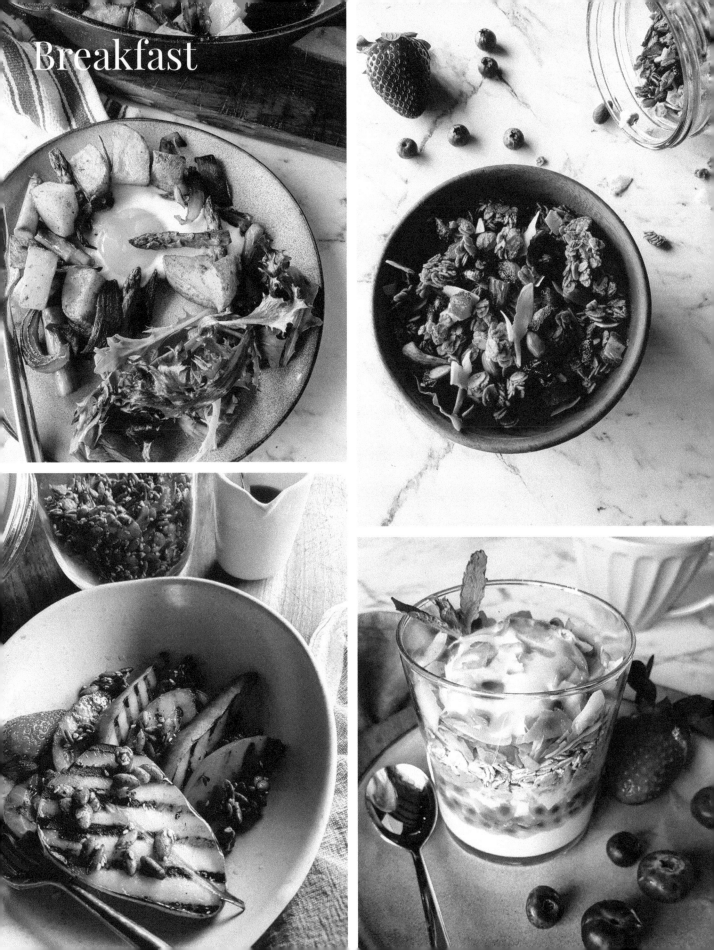

Breakfast

Coconut Ginger & Passionfruit Bircher Muesli

-V -P +K

When it's too hot for porridge, this is the way to go, something I discovered a few years ago that had me wondering where it had been all my life. This tasty overnight oats recipe is great for folks who often run out of time to make breakfast in the morning (and end up starving or eating a ton of junk by lunch time). It's made with all the same stuff that you'd put into traditional hot oats, but the flavors are given hours to "connect". The result is something you've got to try! **Serves 4; Prep + Cooking time: 4-8 hrs (overnight)**

What's in it:

- 4 whole passionfruit, pulp removed
- ½ small pear, grated, skin on
- ½ small apple, grated, skin on
- ½ cup (50g) shredded coconut
- 1 ¾ cup (150g) rolled oats

- 1 cup milk (any kind is fine)
- pinch of cinnamon
- ⅔ cup (150g) yogurt - try the coconut yogurt
- 2 tablespoons uncrystalized ginger chopped

How to make it:

- Combine the oats, milk, yogurt, coconut, passionfruit, ginger, and cinnamon in a bowl and refrigerate overnight.

- In the morning, mix in apple and pear and top with spiced seeds [Pg 230] if you like or a little toasted coconut!

*Vata: Balancing (at room temperature)

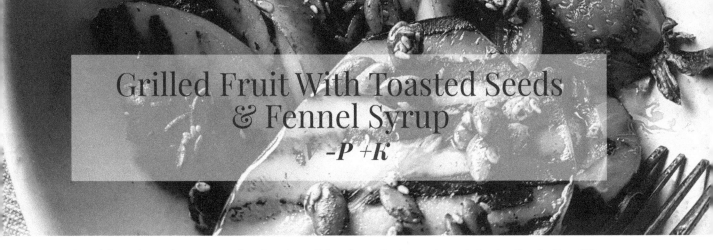

Grilled Fruit With Toasted Seeds & Fennel Syrup

-P +K

Breakfast doesn't get any simpler than this. A perfect way to celebrate the fruits of the season and a clean, luscious breakfast (or snack or dessert) that satisfies with its gentle warmth and beautiful combination of flavors and textures. This is a decadent way to start the day! *Serves 2; Prep + Cooking time: 20 mins.*

What's in it:

- 2 ripe nectarines, halved with pit removed
- 2 ripe plums, halved with pit removed
- 2 medium sized pears, halved and cored

- 1 tablespoon ghee
- Spiced seeds to serve [Pg 230]
- Coconut yogurt to serve [Pg 282]
- Fennel syrup to serve [Pg 281]

How to make it:

- Heat the barbecue grill or a grill pan to medium high heat.
- Brush the surface of the fruit with ghee and place face down on the hot pan or grill. Allow to grill for a few minutes and then cover with a heat proof bowl for a few minutes more

- Remove the bowl and the fruit. Allow the fruit to cool slightly, then top with a dollop of yogurt and a spoonful of seeds. Drizzle with fennel syrup.

Toasted Granola
V -P -K

Granola is a powerful "go to" for snacks, breakfast, and even the occasional dinner. The issue is that the store-bought brands often overdo it with the sugar. This a a simple recipe that takes no time and makes a wonderfully crunchy granola that's low in sugar and free of preservatives. This can be used as a topping (for porridge or puddings), or eaten on its own with warm or cool milk. One of my favorite ways to enjoy it is with golden milk!
Makes 3½ cups; Prep + Cooking time: 40 mins.

What's in it:

- 2 cups rolled oats
- ¼ cup warm water
- 3 tablespoons maple syrup
- 2 tablespoons coconut oil
- 2 tablespoons chia seeds
- ⅓ cup buckwheat groats
- 1 tablespoon vanilla extract

- 1 teaspoon cinnamon
- 1 teaspoon cardamom
- ¼ teaspoon nutmeg
- ½ cup pumpkin seeds/sunflower seeds
- ¼ cup dried fruit (cranberries, apricots chopped, raisins, dates chopped, etc.)
- ¼ cup flaked coconut

How to make it:

- Preheat an oven to 180°C/375°F. Line a large baking sheet with baking paper. Set aside.

- In a small bowl, mix together the water, oil, maple syrup, and vanilla.

- In a separate bowl combine the oats, buckwheat, chia seeds, and spices.

- Add liquids to the dry ingredients and stir to combine and fully coat.

- Spread the mixture evenly on a baking sheet and bake for 20 minutes, stirring every 8-10 minutes. Add the seeds and dried fruit and bake an additional five minutes.

- Finally, add the coconut and bake until the coconut is just brown around the edges.

- Remove from the oven and allow to cool. Store in an airtight container.

*Vata: Balancing (with warm milk)
*Kapha: Balancing (in moderation)

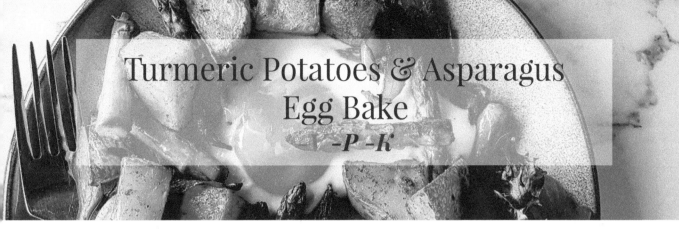

Turmeric Potatoes & Asparagus Egg Bake
-P -K

Deeply satisfying combination of potatoes and greens makes a perfect warm breakfast on a hot summer day. The flavors are simple and fresh, and a perfect balance between grounding and lightness! It's one of those roll out of bed breakfasts that's easy to make and even easier to enjoy! *Serves 2-3; Prep + Cooking time: 35 mins.*

What's in it:

- 1 pound potatoes (any type will do),
- cut into 1-inch chunks
- 1 medium onion, sliced into medium size wedges
- 2 cups asparagus, trimmed and cut into 1 ½ pieces
- 2 cloves garlic, minced
- 1 tablespoon oil or ghee

- 3 tablespoons heavy cream
- 1 tablespoon ground turmeric
- ½ teaspoon ground cumin
- 1 teaspoon freshly ground black pepper
- 2 tablespoons fresh coriander leaves, coarsely chopped.
- ½ teaspoon salt
- 4 large eggs

How to make it:

- Preheat oven to 220°C/400°F. Line a baking sheet with parchment paper.
- Put potatoes, onions, and garlic in a large bowl with turmeric, cumin, salt, and pepper. Toss to coat.
- Spread potatoes and onions on lined baking sheet and bake for 15 minutes until the potatoes are slightly tender.
- Remove the vegetables from the oven and add everything to a large ovenproof skillet on the stove at medium - high heat.
- Cook until the potatoes begin to form a

lightly crispy crust, stirring often (about 6-10 minutes). Add asparagus and toss for a couple minute.

- Remove from heat and make a space amongst the veggies for the eggs. Crack one egg into each of the spaces.
- Sprinkle half of the fresh coriander on top and return the skillet to the oven. Continue cooking for 7-10 minutes or until the eggs are cooked to your desired texture.
- Remove pan from the oven and allow to cool slightly. Top the eggs with the remaining coriander leaves and serve.

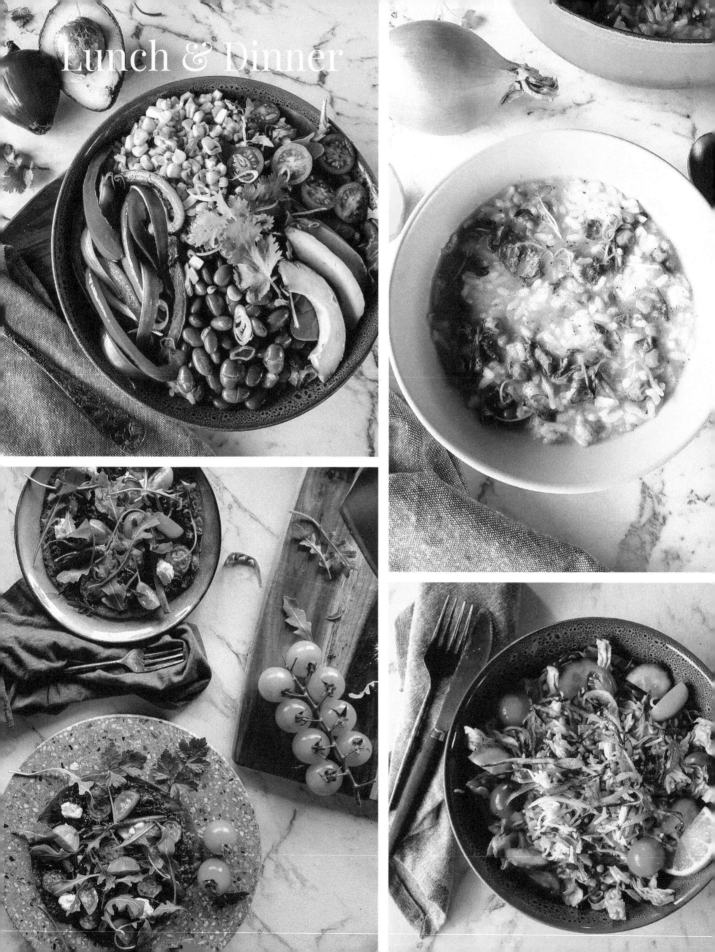

Creamy Beet Soup
-P +K

Beets are one of the most beautiful vegetables, in part because of their deep red color, which highlights the fact that they are great for cleansing the blood. They're high in vitamins A and C and nutrients like magnesium and potassium. They are slightly warm, but the sweetness that comes out from cooking them makes them a beautiful balancing food for summer pitta. Adding cooling coconut to this soup ups the flavor factor and further balances out the heating qualities of the beets. *Serves 4-6; Prep + Cooking time: 45 mins.*

What's in it:

- 4 cups fresh beets, peeled and diced
- 1 onion, chopped
- 1 tablespoon olive oil
- 6 cups water OR vegetable stock
- 2 cups full fat coconut milk
- 1 tablespoon lime juice (~1 lime) + more to squeeze over top as you like
- 2 cloves garlic, minced

- 2 inch-sized pieces of ginger, peeled and coarsely chopped
- 1 tablespoon ground coriander seed
- 2 teaspoons ground cumin seed
- 1 teaspoon freshly ground black pepper
- 1 teaspoon salt
- handful chopped cilantro, to garnish
- coconut yogurt, to garnish

How to make it:

- Line a baking sheet with baking paper. Preheat the oven to 180°C/350°F.
- Toss the beets in a bowl with a tablespoon of oil and a pinch of salt and pepper. Spread them out on the baking sheet. Roast for 25-30 minutes.
- In a soup pot, set on medium high heat, saute the onions in 1 tablespoon of oil until they become translucent and lightly browned. Add the beets, stock (or water), garlic, ginger, and spices,

and bring to a low boil.

- Reduce the heat and add the coconut milk and lime juice. Stir to incorporate and then take off the heat. Use a hand blender (or regular blender) to blend until smooth and creamy. Add salt and pepper to taste.
- Divide the soup into bowls and top with chopped coriander leaves and a swirl of coconut yogurt.

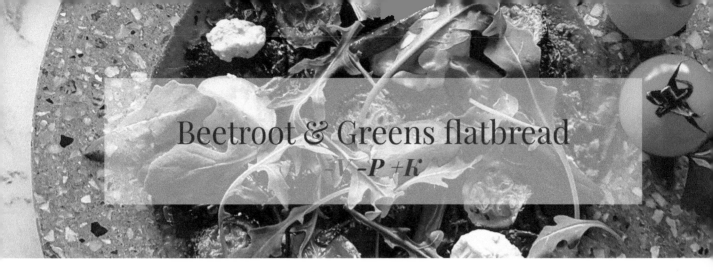

Beetroot & Greens flatbread
-V -P +K

This summer flatbread is a color and taste extravaganza! I've added beets to the flatbread to take advantage of their sweetness and their health giving (and pitta balancing) goodness. We're topping this pizza with a bit of lightness in the way of leafy greens and a delicate mint and lemon ricotta! This dish will be a treat for the eyes (also good for pitta) as well as for the belly. *Serves 4; Prep + Cooking time: 60 mins.*

What's in it:

Flatbread base:

- Start with Simple Flatbread Recipe { Pg 289]. Substitute: beet juice for water.
- Use the dough to make 4 medium sized rounded flat breads.

Toppings:

- ¾ cup ricotta cheese
- 2 teaspoons fresh mint, finely chopped
- ½ teaspoon lemon zest
- 1 teaspoon salt
- Pinch of black pepper
- 2 tablespoons Spring Pesto Pg 229]
- 1 cup of baby spinach leaves
- 2 cups kale leaves, washed, trimmed, and sliced into strips
- ½ cup roasted zucchini slices
- 2-3 sweet grape tomatoes, sliced [optional]
- 1 cup rocket leaves
- 2 teaspoons ghee

How to make it:

For the base:
- Make flatbreads as directed and set aside.

For the toppings:
- In a small bowl, combine ricotta, mint, lemon zest, and a pinch of pepper. Stir to combine and refrigerate until needed.

- Add a teaspoon of ghee to a skillet and throw in the kale leaves. Saute the kale with a pinch of salt and pepper until soft. Set aside to cool.

To assemble the flatbread:
- Working one at a time, top the flatbread with a thin layer of pesto, and top with generous amounts of the kale and spinach leaves, and a few small dollops of the ricotta.

- Bake until the toppings are sizzling and the ricotta is lightly browned on top. Remove from the oven, allow it to cool for a minute and scatter rocket leaves over the top to serve!

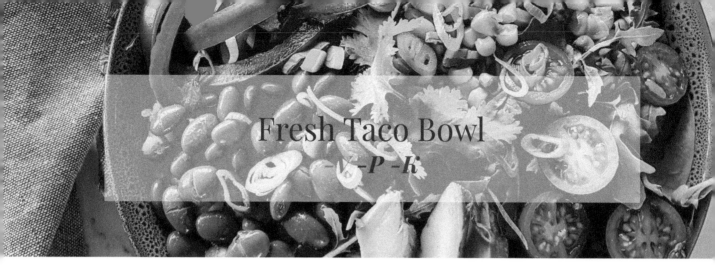

Fresh Taco Bowl
- V - P - K

Growing up in Southern California meant that we ate a lot of beautiful Mexican food. This fresh and simple bowl is something of a throwback to my youth reflecting the fresh and vibrant flavors of the SoCal summer! There's a balancing mix of sweet, warm and astringent, slightly heavy and a little dry. A delicious and powerful combination to keep the summer aggravation at bay, not least because it feels like a Mexican holiday on a plate! ***Serves 4; Prep + Cooking time: 40 mins + beans cooking time***

What's in it:

- 3 cups cooked rice, medium grain,
- 1 cup whole pinto beans soaked overnight
- 1 medium-sized red bell pepper, seeded and sliced into thin strips
- 1 medium-sized yellow bell pepper, seeded and sliced into thin strips
- 2 medium red onions, sliced into thin strips
- 2 cups romaine lettuce, shredded
- 1 cup sweet grape tomatoes diced

- 1 teaspoon asafoetida
- 2 cups fresh corn kernels (or approximately 3 fresh ears of corn)
- 1 green onion (scallion) thinly sliced
- Flesh of one avocado diced
- 3 tablespoons ghee
- 2 tablespoons ground cumin
- 1 teaspoon ground coriander
- 1 medium-sized lime, cut into wedges
- ½ teaspoon garlic powder
- ¼ teaspoon dried oregano

How to make it:

- Add the pinto beans, four cups of water, cumin, and asafoetida to a pressure cooker, cook on high pressure for 15 minutes. Remove beans from the pot and set aside. Alternatively, you can cook the beans on the stove using the same amount of water at a simmer for 1 ½ to 2 ½ hours.

- Melt one tablespoon of butter in a large skillet over medium heat. Add the corn kernels and a pinch of salt.

- Stir slowly, moving the corn around the pan to avoid it sticking (about 10 minutes). The corn will darken on the edges, which is perfect.

- Once this starts to happen throw in half of the sliced green onions and continue stirring until the onions have softened.

- Remove the roasted corn from the pan to a bowl and cover to retain the heat and moisture.

- Add the ghee to the skillet and throw in the peppers and onions. Saute until soft. Add the spice mix and stir to coat. Cover the vegetables and set aside.

- Divide the rice among four bowls. Top each portion with a scoops of beans, a good helping of peppers, and a few spoons of roasted corn.

- Sprinkle shredded lettuce, chopped tomatoes and diced avocado on top. Finish with a squeeze of lime and enjoy!

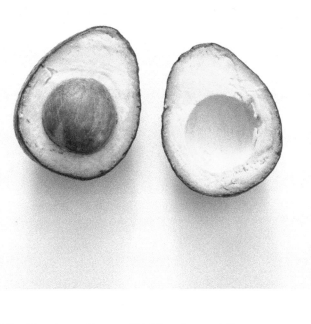

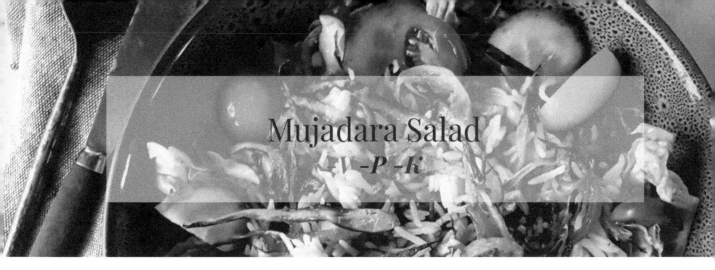

Mujadara Salad
V –P –K

Cooked lentils with caramelized onions mixed with rice and greens. This beautifully rich and flavorful Lebanese dish is packed full of the tastes that bring balance to the summer heat. The sweetness of the rice and onions, brought together with the astringency and slight bitterness of the lentils and greens, makes a winning combination to cool the heat of pitta inside and out. ***Serves 4***

What's in it:

- 1 cup cooked brown or green lentils (not Puy lentils),
- 2 tablespoons olive oil
- 1 teaspoon cumin seeds
- ½ teaspoon cracked black pepper
- 3 medium red onions, thinly sliced
- ¾ cup basmati rice
- ½ teaspoon ground cumin
- ¼ teaspoon smoked paprika
- 1 (1-inch) cinnamon stick

- 4 cups romaine lettuce, shredded
- 2 cups sweet cherry or grape tomatoes, diced
- Salt to taste

For dressing:
- 3 tablespoons lime juice
- 1 teaspoon fresh mint, chopped
- Pinch of salt and pepper

How to make it:

- Add olive oil to a skillet over medium-high heat. Add the cumin seeds and black pepper and cook until the seeds start to darken.

- Lower the heat to medium, throw in the onions with a pinch of salt and cook for about 10-15 minutes until they begin to caramelize and turn slightly crispy, stirring often.

- Remove about half the onions from the pan and set aside on a paper towel lined plate.

- Add the rice, ground cumin, paprika, and cinnamon stick to the pan and saute them for a minute or two.

- Add the lentils, two cups of water, and 1 teaspoon of salt to the pan and stir to combine. Bring the mixture to a boil and then reduce to simmer. Cover and cook for 30 minutes or until the water is evaporated and the rice is tender.

- Turn off the heat and allow the rice to steam for another few minutes. Allow to cool to room temperature.

- While that's happening, make the dressing by mixing all the ingredients in a jar or bowl and whisking (or shaking) until well combined.

- To assemble the salads, place a serving (approx 1 cup) of the rice and lentils mixture in a shallow serving bowl. Top with the shredded lettuce, tomatoes, and some of the leftover onions. Drizzle with salad dressing.

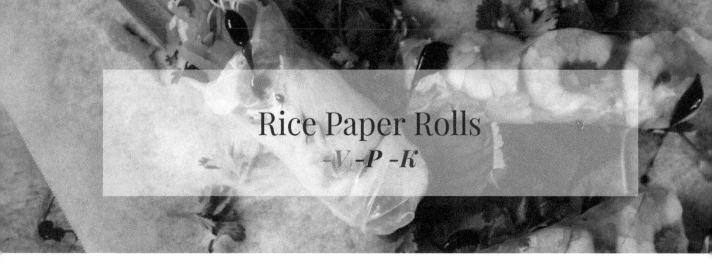

Rice Paper Rolls
-V -P -K

These are a favorite in our home, in large part due to the fact that they are nearly 100% customizable. With a variety of different fillings and dipping sauces to choose from, rice paper rolls make a lovely light lunch or dinner to delight the entire family! ***Serves 4: Prep + Cooking time 60 mins.***

What's in it:

- ½ pound cooked shrimp, peeled and deveined (optional)
- 4 ounces rice vermicelli
- 1 package (12 ounces) 8 1/2-inch rice paper wrappers
- 5 ounces (150g) firm tofu, cut into ¼ inch slices
- 1 cup carrots, cut into matchsticks
- 1 cup cucumber, cut into matchsticks

- 1 cup fresh bean sprouts
- ½ cup fresh mint
- ½ cup fresh Thai basil
- ½ cup fresh coriander leaves (cilantro)
- 1 green onion (scallion), thinly sliced
- 2 tablespoons soy sauce
- 2 teaspoons toasted sesame oil
- hoisin sauce for dipping
- salt and pepper to taste

How to make it:

- Add the sesame oil to a skillet on medium high heat. Fry the tofu pieces until lightly browned on both sides (about 4-5 mins/side). Add the soy sauce and flip each piece to coat. Remove the tofu from the pan and allow to cool. Once cooled, cut the tofu into matchstick-sized pieces.

- Slice the prawns in half lengthwise and set aside.

- Place the rice noodles in a large bowl. Cover with boiling water and allow to sit until the noodles are tender (2-4 minutes). Drain and rinse the noodles

*Vata: Balancing in moderation

in cold water and set aside.

- Assemble all ingredients nearby along with a bowl of warm water. Immerse a rice paper wrapper in the warm water and place on a plate or cutting board. Starting with the rice noodles place a small portion of your selection of ingredients in a pile at the center of the wrapper.

- Fold the top and bottom edges of the wrapper into the center. Fold one of the side edges into the center and roll the roll toward the other edge to seal.

- Serve with hoisin or plum sauce.

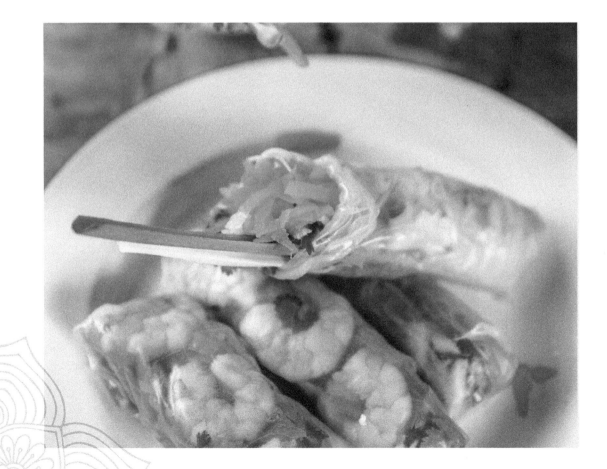

Summer Squash Couscous Salad
-P =K

This is a gorgeous, simple salad that features seasonal veggies that are cooked, but served at room temperature. The warmth of the citrus is offset by the cooling vegetables and couscous. This salad is substantial enough to serve as a light dinner option or a lunchtime side dish. You can make it slightly more substantial (as a lunchtime meal) with the addition of leafy greens tossed into the mix). *Serves 4; Prep + Cooking time: 20 mins.*

What's in it:

- 2 teaspoons lemon zest
- juice of one lime
- ½ teaspoon honey
- olive oil
- 3 garlic cloves, smashed
- (just to open and break the skin)
- 1 ¼ cups vegetable stock
- 1 cup couscous
- ½ cup diced yellow squash

- ½ cup diced zucchini
- 1 medium shallot, finely chopped
- ½ cup golden raisins/dried cranberries
- ¼ cup chopped pistachios
- salt to taste
- 2 tablespoons chopped fresh mint
- freshly ground black pepper

How to make it:

- In a small bowl, whisk the lemon zest, lime juice, honey, and three tablespoons of olive oil. Add the garlic and set aside.

- In a medium saucepan, bring the veggie stock to a boil. Stir the couscous through, cover and remove from heat. Let it stand for 5 mins (or until all the water is absorbed) before removing the cover. Remove the cover and fluff the couscous with a fork to separate the grains. Set aside.

- Add 1 tablespoon of olive oil and the shallots to a fry pan over medium heat. Cook until just soft and then add the zucchini, squash, raisins and pistachios along with a pinch of salt and pepper.

- Cook, stirring or tossing often until the vegetables are slightly tender. Set aside and allow to cool to room temperature.

- Once the veggies are cooled, combine them with the couscous in a medium sized bowl. Remove the smashed garlic cloves from the dressing and add as much dressing as you need to coat the couscous. Toss to combine and coat. Add the mint and lightly toss to distribute it through.

- Salt and pepper to taste. Serve at room temperature.

Fresh Pea & Watercress Rice Soup
-P -K

When you need something fresh, soothing, slightly sweet, and slightly bitter, this is the recipe for you. A simple, creamy rice soup (a thinner version of risotto) that combines the sweetness of peas with a light peppery flavor of watercress, a seasonal green that stimulates the digestion and awakens the senses. ***Serves 4; Prep + Cooking time: 25 mins.***

What's in it:

- 2 ½ cups peas (fresh or frozen)
- 1 tablespoon butter
- 2tablespoons ghee
- 2 tablespoons onion, chopped
- 2 cups watercress, coarsely chopped

- 3 cups chicken or vegetable stock
- 1 cup Arborio rice
- ½ teaspoon finely ground pepper
- 1 tablespoon of freshly grated Parmesan cheese for garnish (optional)

How to make it:

- Add the ghee, butter, and onion to a soup pot or Dutch oven over medium heat. Saute until the onion becomes translucent and lightly golden.
- Add the rice and saute for 1-2 minutes, then add the stock and peas and a pinch of salt. Cover the pot and cook

on low boil for about 15 minutes, stirring occasionally until the rice is tender. Add the watercress and allow to cook for a few minutes longer.

- Add a little more stock if the soup is too thick. Finally, stir the Parmesan and black pepper through and serve.

Snacks

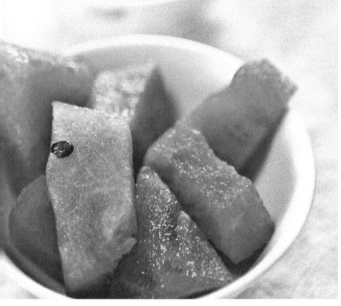

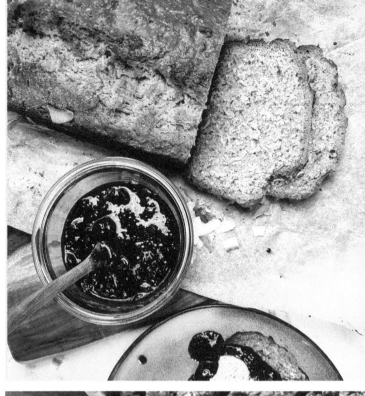

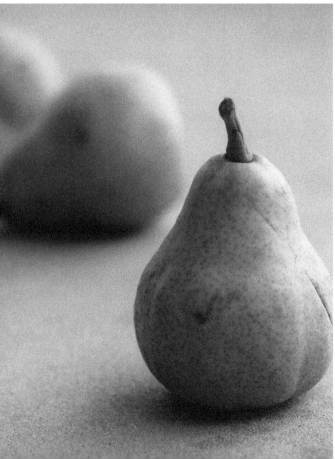

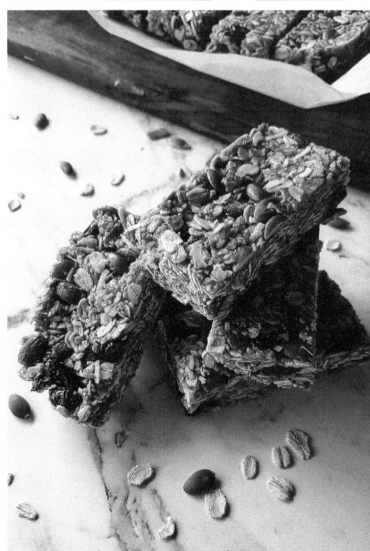

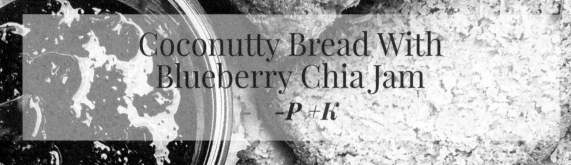

Coconutty Bread With Blueberry Chia Jam
-P +K

This super simple dish brings together two of my favorite flavors of summer. Quick breads are a great solution to avoiding processed junk. This recipe comes together in a flash and pairs moist, decadent coconut with bright and calming blueberries. It's a nourishing combination that rejuvenates the mind and body! A summer holiday in every bite!
Makes 1 loaf; Prep + Cooking time: 90 mins.

What's in it:

- 2 eggs
- 1 ¼ cups milk
- 1 teaspoon vanilla extract
- 2 ½ cups flour
- 2 teaspoons baking powder

- zest of 1 lime
- ¾ teaspoon kosher salt
- 1 cup sugar
- 2 cups unsweetened, shredded coconut
- 6 tablespoons unsalted butter, melted

How to make it:

- Preheat the oven to 180°C/350°F and line an 8 ½ X 4 inch loaf pan with baking paper.

- In a medium-sized pan on low heat, toast ½ cup of coconut until lightly browned. Make sure to watch it while cooking because things can go awry pretty quick! Once it's done, set it aside.

- Whisk eggs, milk, vanilla, and melted butter together in a small bowl.

- In a larger bowl combine the flour, baking powder, lime zest, and salt. Whisk to mix, then add coconut and sugar and whisk to combine.

- Make a well in the center of the dry ingredients and add the wet ingredients. Fold the two together to combine (be careful not to overmix). Gently stir through the toasted coconut.

- Pour batter into the loaf pan and bake for 60 - 70 minutes or until a toothpick inserted into the center comes out clean.

- Remove the bread from the oven when done and allow to cool for 5-10 minutes before removing from the pan.

- Finish cooling on a cooling rack.

- To serve, cut into slices and top with a teaspoon of blueberry chia jam Pg 274

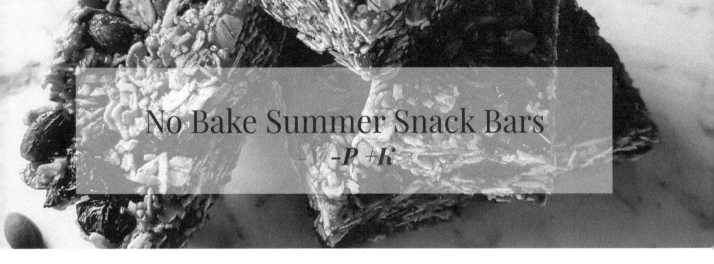

No Bake Summer Snack Bars
–P +K

These snack bars are a simple keep-on-hand snack to prevent the summer "hangries." They take a few minutes to throw together and are pretty forgiving (it's pretty hard to mess them up). Chock full of cooling summer sweetness in the way of fruits and grains, they're perfect for keeping you focused, happy, and calm, even on the hottest days!
Makes about a dozen bars: Prep + Cooking time: 90 mins.

What's in it:

- 2 ½ cups rolled oats
- 1 cup raw pumpkin seeds (pepitas)
- ½ cup golden raisins
- ⅔ cup sunflower seed butter Pg 288
- ½ cup shredded coconut (optional)
- ½ to ⅔ cups date syrup or brown rice syrup (adjust based on how well things stick together)
- ⅛ teaspoon sea salt
- ½ teaspoon cardamom

How to make it:

- Line a 9 X 9 inch baking pan with baking paper.
- Combine the oats, pumpkin seeds, and golden raisins together in a large mixing bowl.
- In a smaller bowl or jug, add the sunflower butter, syrup, salt, and cardamom and mix well to combine them. Pour this mixture over the oats mixture and fold together to coat everything (if it's too dry and the oats aren't sticking together, you can add a little more syrup).
- Pour the mixture into the lined baking pan and spread and press well. Refrigerate for 1-2 hours or until very firm.
- Remove the bars from the pan by lifting the baking paper. Using a sharp knife, cut into desired sized bars. Store in an airtight container in the refrigerator.

Dessert

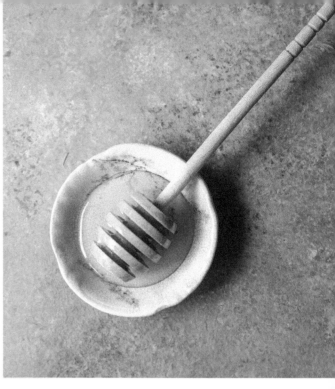

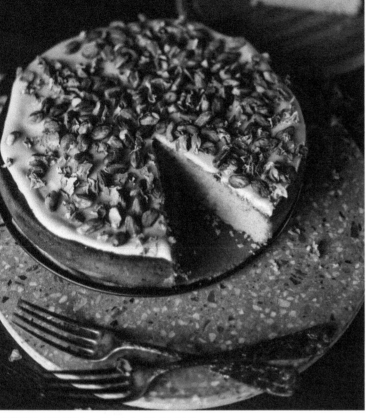

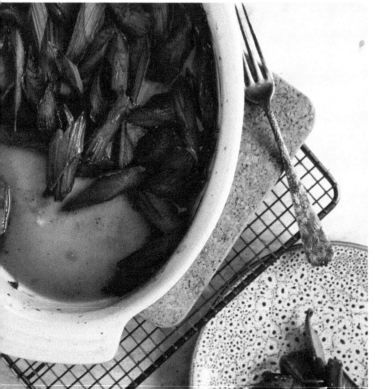

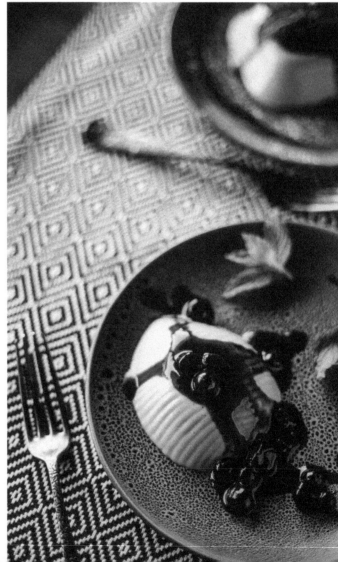

Persian Love Cake
-P +K

This cake looks and tastes like love! Especially when it's made that way. In many ways it reminds me of a simple wedding cake, stripped down to the sweetest foundation of emotion. Maybe it's the addition of roses or the luscious use of simple ingredients. Either way, I invite you to make this cake an expression of the love you feel for yourself and those you share it with! ***Makes one cake; Prep + Cooking time: 60 mins.***

What's in it:

- 200 grams unsalted butter
- ¾ cup baking (caster) sugar
- 4 medium eggs
- 1 ½ teaspoon ground cardamom
- ½ teaspoon nutmeg
- 1 ¾ teaspoons baking powder
- 1 ¼ cup all purpose wholemeal flour
- 1 ¾ cup ground almonds
- zest and juice of 1 lemon

- 1 tablespoon rose water
- pinch of fine sea salt

Icing

- 1 cup cream cheese
- 1 ½ cups icing sugar
- 1 teaspoon rosewater
- Rose petals and pistachios for decorating.

How to make it:

- Grease and flour an 8-inch cake tin or line a springform pan with baking paper.
- Combine flour, baking powder, cardamom, salt and nutmeg in a bowl.
- In a separate bowl cream together butter and sugar until light, fluffy, and pale. Add in the eggs, one at a time.
- Beat the flour and spices mixture into the wet ingredients, and once incorporated, add the lemon zest, juice, and rosewater. Mix until just combined

- Pour the batter into the pan and bake at 160°C/325°F for 30-45 minutes.
- Cake is ready when a toothpick inserted in the centre comes out clean.
- Remove cake from the oven and cool.
- For the icing, soften the cream cheese, add icing sugar and rosewater. Mix until smooth. Ensure that the cake is completely cool before topping with a layer of icing. Sprinkle rose petals and pistachios on top.

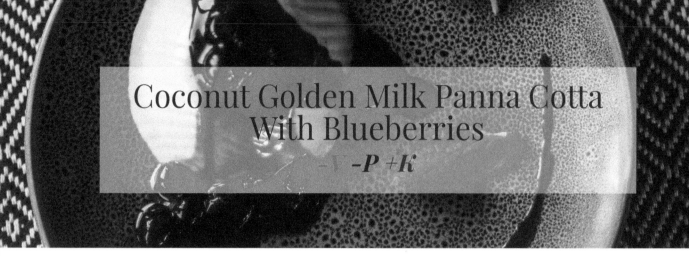

Coconut Golden Milk Panna Cotta With Blueberries
-V -P +K

If you're looking for a simple, beautiful, and healthy dessert, you've found it. Panna cotta is the easiest "fancy" dessert I know. At its very foundation, it's smooth, cooling, and beautiful -- all qualities that are perfect for balancing out the sharp, intense acidity of summer and pitta! So if you've never made panna cotta before, don't worry, it's nearly fool proof, and on top of that, you'll bring joy into the hearts of everyone you share it with! *Makes 6 4-ounce puddings; Prep + Cooking time: 20 mins + 3 hrs. for Cooling.*

What's in it:

- 1 ½ cups coconut milk (you can use whole milk or experiment with soy milk)
- 3 teaspoons powdered gelatin OR 2 tablespoons agar agar
- ¼ cup coconut sugar
- 1 ½ cups coconut cream
- 1 teaspoon vanilla extract
- ½ teaspoon cinnamon
- ½ teaspoon cardamom
- ¼ teaspoon finely ground black pepper
- 1 teaspoon ground turmeric
- pinch salt

Blueberry sauce

- 2 cups fresh or frozen blueberries
- 1 tablespoon sugar (or coconut sugar)
- 2 teaspoons lemon juice
- 2 teaspoons cornstarch or tapioca flour
- 1 tablespoon water

How to make it:

- Lightly grease six small containers (ramekins, small bowls, etc.) with coconut oil by putting a few drops of oil on a paper towel and wiping the insides of the containers.

- Pour the milk into the saucepan and sprinkle the powdered gelatin over top. Let soften until the surface of the milk is wrinkled and the gelatin grains look wet and slightly dissolved.

- Place the saucepan over low heat and gently warm the milk, stirring or whisking constantly (do not allow the milk to boil, simmer, or get hotter than lukewarm).

- Once the gelatin has fully dissolved (you can check by dipping your finger into the milk and watching for grains of undissolved gelatin), add the sugar and allow it to dissolve.

- Next whisk in the spices and warm for another 5 minutes. Then remove from the heat and whisk in the vanilla, salt, and coconut cream.

- To strain the spices before setting, so that they don't settle at the bottom, fill a large mixing bowl about ¼ of the way with cold water and a few pieces of ice. Place another bowl inside and put a strainer with a piece of cheese cloth over that bowl. Pour the warmed milk mixture over the cheesecloth strainer into the bowl below.

- Gently stir the milk to "pre-cool" it [this will prevent it from separating into a milk and cream layer in the fridge].

- Fill each of the greased ramekins with the cooled milk mixture. Cover and refrigerate for around 3 hours (or overnight if you plan to unmold it).

To make the blueberry sauce:

- Place blueberries, lemon juice, and 1 teaspoon of sugar in a saucepan over medium high heat. Allow to cook until the juices release. Thicken the sauce with a slurry of cornstarch or tapioca flour and water. Allow the sauce to cool before serving.

- To unmold, fill a bowl with warm water. Run a knife around the inside of the ramekin to release the pudding (be careful not to cut into the pudding). Hold the ramekin in the warm water just up to its edge for a few seconds. Unmold onto a plate. Top with a spoonful of blueberry sauce.

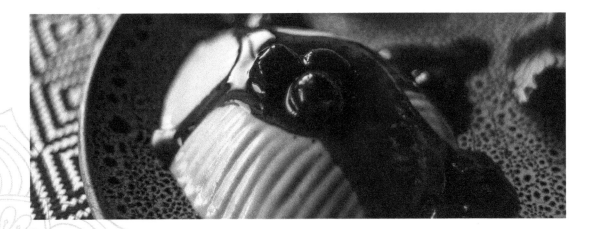

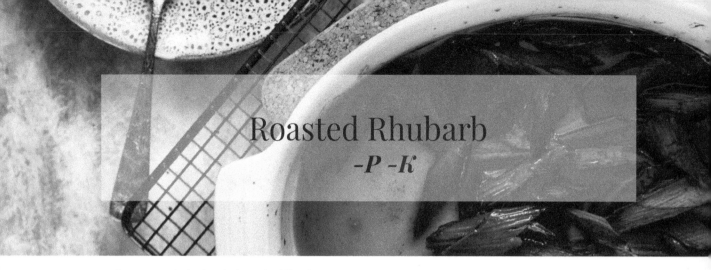

Roasted Rhubarb
-P -K

I discovered rhubarb late in life, but you know what they say: better late than never! Rhubarb is balancing for all of the doshas, so it can be the perfect comfort food for any season of the year. I typically enjoy it in a crumble, but have taken to cooking and eating it this way, which is a bit lighter and definitely more versatile. Have it on toast or porridge or even a little by itself with a dollop of coconut yogurt and cup of warming chai for a light and simple breakfast! *Serves 2-4; Prep + Cooking time: 40 mins.*

What's in it:

- 3-5 rhubarb stalks with leaves and ends removed
- 1 tablespoon coconut sugar or sucanat
- 1 teaspoon ghee
- pinch cinnamon
- pinch cardamom
- pinch fennel powder

How to make it:

- Preheat the oven to 165°C/325°F.
- Slice the rhubarb stalks into small pieces. You can get creative here and slice them in short "sticks" or diagonally into small pieces (go with what feels right).
- Mix the sliced rhubarb with all the other ingredients and combine with your hands to fully coat.
- Add to a small roasting pan. Sprinkle 2 tablespoons of water over the mix and cover with tinfoil. Roast for 20 minutes or until just fork tender.
- Remove foil, and cook for an additional 10 minutes until rhubarb has browned and some of the water has evaporated/absorbed.
- Remove from heat and serve warm over porridge, spread on toast, or on its own with a few spoonfuls of granola on top!

Drinks

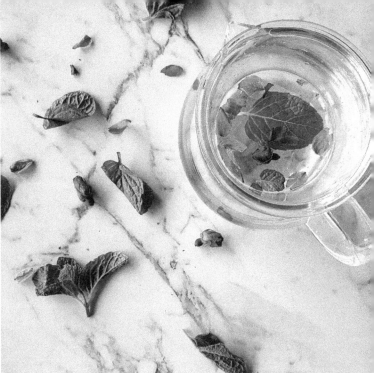

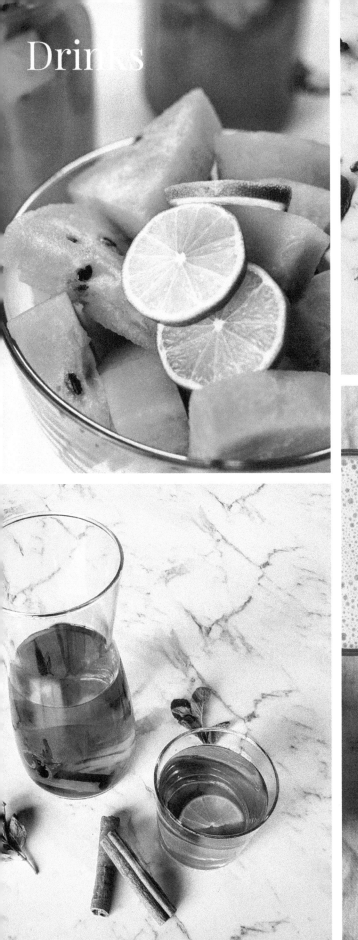

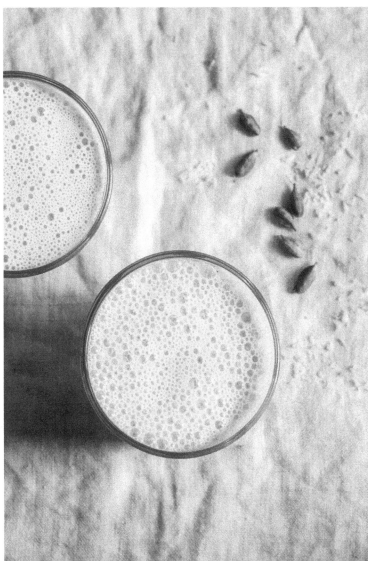

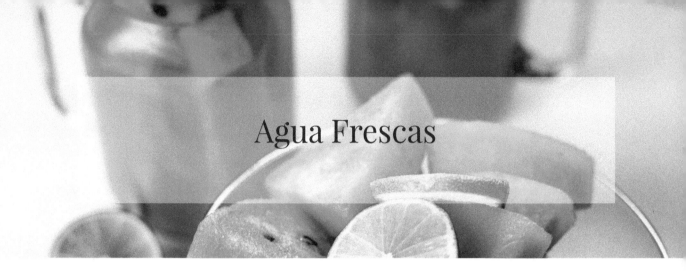

Agua Frescas

Agua frescas are a simple way to enjoy the cooling power of fruit. They're also a great option for combining summer fruits with fantastic herbs and spices that support their power to heal and delight. Here's a selection of recipes that include my favorite fruits of the summer season with some interesting flavor combinations. Need a quick (and delightful) cool down? Get your blender and have a go!

What's in it:

-V -P +K

Cucumber Ginger Cooler
- ¾ liter water (4 quarts)
- 1 English cucumber
- juice of 2 limes
- ¼ cup ginger syrup (you can adjust this to taste)
- 1 handful mint

-V +P -K

Watermelon Lime Fennel
- 2 pounds seedless watermelon (⅛ of a good-sized watermelon)
- 1 cup cold water
- 2 teaspoons lime juice
- 1 tablespoon fennel syrup or agave nectar

-V -P -K

Pineapple, ginger, mint
- 4 cups fresh pineapple with 2-4 cups water to blend
- 8-10 cups water
- ¼ cup ginger simple syrup [Pg 281]
- handful of mint leaves

How to make it:

- Puree the fresh fruit and herbs in a blender with 1-2 cups of water.
- Strain into a pitcher, add the herbal syrup and more water to taste.

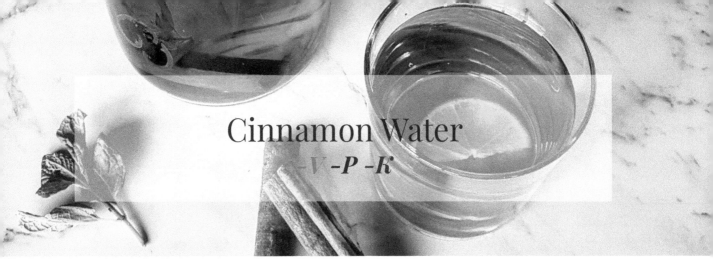

Cinnamon Water
–V –P –K

This beautiful alternative to water is ridiculously simple and satisfyingly good! Cinnamon is probably my most favorite spice ever, which is why I was delighted to discover this refreshing drink in a small cafe in Los Angeles years ago! I don't even think they knew how good it was for us! *Makes 2-3 liters; Prep + Cooking time: 1-4 hrs.*

What's in it:

- 2-3 liters (approx. 2-3 quarts/litres) pure filtered water
- 3 cinnamon sticks

How to make it:

There are two options for making this...

- **As a sun tea** - Combine the water and cinnamon sticks in a glass jar or pitcher. Cover and sit in the sun for approximately 4-5 hours or until the water becomes slightly tinted reddish brown. Refrigerate and serve on the cooler side of room temperature.

- **As a prepared tea** - Combine water and cinnamon sticks in a large, heavy-bottomed pan. Bring to a boil and simmer on medium heat for 3-5 minutes. Allow to cool. Serve on the cooler side of room temperature.

Coconut Mango Lassi
-V -P +K

The perfect cooling beverage for a hot day! Mango lassi is an Indian tradition that cools the body without slowing things down too much (mango is slightly warming). ***Serves 2; Prep + Cooking time: 10 mins.***

What's in it:

- 2 cups cubed ripe mango
- 1 ½ cups plain coconut yogurt [Pg 282]
- ½ teaspoon cardamom powder
- 1 tablespoons honey (optional) (depending on the sweetness of mango)
- handful of ice cubes (optional)

How to make it:

- Add all ingredients into a blender.
- Blend until smooth.
- Pour into a glass and enjoy!

Summertime Tea
-V -P -K

Summertime teas help to cool the mental and physical heat that can lead to things like inflammation, aggravation, diarrhea, and other digestive upsets. Each of the tea combinations below are easily consumed either hot or cooled down to room temperature.

What's in it:

3-Roots Tea
- 2 slices turmeric root
- 1 teaspoon dried licorice root
- 2 slices fresh ginger
- 1 teaspoon rose petals

Rosy-Mint Tea
- 1 teaspoon rosewater or ¼ cup fresh rose petals
- few fresh mint leaves
- 1 piece of sweet orange peel

Fennel Summer Tea
- 1 teaspoon fennel seed
- few fresh mint leaves

How to make it:

- If you plan to make teas regularly (even if you don't), it's best is to invest in a teapot, a tea ball, or tea strainer, as they can be pretty handy.

- Add ingredients to a small tea pot, or large tea ball. Cover with hot water and steep for 5 minutes minimum. Allow to cool slightly or totally. Enjoy!

The Summer Salad System

Summertime is salad season. A trip to your local farmer's market this time of year will definitely confirm that! The large variety and selection of fresh produce available this time time of the year, coupled with rising temperatures, falling appetites, and busy lifestyles, makes salad the perfect "go-to" for just about any meal of the day. But not all salads are created equal

In the age of convenience foods and eating on the go, anything fresh or with vegetables is automatically given the wellness industry "healthy" stamp along with a free ticket to eat all you want! The result is that salads have become the new "junk food" with the potential to cause more problems than they solve.

Salad pitfalls to avoid...

If you're eating to feel light, strong, energized, and calm this summer, the first thing to remember is that portion size matters... and so do ingredients. Meat, oil, vinegar, and cheese can add heaviness and heat at a time when we're most in need of cooling moderation. Traditional salad bar staples like onions, tomatoes, radishes, chilis, and olives have heating qualities that can turn up the internal heat and fuel the fires of anger, indigestion, heartburn, or inflammation!

Eating like you love yourself in summer means...

Choosing foods that are cooling, flavorful, and satisfying, and resisting the urge to overdo it! For salad as a meal, use grains as a "filler" rather than meats. They are cooler, drier, and lighter than meat and are truly satisfying when mixed with a selection of fresh greens and veggies and brought together with a flavorful "glue" of citrus juices and good quality oils.

And if you're not sure how to put together a salad that will have you feeling cool, calm, and satisfied, consider one of these salad "formulas" for bringing together the right ingredients to balance the summer heat inside and out.

Salad Formula:

Choose from the following "summer friendly" ingredients combined
according to the salad formulas below:

Leafy greens

- Kale
- Watercress
- Arugula
- Lettuce mix

Legumes

- Lentils
- Chickpeas
- Mung beans (sprouted)

Veggies

- Cucumber
- Avocado
- Asparagus
- Snow peas
- Peas
- Peppers (sweet)
- Beets (cooked)
- Sweet potato (cooked)
- Carrots (cooked)
- Cauliflower (cooked)
- Red Onions (cooked)

Grains

- Couscous
- Rice
- Quinoa

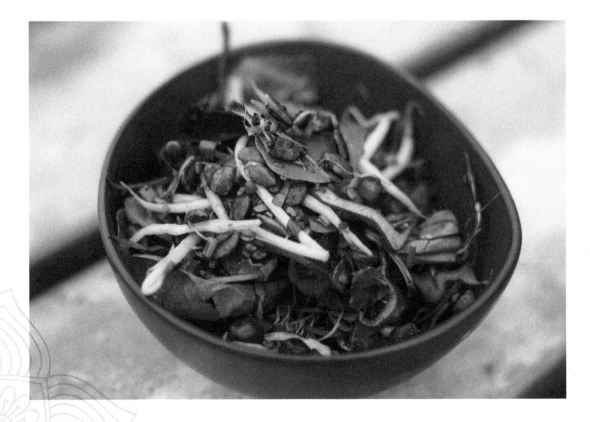

For light to moderately filling salads go with

½ Greens + ½ Veggies
[e.g. watercress + [snow peas + roasted beets]
– Or–
½ Greens + ¼ Veggies + ¼ Grains or Legumes
[e.g. romaine lettuce + couscous + sweet peppers]

For substantially filling salad (i.e. meal) go with

Greens + Legumes + Grains + Veggies
[e.g. kale + rice + lentils + cooked sweet onions]

Dressing things up...

You can "glue" the whole thing together with sauces and dressings that are cooling as well. Try one of these depending on your tastes.

- **Citrus** - Try a squeeze of lime juice (about 3 tablespoons) + a pinch of salt + 1 tablespoon of sunflower oil.
- **Creamy** - Blend ¼ avocado with a small bunch of cilantro + pinch of salt + small garlic clove + 1 tablespoon Greek yogurt.

Let your body be your guide...

If you're not sure how to choose ingredients, consider what you've got on hand and tune in. Learning to create balance with food starts with listening and trusting your inner knowing to steer you in the direction of genuine wellness.

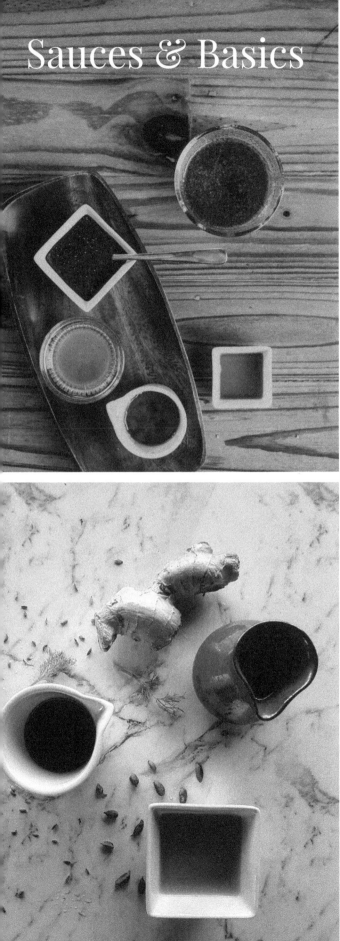
Sauces & Basics
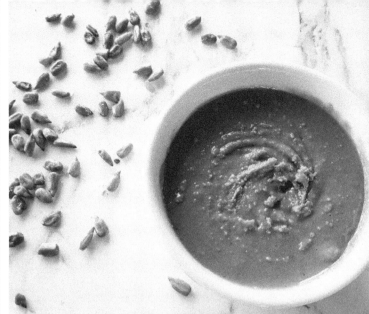
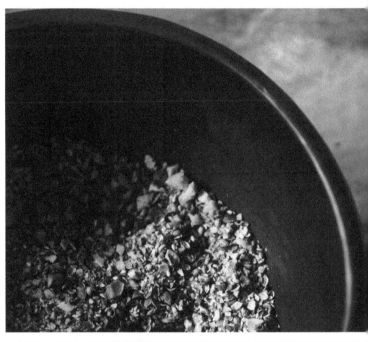
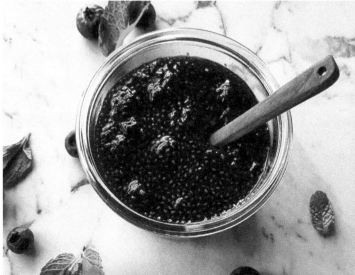

Chia Blueberry Jam
-V -P +K

Making jam is one of the few things that I've kind of sworn against. In part because it can be fiddly (all that sterilizing and handling hot jars) and because it can be time consuming. Enter chia seeds!! Chia is cooling and deeply moisturizing. It's also very high in omega-3s, proteins, vitamins, and minerals. And making jam couldn't be easier than using this recipe. Feel free to experiment with different fruit combinations. ***Makes about 1 ¼ cups***

What's in it:

- 2 cups fresh blueberries
- ½ teaspoon vanilla extract
- 2 tablespoons water

- 3 tablespoons chia seeds
- sugar, honey, or maple syrup to taste

How to make it:

- In a small pot over medium heat, bring blueberries, vanilla, water, and chia seeds to a low boil. Maintain on heat until the fruit has broken down and begun to release its juices.

- Add the chia seeds and continue stirring until the mixture thickens slightly. Add sugar or maple syrup (if adding honey, allow the mixture to cool to lukewarm).

- Remove from heat and allow to cool down. Add additional sweetener if needed.

- Once the jam has cooled to room temperature, transfer to a clean jar with an airtight lid. Refrigerate. Jam will continue to thicken in the fridge and will keep for up to 2 weeks.

- **Note**: If you're not a fan of the chia texture, you can grind the seeds and add them rather than adding whole seeds

Coconut Mint Tzatziki
-V -P +K

Love this simple dip as a cooling accompaniment to spicy dishes or as a snack with crackers or flatbreads. This version uses our homemade coconut yogurt to up the cooling factor and offset a little of the heating qualities of traditional tzatziki, which is made with whole milk yogurt. *Makes about 1 ½ cups*

What's in it:

- 1 cup coconut yogurt [Pg 282]
- ½ cup cucumber, seeded and finely grated (Lebanese or English cucumbers are great for this)
- 1 teaspoon lemon zest
- 1 tablespoon fresh lemon juice
- 2 cloves garlic, finely minced
- 1 tablespoon freshly chopped dill
- 1 tablespoon freshly chopped mint
- salt and freshly cracked black pepper to taste

How to make it:

- To drain the cucumber, place on top of a few paper towels or a piece of cheesecloth and squeeze the water out. Set aside.
- Whisk the yogurt, cucumber, garlic, lemon zest, lemon juice, dill, and mint together in a bowl. Add salt and pepper to taste (I usually add a couple of pinches of each). Transfer to an airtight container and chill until needed. Can keep refrigerated for up to two days.

Coriander & Coconut Chutney
-V -P +K

Makes 6 servings

What's in it:

Chutney
- ½ cup grated fresh coconut
- ¼ inch piece of fresh ginger, peeled
- 2 garlic cloves
- 1 green chili, coarsely chopped
- ½ cup chopped coriander (cilantro), stems and leaves included
- 1 tablespoon roasted chana dal or peanuts

- 1½ teaspoon lemon juice
- 4 tablespoons water
- salt

Tempering oil
- 2 teaspoons ghee or vegetable oil
- ¼ teaspoon mustard seeds
- ¼ teaspoon cumin seeds
- few small curry Leaves

How to make it:

- Combine ginger, coconut, garlic, chili, and roasted peanuts/dal in a food processor or mortar and pestle. Process (or grind) until they come together in a coarsely textured mixture.
- Add coriander and half of the lemon juice and continue processing/grinding to combine. Add the rest of the lemon juice and water and process or grind into a smooth paste. Transfer it to bowl.

- Heat ghee in a small pot or pan. Add the cumin and mustard seeds. When the seeds begin to sizzle, add the curry leaves, and sauté for few seconds.
- Pour the hot oil over the chutney and mix to combine.

Dukkah

-V +P +K

I discovered this beautiful Egyptian treat about a decade ago and have never looked back. It's a beautiful and incredibly tasty way to incorporate warming spices (and foods) into just about anything (it's also a great to give away as gifts during holiday season). I originally started with a simple recipe and have customized it somewhat to suit the tastes that I like (and need) most and I definitely recommend that you do the same. All of the ingredients in this one are warming. Some are heavier than others (i.e. the nuts are heavy the spices lighter). I use this as an accompaniment for salads, soups, just bread and oil, and anything else I can think of! If you need a hit of heat that's not too heavy, try this! ***Makes 1¾ cups***

What's in it:

- ½ cup almonds (best with skins removed)
- ½ cup macadamia nuts
- ½ cup coriander seeds
- ⅓ cup sesame seeds
- 2 tablespoons cumin seeds
- 2 teaspoons flaked sea salt (I use Maldon)
- 1 ½ teaspoons sumac

How to make it:

- In a large frying pan over medium-high heat, combine nuts and toast until lightly brown (make sure to move them around or they will scorch).
- Remove nuts from the pan and coarsely chop them (you can use a processor or just a knife). Add to a bowl.
- Toast the sesame seeds in the same way and add to the bowl with the chopped nuts.
- Lightly toast the cumin and coriander seeds and coarsely crush them in a mortar and pestle or processor. Add to the bowl
- Add the salt, and sumac to the bowl with the other ingredients and stir to combine well.
- Store the mixture in an airtight container. Use dukkah as seasoning in cooking, a topping for salads and soups or serve as an accompaniment with bread and olive oil.

Dressings

Make-ahead dressings for salads or accompaniments to meats and other dishes that can keep for up to 3 weeks in the refrigerator. Putting these together in advance and storing them in airtight jars or bottles can help take some of the time out of homemade meal prep.

What's in it:

$-V +P +K$ **Ginger Dressing**
- 3 tablespoons finely grated ginger
- ½ cup mirin
- ⅔ cup rice wine vinegar
- ¾ cup olive oil
- 2 tablespoons light soy sauce

Add all ingredients to a jar and shake to emulsify. Store in the jar so that you can emulsify again before using.

$-V -P +K$ **Beetroot Dressing**
- 1 medium sized beet, finely grated
- ⅔ cup red wine vinegar
- ¾ cup olive oil
- pinch of salt
- pinch of black pepper

Add all ingredients to a bowl or large jar and mix well. This dressing can be used for salads or as a tasty accompaniment to fish, meat, cheese or even on avocado toast!

$-V +P -K$

Black Sesame Dressing
- 2-3 tablespoons. rice vinegar
- 1 tablespoon soy sauce
- 2 teaspoons sugar
- 1 teaspoon sesame oil
- 3 tablespoons black sesame seeds
- 1 clove garlic

Mix rice vinegar, soy sauce, and sugar in a small bowl. Using a food processor or a mortar and pestle, grind the sesame seeds until smooth. Combine all the ingredients in a bowl and whisk everything together.

Lemon Dressing

$-V +P -K$

- 4 tablespoons fresh lemon juice
- 4 tablespoons white wine vinegar
- ½ teaspoon dijon mustard
- ½ teaspoon honey
- ¼ cup olive oil

Add all ingredients to a bowl and whisk together to combine. Dressing can be stored in an airtight jar and refrigerated for up to 2 weeks.

Fresh Garden Pickles
-V +P +K

Pickles are a lovely way to make the most out of seasonal produce and are best suited to the late summer and autumn seasons as their sweet and sour flavors balance vata dosha. They can be aggravating for pitta and kapha, so it's important to eat them in small, manageable quantities (i.e. more like a condiment than a side-dish). The pickling process extends the life of the foods and retains some of the energy as well. So don't be discouraged by an overabundance of tomatoes, cucumbers or even carrots and radishes from your garden this year. Check out this super simple recipe for creating luscious pickles that you can enjoy through the harvesting season and beyond! *Makes 2 quarts (2 liters) of pickles*

What's in it:

- 1 ¼ cups vinegar
- ½ cup of sugar
- 2tablespoons. mustard seed
- 1 tablespoon. coriander seed
- 2 teaspoons. celery seed
- 2 teaspoons . black peppercorns

- 1 tablespoon - fennel seeds
- 3 tablespoons pickling salt
- 8 cups of vegetables of your choosing- cucumbers, bell peppers,
- carrots, celery, onions, tomatoes are all good choices.
- 5-8 whole garlic cloves

How to make it:

- Add vinegar, spices, salt and 3 cups of water to a large saucepan over medium heat. Bring to a gentle simmer and leave on low for 5-7 minutes.
- Remove from the heat and allow to cool slightly.
- Place the cleaned and sliced vegetables into two 1 quart (1 liter) sealable jars.

- Cover the vegetables with the warm pickling liquid and allow them to sit uncovered until they've cooled to room temperature.
- Allow the pickles to sit at room temperature for about two hours. Serve or cover and refrigerate until you're ready to enjoy them.
- Pickles can be stored in the refrigerator for up to one month.

Herbal Simple Syrups
-V -P +K

Herbal syrups are another simple (and delicious) way to incorporate the healing power of herbs into your diet. They can be used in cool drinks, baking, coffees, and teas, or as toppings for some of your favorite dishes, or just about anywhere you need a little balancing sweetness. All are balancing for all the doshas (in moderation for kapha due to the sugar medium). You can also vary the sugars used for different flavors.

What's in it:

Ginger Simple Syrup [sweet, pungent, heating, wet, heavy]

- ¾ cup sugar
- 1 cup water
- 4 pieces fresh ginger, cut into slices

Bring water and sugar to a boil and then add the pieces of ginger. Remove from heat and let cool completely. Strain and discard the ginger.

Fennel Syrup [sweet, pungent, bitter, heating, light, dry]

- 1 ½ tablespoons fennel seeds
- ¾ cup granulated sugar
- 1 cup water

Gently crush the fennel seeds in a mortar and pestle. Bring water and sugar to a boil and then add the fennel seeds. Remove from heat and let cool completely. Strain and discard the fennel seeds.

Cardamom Simple Syrup [sweet, pungent, cooling, light, dry]

- 25 lightly crushed green cardamom pods
- 1 cup sugar
- 1 cup water

Bring water and sugar to a boil and then add the cardamom. Remove from heat and let cool completely. Strain and discard the cardamom.

Homemade Coconut Yogurt
-V -P +K

Coconut yogurt was for a long time something of an indulgence in part because it's pretty expensive relative to regular yogurt (usually at least twice the price). And then I found out how easy it is to make it! As a fermented product, yogurt is heating and a little heavy and the coconut version is no different, but as coconut is cooling, the yogurt made from it's milk is a better for balancing pitta and to have during the summer time. ***Makes 1 cup***

What's in it:

- 1 400ml (13.5oz) can full fat coconut cream
- 4 probiotic capsules (minimum 30 billion CFUs)

How to make it:

- Empty the can of coconut cream into a clean jar.
- Pull apart the capsules and sprinkle the contents over the top of the coconut cream.
- Stir to incorporate (make sure the powder is well incorporated).
- Cover the jar with a piece of cheesecloth (you can seal it by putting a rubber band around the jar lid).
- Set in a warm place in your kitchen or home for up to 48 hours (the longer you leave it, the more sour the taste. I usually leave it a minimum of 24 hours).

- Test the yogurt for taste after 24 hours. Refrigerate it once you've achieve the level of sourness you desire (but not longer than 48 hours).

FOR THICKER YOGURT:

- You may find after refrigerating that a decent amount of liquid has settled to the bottom of the jar. This can be drained off and you will be left with a thick, Greek style yogurt) or stirred in for a thinner style yogurt.

Honey Ginger Nut Butter
-V +P +K

One word...yum. This simple spread combines so much warming goodness! It's a bit of a throwback to the peanut butter and honey sandwiches of my youth, with a little bit of ancient wisdom thrown in. If you're in the habit of buying nut butters from the supermarket, I can almost guarantee that you'll never want another jar of processed nut butter again.
Makes 2 ¼ cups of nut butter

What's in it:

- 1 cup almonds (dry roasted or raw with skins removed)
- ¾ cup cashews (raw or dry roasted)
- ½ cup macadamia nuts (optional - roasted or raw)

- A pinch of salt
- 2 tablespoons of raw honey
- 1 tsp of ginger powder

How to make it:

- Add nuts, salt and ginger to a food processor or high speed blender. Process until smooth. Keep an eye on this as the consistency can change quickly. Consider first the texture that you like your nut butter and keep checking on the butter until it reaches your desired consistency.

- Add honey and process just to mix (avoid heating the honey).
- Store in an airtight container in a cupboard or fridge. Enjoy on EVERYTHING!

"Magic Dust" - Spice Mix
-*V* -*P* -*K*

The first time I made this and gave a little to my daughter, her response was, "This is EVERYTHING!" If you're a fan of cinnamon and cardamom, or are having any digestive issues, then this just may be everything for you. Not only that, but it's an all purpose sweet spice mix that can be USED with nearly everything! Each of the three spices that make up this gorgeous mix have properties that promote healthy digestion. When you combine them , they also have the power to make you smile. My favorite ways to use this mix are:

- *On buttered toast - a whole new take on cinnamon toast*
- *On popcorn - Yum. Just. Yum.*
- *On hot chocolate, coffee, or chai - Adds depth and intrigue*

What's in it:

- 1 teaspoon ground cinnamon
- ¾ teaspoon ground cardamom
- ¾ teaspoon ground fennel

How to make it:

- Add spices to a small bowl and mix together to completely combine.
- Use as needed, store in an airtight container.
- This mixture does not need to be refrigerated. We typically store it in a spice shaker in our pantry.

Basic Ghee
-V -P =K

Ghee is a fixture in an Ayurvedic approach to cooking and eating. A form of clarified butter (made with love), ghee is a wonderful cooking oil with a high smoke point and a terrific substitute for butter in cooking. Ghee is a great support to a healthy digestive system as it enhances absorption and assimilation of nutrients in the GI tract. It has soothing effects that can help to heal intestinal walls and lubricate joints and soft tissues. Ghee is also said to help improve and maintain memory function. It's balancing for vata and pitta and in moderate quantities, kapha. It's also easy to make at home, which means you can be sure to include a little extra love! ***Makes 1 pint (about ½ liter); Prep + Cooking time: approx 30mins.***

What you need:

- 500g (or 1 lb) unsalted butter
- cheese cloth
- Clean dry jar or container (glass is best)

How to make it:

- Cut butter into chunks and place into a heavy bottomed medium sized pot or medium heat.
- Cook the butter uncovered until ust under the boil and allow to simmer slowly. You'll notice that a foam develops on top and as the butter cooks the dairy solids will form small clumps that sink to the bottom of the pan.
- As it cooks gently skim off some of the foam that forms on top, leaving a golden liquid that smells like a movie theater (popcorn butter).
- Make sure to watch the ghee so that it

doesn't burn (it'll turn brown and smell more nutty than like popcorn).

- All of the water will have been burned off once the butter is clear, free of foam and no longer sputters. By this point the dairy solids will have sunken to the bottom of the pot. Remove from the heat and allow to cool slightly before straining through the cheesecloth into a clean, dry jar or container.
- Ghee can be stored at room temperature in a pantry or on a shelf. It doesn't need refrigeration. As the ghee cools it will look golden and opaque, but it will be soft.

Pitta: & kapha balancing (in moderation)

Seasonal Churnas (Spice Mix)
-P -K

Churna is a Sanskrit word that means a mixture of powdered herbs. Traditionally ayurvedic herbal formulations are given out in this powdered form. One of my best memories from working in ayurvedic clinics was watching the vaidya (ayurvedic doctor) put together individual formulations for each patient as they watched, sitting across the desk. Creating spice mixes is something of a seasonal tradition in parts of India where families (most often the women) will choose, toast, and grind the spices into a churna that can be used all season to ward off imbalances.

I love the idea of making it a seasonal ritual and definitely recommend starting with whole spices where you can and making small batches of the mix to use throughout the season or for addressing particular imbalances.

What's in it:

Vata Churna
Good for vata imbalance or for use from late summer through early winter

- 2 tablespoon cumin seeds - toasted and ground
- ½ teaspoon ground cardamom
- ½ teaspoon ground ginger
- ¼ teaspoon asafoetida (sometimes marketed as 'hing." It's often mixed with other things like rice flower and turmeric, so buy the simplest mix (i.e. one with the fewest ingredients) you can find)

Pitta Churna
Good for pitta imbalances or for use in summer and early autumn

- 2 tablespoons coriander seeds, toasted and ground
- 2 tablespoons fennel seeds, toasted and ground
- 1 teaspoon ground cinnamon
- ½ teaspoon ground ginger
- ½ teaspoon ground turmeric
- ¼ teaspoon black pepper

Kapha Churna
Good for kapha imbalances or for use in late winter and spring

- 2 tablespoons coriander seeds, toasted and ground
- 1 tablespoon ground ginger
- 1 tablespoon ground turmeric
- 1 teaspoon ground cinnamon
- ½ teaspoon black pepper

How to make it:

- Throw the whole spices in a warm skillet or pan and heat until they are aromatic (you can smell them!). Remove from the heat and allow them to cool slightly before grinding them in a spice grinder, high speed blender, or by hand in a mortar and pestle.

- I like to combine all the ingredients and throw the mixture into an airtight container (saved spice bottle from store bought ground spices will do wonderfully), and store them in the pantry until they're all gone. Best to use them within 3 months!

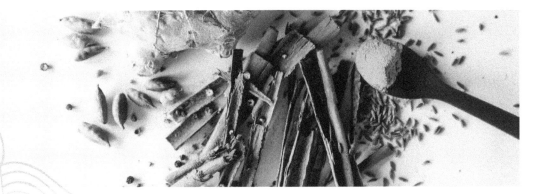

Sunflower Seed Butter
-V -P +K

Tired of the same old almond or peanut butter? Why not give this one a try? Sunflower seeds are sweet, a little bitter, and cooling. They are balancing for all the doshas and help to cleanse the lungs and lymphatic system. This butter is a great nut butter option for kapha and a terrific choice for any of the doshas any time of the year! ***Makes about 2 cups of butter***

What's in it:

- 6 cups raw sunflower seeds
- 1 teaspoon sunflower oil (optional)
- ½ teaspoon salt (optional)
- ½ teaspoon cinnamon

How to make it:

- Preheat oven to 180°C/350°F. Line a baking sheet with baking paper and spread the seeds in an even layer.

- Roast the seeds for 20 - 25 minutes, gently stirring them occasionally to ensure an even roast. Remove the seeds when they are golden brown and fragrant.

- Transfer the seeds to a blender or food processor along with the salt and cinnamon. Process for 10 - 15 minutes, stopping occasionally to scrape the sides down into the middle.

- Don't get discouraged if you've never made nut butter before. It can take a few good minutes of processing before the seeds release their oils and begin to liquify.

- Once the mixture becomes liquid, process until you reach the consistency you're looking for (some like it a little crunchier, some like it super smooth and creamy).

- Once done, transfer butter to a jar with an airtight lid. This butter will last refrigerated for 2 - 3 weeks.

Simple Flatbread (roti)
-V -P -K

My take on the Indian chapatis that were a part of nearly every meal during my studies in India. Chapatis are simple (even fun) to make, and can be thrown together in a pinch as an accompaniment to curries and soups or as a base for pizzas (as we're using them). You can also add fresh herbs or chopped greens to them for a small meal option! ***Makes 10; Prep + Cooking time about 30 mins***

What's in it:

- 2 cups (250g) flour - Wholemeal, gluten free or any preferred type
- 1 teaspoon salt
- 2 tablespoons ghee
- 3/4 cup (185ml) hot water or as needed

How to make it:

- Add flour and salt to a bowl and mix well to combine. Mix in the ghee and add water bit by bit to create a soft dough.

- Knead the dough on a lightly floured surface until it is smooth and cut it into 10 pieces, or fewer if you want larger breads.

- Roll each piece into a ball, cover the balls with clingfilm or a damp tea towel and leave to rest for a 10-15 minutes.

Okay for Kapha in moderation

- Heat a frying pan on medium heat. Roll out the balls of dough with a rolling pin until nice and thin.

- Lightly grease the warm frying pan and place the roti in the pan, heating each side for about 30 seconds or until done.

- Place the finished rots in a warm oven or a tortilla warmer. Repeat with all the remaining balls of dough.

Chapter 14

Ayurvedic Cleansing for Self Renewal

Ayurveda says that one of the biggest factors holding us back from experiencing our true potential is our inability to let go of what we really don't need any more: the basement full of junk, the extra weight, unhealthy eating habits, self-criticism and judgment, and that enduring belief that who we are is never going to be enough.

This physical, mental, and emotional "residue" of unresolved and undigested life is what lies between us and the truest and healthiest expression of ourselves. The more we accumulate, the more we compromise our ability to be our authentic selves. And eventually we feel overburdened, unclear, complacent, jaded, and just plain sick and tired.

The primary purpose of Ayurvedic cleansing is to ease the burden on our systems of digestion and assimilation, allowing time and space to refocus the mind and body, revisit what we're committed to in life, and re-align ourselves with the cycles of nature. Cleansing also creates a clarity of mind and body that makes us feel renewed and reconnected to ourselves and the joy of living.

When you cleanse on a regular basis, you clear away some of what holds you back and slows you down in life, giving you access to the healthiest, happiest, and most powerful expression of you. It will also amplify your gifts and allow you to dedicate more of you to what really matters.

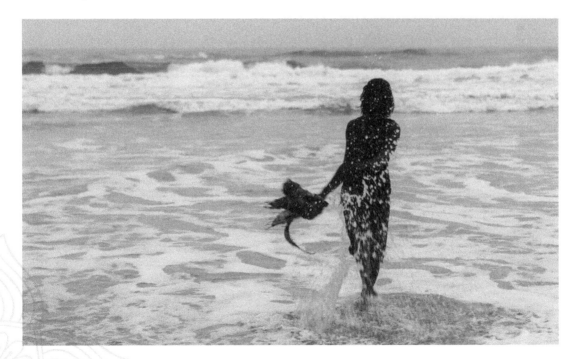

How toxic are you?

Signs of toxic build up in the body-mind include:

- Thick white coating on the tongue
- Feeling sluggish, bloated, or sleepy, especially after a meal
- Skin breakouts
- Foul-smelling breath, sweat, gas or stools
- Lusterless skin, whites of the eyes, or yellow teeth
- Clouded thoughts, feeling unable to focus or generally unmotivated
- Lethargy or feeling of heaviness in the body
- Irregular appetite or reduced appetite
- Generalized body and joint pains
- Bloated stomach, gases, flatulence
- Constipation or sticky stools
- Lack of mental clarity and energy
- Weary and unenthusiastic feeling

Some of the benefits of Ayurvedic cleansing include:

- More energy
- Weight loss
- Mental clarity
- Happier mood
- More confidence
- Better digestion
- Decreased cravings
- More restful sleep
- Glowing skin and eyes
- Connection with your physical, emotional, and spiritual well-being
- Clarity about what you're committed to in life
- Feeling motivated and inspired

What to know about cleansing, and a few things we can do without...

The focus of cleansing is to reduce the amount of toxins coming into your body and increase the amount of fresh air, water, sunlight, and rest that you receive so that your body's own natural cleansing and detoxification process can happen as effectively as possible.

The best part about Ayurvedic cleansing is that it's simple. It can be done for one or two days regularly or anywhere up to around 30 days a couple of times a year. But is NOT recommended for individuals who are infirm or pregnant or for children.

Spring and Fall are the recommended seasons for cleansing, and I usually do a regular 7-10 day program during these seasons.

While Cleansing you'll want to avoid:

- Processed foods
- Processed Sugar
- Caffeine
- Soft Drinks
- Dairy products
- Refined flour

- Meat, seafood & Eggs
- Alcohol
- Excess television, radio and social media
- Recreational drugs

What to eat while cleansing

The process of cleansing is simple and typically includes adopting a simple ama-reducing diet :

- Fresh vegetables cooked w/spices
- Limited amounts of fruit (bitter, astringent fruits are best)
- Limited quantities of ghee
- Fresh grains (primarily rice)

- Warm drinks (no cold drinks, or fruit juices)
- Limited legumes (mung beans)

What to do while cleansing...

Cleansing is a great opportunity to put yourself onto an Ayurvedic daily routine , but before starting, I always recommend setting an intention. Take a moment to consider what's going on in your life. How well is your experience of life feeding your soul?

Understand that no matter what your experience of life, taking time (even one day) to ease the burden on your mind and body is a powerful step toward living your bliss. So to make the most of it...:

Know why you're cleansing – Consider why you're taking the time out to lighten up and let go, and remind yourself why you're worth it (because you are SO worth it!).

Make a commitment – Commit yourself fully to the process of cleansing by getting clear on who you need to be in order to support yourself through to the end, and who you want to be as a result. Consider committing to the following every day of your cleanse, and your life!:

- *Joyful Energetic Body*
- *Loving compassionate heart*
- *Restful reflective alert mind*
- *Lightness of being...Total Ease*

A typical *cleansing day routine*:

- **Wake up early** – An inspired day begins at an inspiring time. Wake up before dawn and take a few moments to enjoy the stillness in your mind, body, and environment. Remind yourself of who you are and what you're committed to for the day.

- **Warm water with lemon and ginger** – Kick-start your digestive fire first thing in the morning with this simple warming drink, giving your digestion the boost it needs to efficiently process what you're taking in today and every day.

- **Yoga and meditation** - Take some time to mindfully move your body and then listen to it by sitting in meditation for 5-10 minutes...or more!

- **Eat light** – Keep breakfast light [Try the Yogi Breakfast - (Pg 306) and enjoy lunch as your largest meal of the day today. Try kitchari (Pg 301) the traditional Ayurvedic cleansing dish). Take a light dinner before the sun goes down.

- **Rest your mind and your body** – Resist doing more work or critical thinking than is absolutely needed, and keep interactions with electronics to a minimum. Rest your body and your mind deeply. Turn your thoughts inward to how your mind and body feels and just notice what comes up. Consider writing some of your thoughts down.

- **Hydrate** – Make sure to get plenty of water, and support digestive fire by sipping warm Ayurvedic tea throughout the day.

- **Let go of the day** - Wind down your day starting in the early evening and get to bed by 10pm. As you lie in bed before falling to sleep, take a moment to digest your day, connect with how it nourished you... and let it go!

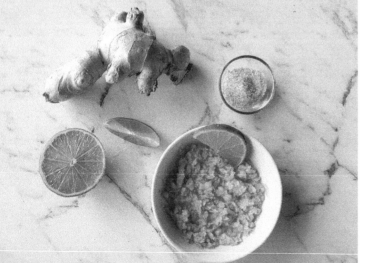

Detox & Healing recipes

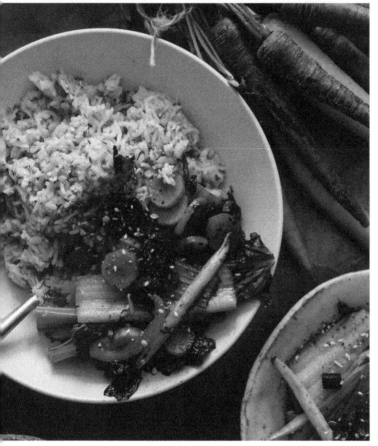

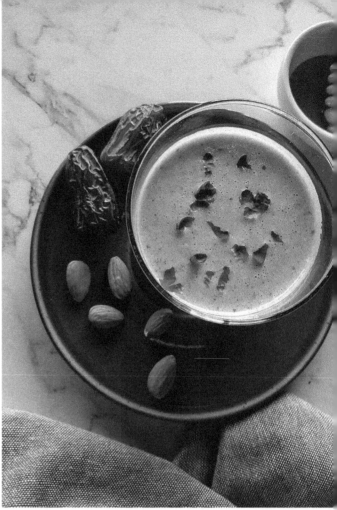

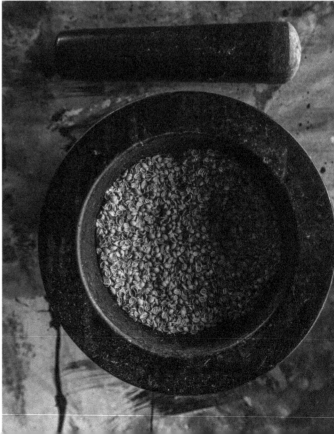

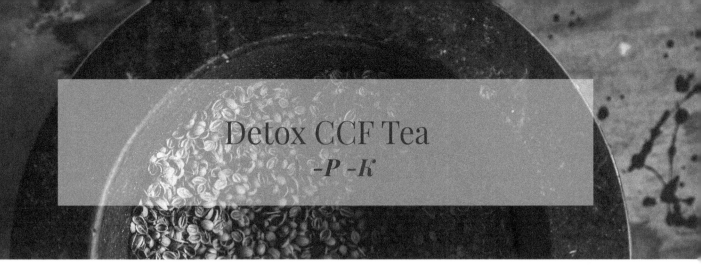

Detox CCF Tea
-P -K

Sometimes referred as "agni tea", CCF stands for the three primary digestive spices that lend their powers to this simple, tasty tea. Balancing to the digestive system, this tea supports the absorption of nutrients in the body and balances all the doshas. It also stokes metabolism and the digestive fire, restoring vitality where sluggishness abounds. Its mild bitterness also revs up the detoxification process and purifies the blood. CCF is a soothing formula that reduces agitation and inflammation. It restores a calm clarity and spaciousness to a tense mind. *Makes 1 serving; Preparation + Cooking time: 10mins*

What's in it:

- 1 teaspoon cumin seeds
- 1 teaspoon coriander seeds
- 1 teaspoon fennel seeds
- 1-2 cups of boiling water

Optional extras: Additional add-ins for a seasonal balancing boost
- 1-2 small mint leaves - *summer or spring*
- small slice fresh ginger - *autumn or spring*
- ½ cinnamon stick - *great any time of the year!*

How to make it:

Gently crush seeds (best to use mortar and pestle), then add to 1 cup of hot water (along with any optional herbs or spices). Steep for 5 minutes. Enjoy!

Detox Juices
-V -P -K

Juicing is great for reducing kapha (heaviness, dullness) and ama (toxins). The qualities of juice are cold, light, and dry. So counteract the cold qualities by juicing veggies and fruits at room temperature. Organic ingredients are especially important in juicing recipes because the juice is potent and highly concentrated. Although most people typically enjoy fruit-based juices, juice for cleansing should contain at least 70% vegetables (make sure to include bitter veggies).

What's in it:

Celery, beet, and carrot detox juice
- 1 medium sized carrot, peeled
- ¼ cup celery stalks
- ¼ teaspoon black pepper
- 1 cup fresh raw beets
- 2 small radishes
- ¼ cup fresh parsley
- 1 clove garlic (raw)

Green apple cleanser
- 4 sprigs (handful) parsley
- 1 medium sized green apple
- 2 cups spinach
- 1 lemon or lime (peel removed)

Detoxifying green juice
- 1 cup (loosely packed) leafy greens (spinach, lettuce, kale, celery, beet greens/carrot tops)
- 1 medium sized apple
- 2 medium sized carrots
- 1 small beet or ½ of a medium to large beet
- 3 inch chunk fresh ginger
- 1 whole organic lemon (peel removed)

How to make it:

- Wash, trim, and peel all fruits and veggies before juicing.
- Juice per your juicer's instructions. If you're using a blender, add fruit to the blender with ½ cup of water. Blend fully and then strain the pulp from the juice before drinking.

Digestive Elixir
-V +P -K

This is a bit like adding lighter fuel to the fire, so be mindful when taking (pay attention to how it makes you feel). It's particularly good if you're feeling heavy or have digestion that can be variable or slow. I often recommend this during the holidays when we tend to eat foods that are heavier, colder, and a little harder to digest.

What's in it:

- 2 tablespoons finely grated fresh ginger root
- 1 pinch Himalayan pink salt
- 1 tablespoon lime juice

How to make it:

- Mix all ingredients together in a clean dish (with a lid).
- Take a small (pea-sized) portion 1 hour to 10 minutes before a meal to give your digestion a BOOST!

- Tune in to how this makes you feel. If you experience overheating, burning, or anything that's uncomfortable, stop taking.
- This will last covered in the refrigerator for 1-2 weeks.

Medicinal Teas

Simple Calming Ginger Tea (Anxiety Tea)

A super simple brew to calm the mind and body.

What's in it:

- 1 teaspoon fresh ginger
- 4-6 cups fresh water
- 1 cardamom pod
- pinch nutmeg
- maple syrup to taste (optional)

Garlic Ginger Tea

This lovely tea is just the thing for when you feel a cold or flu coming on, or are in the throes of one and are looking for a little bit of relief from congestion and aches,

What's in it:

- 4 cloves garlic
- 1 small piece turmeric root
- 4 teaspoons chopped fresh ginger
- 4-6 cups water
- pinch cayenne pepper
- honey to taste (local honey is best)
- lemon juice to taste

How to make it:

- Add everything to a medium-sized saucepan.
- Bring to a boil and then reduce to simmer for 30 minutes.
- Strain, allow to cool, and serve with honey and a squeeze of lemon.

Kitchari
-P -K

Often referred to as Ayurvedic Chicken Soup, Kitchari is easy to digest and uses warming spices to gently stimulate the digestion. It's also a complete protein that is simple to make, delicious, and nourishing for the body! It's often eaten with vegetables that can be added in while cooking or cooked and eaten alongside. **Serves 3-4**

What's in it:

- 1 cup moong dal/moong dal, split yellow lentils (NOT the whole green ones)
- 1 cup basmati rice
- 4 cups water (if you want it more moist/soupy, use more water)
- 3 tablespoons ghee
- 1 teaspoon mustard seeds
- 1 teaspoon cumin seeds

Optional:

- 1 inch piece fresh ginger (root), peeled, and finely diced
- ¼ teaspoon ground turmeric

How to make it:

- Wash and strain the mung dal and the rice. Then heat the ghee gently in a pot and add spices. Once mustard seeds begin to pop (like popcorn), add the rice and dal mixture.
- Sauté for 2-3 minutes, then add water. Stir. Cover. Turn on low heat and cook until all water is absorbed. Serve with ghee and you can add a little salt.

Adding vegetables:

- You can add seasonal vegetables to this (2 cups of veg for this recipe) half way through cooking. Ok roast, saute or steam vegetables separately to eat alongside.
- Great vegetable options for cleansing includ: Green beans, carrots, asparagus and leafy greens like spinach or kale.

Nutmeg Milk for Insomnia
-*V* -*P* -*K*

Here's something for sleepless nights! Nutmeg is a nervine agent that calms the agitated mind. It's pungent, heating, oily qualities make it perfect for balancing the subtle active-ness of vata. This is best for transient insomnia that is more related to active mind, and should not be taken continually. Nutmeg is also good for digestion. *Serves 1*

What's in it:

- ⅛ teaspoon finely ground nutmeg
- 1 cup soy, cow or nut milk
- Pinch of cardamom
- Honey to taste (optional)

Add a little ghee if you're experiencing constipation.

How to make it:

- Heat milk on medium heat until warm. Whisk in spices and ghee (if adding).
- Allow milk to cool before adding honey.

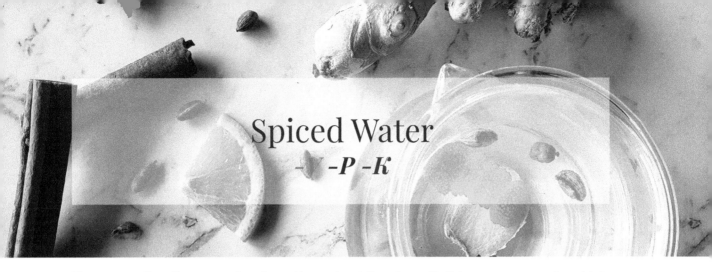

Spiced Water
-P -K

Keep your digestion on a slow burn throughout the day with this yummy warming drink. GREAT if your digestion is a bit variable, particularly if you're experiencing any feelings of heaviness before or after meals or constipation. If you're particularly susceptible to the cold, this will change your life (and the lives of the people around you). This is great for sipping throughout the day. I often make a double or triple recipe and keep it in a warm cup. **Serves 1**

What's in it:

- 2 cups pure water
- 1 cinnamon stick
- 2 cardamom pods
- 1 star anise
- ½ inch piece of orange peel
- ½ inch piece of lemon peel
- small slice of ginger
- honey to taste (optional)

How to make it:

- Bring water to a boil (or boil in kettle). Add spices and ginger to a cup or teapot.
- Cover with boiling water and allow to steep for 3-5 minutes.
- Allow to cool before adding honey.

Turmeric Cold & Flu Elixir
-V -P -K

The bitter and pungent qualities of turmeric make it great for cleansing the channels and warming the body from the inside out. And when you add the additional warming and soothing qualities of honey, ginger, and cinnamon, it makes a perfect combination for calming inflammation (as in sore throats, allergies, and some infections), and clearing the sinuses with the added bonus of being a great booster for immunity! This simple, luscious elixir is something you can make and take ahead of the first sniffle or cough, or as soon as you start to feel a tickle.

What's in it:

- 1 tablespoon finely ground dried turmeric
- 3- 4 tablespoons local raw honey
- 1 teaspoon dried ginger powder
- 1 teaspoon black pepper (finely ground)

How to make it:

- In a small bowl with a lid, whisk spices together to combine fully. Add honey and mix completely to combine.
- Store spiced honey in a cool, dry place.

To Use:
- Cold and flu tonic - Mix 1 teaspoon of elixir with warm water and a tsp of lemon juice.
- Preventative jam - Enjoy as a spread on toast or bread.
- Immunity building elixir - Mix 1 teaspoon with 1 cup of warm milk.

*Can also be added to smoothies!

Vitality Boosting Elixir
-V -P +K

Ojas is a Sanskrit word that translates to mean vigor or vitality. And it's sometimes referred to as our natural honey. Ojas is a major factor in our immune system function as well as the healthy functioning of our endocrine, nervous, and digestive systems. It is considered vital to our experience of wellness, vitality, and "juiciness"! *Serves 2*

What's in it:

- 10 raw almonds, soaked (overnight) and peeled
- 1 cup pure water
- 1 cup milk (nut, soy, cow)
- 3-4 dates (pitted)
- 1 tablespoon. organic rose petals (dried or fresh)
- ⅛ teaspoon ground cardamom
- ⅛ teaspoon ground ginger powder
- 1 tablespoon. honey
- pinch of saffron (optional)

How to make it:

- Soak dates in 1 cup of water either overnight or for several hours.
- In a blender, add the dates AND their soaking water with the drained and peeled almonds.
- Add rose petals, honey, saffron, cardamom, and ginger. Blend until smooth.

Yogi Breakfast
-*V* -*P* -*K*

Ayurvedic cleansing day begins before dawn - Brahmamurhuta (Sanskrit for "The Godly hour") - sacred time for yogis - peace, purity, calm pervades. Digestion is like the sun, low and slow. Lemon with water is great to kickstart your digestion, followed by this light and lovely breakfast. This one is a real crowd pleaser! ***Serves 1***

What's in it:

- 8 almonds (soaked, peeled)
- 1 cup soy milk, almond milk, or rice milk
- pinch nutmeg
- pinch cinnamon
- pinch cardamom
- pinch turmeric
- pinch ginger
- 1 teaspoon ghee (optional)
- 1 teaspoon honey (optional)

How to make it:

- Place the almonds in the bottom of a small pan. Pour the milk over and heat on low until milk is warm and bubbles just on the edge. Whisk in spices and remove from heat.
- Pour into a mug and allow it to cool before adding honey.

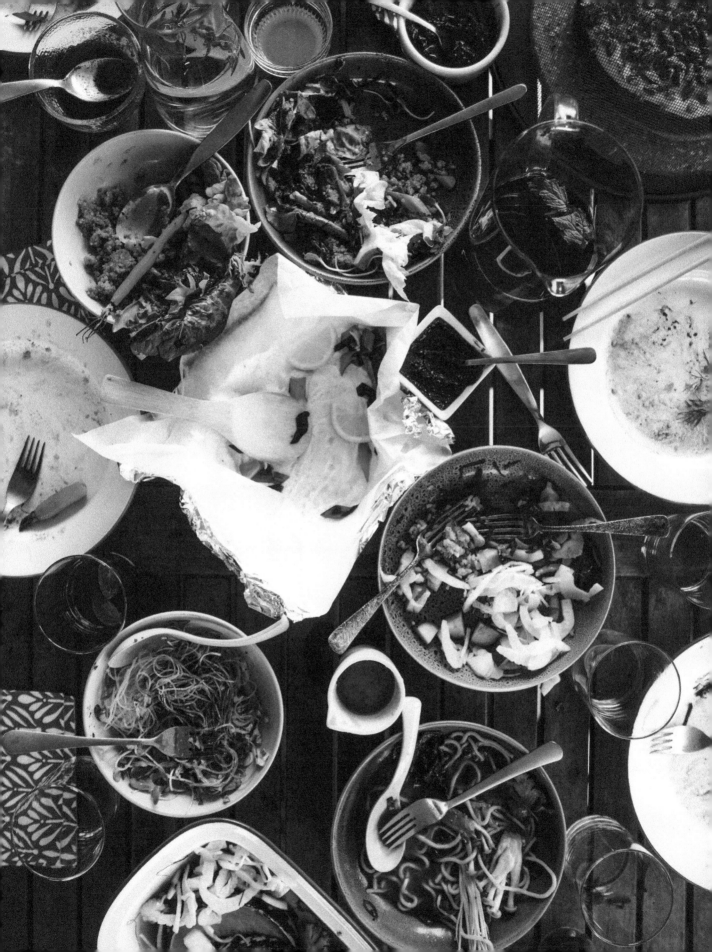

Appendices

- Ayurvedic Pantry Items
- Recipes For Healing
- Shopping Lists (For Each Season)
- Seasonal Foods And Produce Lists
- Food Combining Guidelines
- Food Qualities List
- Ama Test
- Dosha Test
- One Day Detox Guide

Grains

Rolled oats
Basmati rice
Brown rice
Quinoa
Millet
Cornmeal
Buckwheat
Couscous
Amaranth

Legumes

Mung Dal (green)
Split mung dal (yellow)
Aduki beans
Pinto beans
Red lentils
Kidney beans
Chickpeas

Condiments

Soy sauce
Harissa
Apple cider vinegar
White vinegar
Dijon mustard
Chutney
Tahini

Herbs & Spices

Cumin
Coriander seed
Cardamom
Fennel seed
Ginger
Turmeric
Black pepper
Cinnamon
Paprika
Star anise
Nutmeg
Red pepper flakes
Asafoetida (hing)
Himalayan pink salt

Seeds & nuts

Almonds (whole raw)
Cashews([whole raw)
Coconut (unsweetened, flaked)
Chia seeds
Flax seeds
Sesame seeds
Popcorn [organic kernels]

Oils

Sesame oil [non-toasted]

Olive oil
Ghee
Coconut oil
Sunflower
Butter (fresh, organic)

Teas & Herbal Teas

Dandelion
Hibiscus
Black tea
Green tea
Jasmine tea

Sweeteners

Honey [raw local is best]
Jaggery
Maple syrup
Molasses
Rice syrup
Coconut sugar
Raw cane sugar

Supplements

Aloe vera juice
Vitamin C
Triphala
Shilajit
Ashwaghanda

Recipes for healing
Ayurvedic home remedies from your kitchen and garden

Please note that the information provided here should not be considered medical advice. This information has been provided for educational purposes only. I make no clairms of the particular healing qualities or efficacy of these recipes as they relate to any specific symptoms or issues you may be experiencing. So please be sure to consult with your health professional before following any of the advice in this book.

Common issue	Generally Suggested remedy
Acne	**Turmeric Sandalwood** - Mix ½ tsp each of turmeric and sandalwood powder with purified water to make a paste. Apply to affected area 2x/day. **Diet:** Avoid sugar, sweets, starchy, greasy foods. Choose leafy greens, fermented foods, turmeric.
Anger/hostility	**Oiling** - Rub coconut oil on the scalp and soles of the feet; **Cooling drink** - 1 cup of grape juice with ½ teaspoon cumin, ½ teaspoon fennel, and ½ teaspoon sandalwood powder; **Nasya** - 2-3 drops of liquified ghee in the nose (ensure it is not hot)
Anxiety	**Ginger bath** - Warm bath with ⅓ cup ground ginger and ⅓ cup baking soda.
Backaches	**Ginger paste + oil** - Make a paste from ground ginger and purified water and apply to the area. Then rub the area with eucalyptus oil.
Bites and stings (insects)	**Coriander (cilantro) juice** - blend a handful of leaves with ⅓ cup of water. Strain and drink the juice and apply the pulp to the sting.
Burns	**Aloe turmeric** - Mix fresh aloe gel with a pinch of turmeric to make a paste. Apply to the burned area. Ghee or Coconut oil - Apply ghee or coconut oil to the area.
Common colds/flu	**Ginger cinnamon teas** - 1 tsp cinnamon + 1 tbsp fresh grated ginger + 1 tsp licorice - boil in 4 cups of water for 10 mins (drink 1 cup 3x/day); OR ½ tsp ginger + ½ tsp cinnamon + 1 tsp lemon grass in 1 cup of hot water (steep for 10 mins); **Diet:** Avoid dairy, sugary foods, deep fried foods, choose ginger, tulsi, garlic, cayenne, oregano taken with honey.
Cold sores	**Turmeric and honey paste** - 1 tsp honey + ¼ tsp turmeric - apply to the sore.
Conjunctivitis	**Coriander tea** - 1 tsp coriander seeds in 1 cup of hot water. Steep and allow to cool. Apply to closed eyes with cotton ball. **Goat milk compress** - Sterile cotton ball in goat's milk, apply to closed eye.

Common issue	Generally Suggested remedy
Constipation	**Mild:** 1 tsp ghee in a cup of warm milk before bed. **Moderate:** Boil 1 tbsp flax seeds in 1 cup of water. Drink. Severe: Warm water enema, followed by a focus on prevention **Diet:** Avoid junk food, deep fried foods; Choose fatty soups, stews, garlic, fennel, ginger, fermented foods.
Cough	**Dry cough** - chew ¼ teaspoon ajwain seeds mixed with 1 teaspoon of organic raw sugar. **Banana honey** - Ripe banana with 1 tsp honey and 2 pinches finely ground black pepper.
Congested sinuses	**Ginger paste:** Make a paste with ground ginger and purified water. Apply the paste to the affected area (external only). **Ginger honey** - Mix 1 tsp fresh ginger juice (or grated fresh ginger) with 1 tsp honey. Take 2-3x per day.
Dehydration	**Lime wate**r - Add 1 tsp lime juice, 1 tsp raw cane sugar, a pinch of salt to 2 cups of room temp water and sip throughout the day.
Diarrhea	**Spiced apple** - Cook 1 apple with a little water until it is soft. Add 1 tsp ghee, a pinch of cardamom, and a pinch of nutmeg; **Yogurt and ginger** - ½ cup yogurt + ½ cup water + ⅛ tsp fresh grated ginger. Drink. **Diet:** Avoid spicy, greasy food, choose broths, light rice dishes (kitchari, rice soups), choose fennel, ginger, cardamom, asafoetida, cinnamon, coriander, rock salt.
Earache	**Garlic oil** - Gently heat 2 tbsp of sesame oil with 2 whole garlic cloves until the cloves become lightly brown. Add a drop of oil to affected ear.
Eyes (red or burning)	**Rosewater eye wash** - 2 tbsp purified water + 5 drops of rosewater (NOT rose essential oil) - Rinse the eyes using an eye cup.
Gas (bloating)	**Cumin-fennel-ajwan** - Combine 1 tsp each of cumin, fennel, and ajwan seeds. Chew ½ tsp of the seed mix, follow with a ½ cup of water. **Cardamom - fennel - ginger** - Make a tea with equal parts of each herb - add 1 tsp of the tea to 1 cup of fresh water + pinch of asafoetida.

Common issue	Generally Suggested remedy
Heartburn/acid indigestion	**Aloe vera** - 2 tbsp aloe vera gel with pinch of baking soda; **Papaya Juice** - 1 cup papaya juice + 1 tsp raw organic sugar + ¼ tsp cardamom [NOT for PREGNANT WOMEN] **Diet:** Avoid hard to digest foods, sweets, greasy foods, alcohol and spicy herbs (garlic, peppermint, ginger). Choose simple rice dishes and light soups, high fiber
Hangover	**Spiced orange juice:** 1 glass of orange juice + 1 tsp lime juice + pinch of ground cumin. **Soothing lassi:** I tbsp fresh plain yogurt + 1 cup of fresh water + pinch of cumin (drink 3-4x/day); **Rehydration Lime drink** :1 glass of water with 1 tsp lime juice + ½ tsp sugar + a pinch of salt. Add ½ tsp baking soda just before drinking.
Headaches	**Vata type [Back of the head (occipital)]: Massage** - Sesame oil to the back of the neck followed by a warm shower; **Nasya** - 2-3 drops liquified ghee in the nose; **Pitta [temporal]: Aloe vera gel:** 2 tbsps 3x/day; **Cumin coriander tea** - ½ tsp of each in 1 cup of hot water - allow to cool before drinking. **Kapha[sinuses] - Ginger paste** - make a paste from ground ginger and water. Apply to sinuses area (external); **Neti pot** - Saline flush of the sinuses; **Cinnamon paste** - ½ tsp of cinnamon with water. Apply to sinuses area
Hemorrhoids	**Aloe vera drink:** ½ tbsp aloe gel in water or ½ cup aloe juice with a pinch of ginger, 2x/day. **Carrot Coriander:** 1 cup carrot juice mixed with 2 tsp coriander leaf (cilantro) juice 2x/day on an empty stomach.
Insomnia	**Nutmeg milk** - Add ⅛ tsp nutmeg to 1 cup of warm milk. **Oil massage** - Massage the scalp and soles of the feet with warm sesame oil before bed.
Jet lag	**Before flying:** 2 capsules of ground ginger; **In-flight:** Drink plenty of water (2-3 cups every 1-2 hrs), avoid coffee/caffeine; **In destination:** Massage feet and scalp with sesame oil, warm milk with pinch of nutmeg + pinch of ginger.
Muscle strain	**Ginger turmeric paste:** Make a paste with 1 tsp of ground ginger + ½ tsp of ground turmeric + purified water. Apply to the affected area 2x/day.

Common issue	Generally Suggested remedy
PMS/Menstrual cramps	**Aloe black pepper:** 1 tbsp aloe vera gel + ¼ black pepper 3x/day; **Roasted cumin seeds:** Dry roast 1 tsp of cumin seeds, cool them and chew them slowly, follow with a tbsp of aloe vera juice. **Diet:** Choose omega-3 rich foods, high fat, high protein foods. Reduce sugary, deep fried, or processed foods. Choose turmeric, ginger, rose.
Rash	**Coriander leaf pulp:** Make a pulp from a handful of coriander (cilantro) leaves. Apply to the affected area; **Coriander tea:** Drink tea made from 1 tsp of coriander seeds steeped in 1 cup of water.
Sore Throat	**Gargle:** Add ½ tsp ground turmeric + ½ tsp salt to 1 cup of warm water. Gargle morning and evening; **Turmeric milk** - 1 cup hot milk + ½ tsp ground turmeric. Drink.
Sunburn	**Coconut oil:** Apply directly to the affected area; **Milk:** Apply cows milk or goat's milk to affected area (use a gauze pad); **Lettuce pulp** - Mash lettuce in a mortar and pestle. Apply to the affected areas.
Toothache	**Clove or tea tree oil:** Use a cotton bud to apply a drop or two of clove or tea tree oil to the affected area.
Yeast infection	Avoid sugar, fermented foods, yeast breads; Licorice tea douche: 1 tbsp ground licorice + 1 liter water - boil, cool, strain, douche.

Seasonal Foods & Produce

Not sure what's seasonal where you are? No farmer's market near enough to visit on a regular basis? Here's a list of seasonal produce and pantry items that you can use as a guide for supermarket shopping and meal planning.

Autumn/Early Winter

VEGETABLES

Cook all vegetables and add a healthy oil, such as ghee, and warming spices. Favor root vegetables:

Artichokes, hearts
Avocadoes
Beets
Brussels Sprouts
Carrots
Chilis
Corn
Fennel
Eggplant, cooked
Garlic
Ginger
Hot Peppers
Leeks
Okra
Onions
Parsley
Potatoes, mashed
Pumpkins
Seaweed, cooked
Squash, Acorn
Squash, Winter
Sweet Potatoes
Tomatoes
Turnips

OILS

Almond
Avocado
Canola
Coconut
Flax
Mustard
Olive
Peanut
Safflower
Sesame
Sunflower

FRUITS

Favor sweet, sour or heavy fruits. Eat fruit separately from other foods. Serve warm:

Apples, cooked
Apricots
Bananas
Blueberries
Cantaloupe, with lemon
Cherries
Coconuts, ripe
Cranberries, cooked
Dates
Figs
Grapefruit
Grapes
Guava
Lemons
Limes
Mangoes
Nectarines
Oranges
Papayas
Peaches
Pears, ripe
Persimmons
Pineapples
Plums
Prunes (soaked)
Raisins (soaked or cooked)
Strawberries
Tangerines

MEAT & FISH

All meat, eggs and fish are good:

Beef
Chicken
Crabs
Duck
Eggs
Fish, freshwater & ocean
Lamb
Lobster
Oysters
Pork
Shrimp
Turkey
Venison

SPICES

Most spices and herbs are good, hotter spices are best in moderation.

Anise
Asafetida
Basil
Bay Leaf
Black Pepper
Caraway
Cardamom
Cayenne
Chamomile
Cinnamon
Clove
Coriander
Cumin
Dill
Fennel
Fenugreek
Garlic
Ginger
Horseradish
Marjoram
Mustard
Nutmeg
Oregano
Peppermint
Poppy Seeds
Rosemary
Saffron
Sage
Spearmint
Tarragon
Thyme
Turmeric

CONDIMENTS

Favor sweet, sour and salty tastes

Carob
Dulse
Fermented foods
Lemon or Lime
Mayonnaise
Pickles
Salt
Vinegar

NUTS & SEEDS

Most nuts and seeds are good:

Almonds
Brazil Nuts
Cashews
Filberts
Flax seeds
Lotus Seed
Macadamias
Peanuts, raw
Pecans
Pinons/Pine nuts
Pistachios
Pumpkin seeds (pepitas)
Sunflower seeds
Walnuts

DAIRY

All dairy is good, ideally at room temperature or warm (such as boiled milk). Favor raw or vat-pasteurized.

Butter
Buttermilk
Cheese
Cottage cheese
Cream
Ghee
Kefir Milk, not cold
Non-Dairy substitutes
Sour Cream
Yogurt

SWEETENERS

Most natural whole foods sweeteners, in moderation:

Honey - Raw
Jaggery
Maple Syrup
Molasses Sugar, Raw
Rice Syrup

LEGUMES

Mung – split, yellow
Tofu

BEVERAGES

Favor warm-hot drinks that are low in caffeine and alcohol:

Alcohol (moderation)
Black Tea (moderation)
Coffee (moderation)
Water (warm or hot)

HERB TEAS

Choose warming and/or calming teas, such as:

Cardamom
Chamomile
Cinnamon
Cloves
Ginger
Orange Peel

WHOLE GRAINS

Most grains are good. Best eaten warm, moist and with a healthy oil:

Amaranth
Buckwheat (moderation)
Millet (moderation)
Oats
Quinoa
Rice
Rice, Brown
Rye (moderation)
Wheat

Late Winter/Spring

VEGETABLES

Warm/cooked is best. Avoid preparing these with creamy, cheesy dressings or sauces.

Alfalfa Sprouts
Artichokes
Asparagus
Bean Sprouts
Beets
Bell Peppers
Bitter Melon
Broccoli
Brussels Sprouts
Cabbage
Carrots
Cauliflower
Celery
Chicory
Chilies, dried
Cilantro
Collard Greens
Corn
Dandelion
Endive
Fennel
Garlic
Ginger
Green Beans
Hot Peppers
Jicama
Kale
Leeks
Lettuce
Mushrooms
Mustard Greens
Onions
Parsley
Peas
Potatoes, baked
Radishes
Seaweed
Snow Peas
Spinach
Swiss Chard
Turnips
Watercress

FRUIT

Warm or cooked is great. Can also do raw fruits that are ripe (eaten on their own)

Apples
Blueberries
Dried Fruit (all)
Grapefruit
Lemons, Limes
Papayas
Pears
Pomegranates (sour)
Raspberries
Strawberries
All Berries

DAIRY

Favor raw or vat pasteurized.

Ghee (moderation)
Low Fat yogurt (moderation)
Rice/Soy milk
Goat milk

OILS

Flax
Hemp
Sunflower
Coconut Oil

SWEETENERS

Favor natural whole foods sweeteners, in moderation:

Honey - Raw, local if possible
Maple Syrup
Molasses

HERBS & SPICES

Anise
Asafoetida
Basil
Bay Leaf

Black Pepper
Chamomile
Caraway
Cardamom
Cayenne
Cinnamon
Clove
Coriander
Cumin
Dill
Fennel
Fenugreek
Garlic
Ginger
Horseradish
Marjoram
Mustard
Nutmeg
Oregano
Peppermint
Poppy Seeds
Rosemary
Saffron
Sage
Spearmint
Thyme
Turmeric

CONDIMENTS

Carob
Pickles

BEANS & LEGUMES

All Sprouted Beans
Adzuki
Black

Gram
Garbanzo
Fava
Kidney
Lentils
Lima
Mung
Split Pea

LEAN MEAT & FISH

Chicken
Duck (moderation)
Eggs (moderation)
Freshwater fish
Lamb (moderation)
Ocean fish (moderation)
Turkey

NUTS & SEEDS

Filberts
Pine nuts
Pumpkin seeds
Sunflower seeds

WHOLE GRAINS

Amaranth
Barley
Buckwheat
Corn
Millet
Oats, dry
Quinoa
Rice, Brown, long grain
Rye Alfalfa

HERBAL TEAS

Cardamom
Chicory
Cinnamon
Cloves
Dandelion
Ginger
Hibiscus
Orange Peel
Strawberry Leaf

BEVERAGES

Black Tea (moderation)
Coffee (moderation)
Water (room temp. to hot)

Summary

VEGETABLES

Alfalfa Sprouts
Artichokes
Asparagus
Avocados
Bean Sprouts
Beet greens
Bell Peppers
Bitter Melon
Broccoli
Cabbage
Cauliflower
Celery
Chicory
Cilantro
Collard Greens
Corn
Cucumbers
Dandelion
Eggplant
Endive
Fennel
Green Beans
Jicama
Kale
Lettuce
Mushrooms
Mustard Greens
Okra
Parsley
Peas
Pumpkin
Radishes (moderation)
Seaweed
Snow Peas
Spinach (moderation)
Squash, Acorn Squash, Winter
Sweet Potatoes
Swiss Chard
Tomatoes (sweet)
Turnip Greens
Watercress
Zucchini

FRUIT:

Cooked and cooled is best. Raw fruit okay. Preferably eaten on it's own

Apples
Apricots
Blueberries
Cantaloupe
Cherries (ripe)
Cranberries
Coconut
Dates
Dried Fruit
Figs
Grapes
Guavas
Mangoes
Melon
Nectarines
Oranges
Papayas (small amounts)
Peaches (ripe and/or peeled)
Pears
Persimmons
Pineapple (sweet)
Plums (ripe)
Pomegranates
Raspberries
Strawberries
Tangerines

MEATS

Beef (moderation)
Chicken
Duck (moderation)
Eggs (moderation)
Freshwater Fish
Lamb (moderation)
Pork
Shrimp (moderation)
Turkey

BEANS & LEGUMES

Adzuki
Bean Sprouts
Black Gram
Fava
Garbanzo
Kidney
Lentils
Lima
Mung
Split Pea
Tofu

CONDIMENTS

Carob
Mayonnaise
Sweet mango chutney
Tamari

OILS

Sunflower
Avocado
Coconut
Flax
Olive
Ghee

HERBS & SPICES

Anise
Asafoetida
Chamomile
Coriander
Cinnamon
Ginger (fresh)
Saffron
Cumin
Fennel
Peppermint
Saffron
Spearmint

WHOLE GRAINS

Barley
Oat
Rice
Rye
Wheat
Chicory
Dandelion
Hibiscus
Mint

BEVERAGES

Water (room temp or cool)
Coconut water
Fruit juices (apple, grape, berry, apricot, peach, pear, mango, cherry, pomegranate)
Grain coffee
Dandelion "coffee"
Aloe vera juice

SWEETENERS

Favor natural whole foods sweeteners, in moderation:

Maple Syrup (small amounts)
Raw Sugar
Rice Syrup

NUTS & SEEDS

Almonds
Flax
Macadamias
Pine Nuts
Pumpkin seeds
Sunflower seeds

DAIRY

Favor raw and vat-pasteurized.

Butter
Cheese (moderation)
Cottage Cheese
Ghee
Ice Cream
Milk
Rice/Soy Milk

Food Combining Guidelines

According to Ayurveda, each food has its own taste, energy and effect. Combining foods who's qualities or effects aggravate or intensify each other can challenge and compromise the digestive system. For that reason it's important to pay attention to how you feel before and after eating and to consider the chart below when it comes to combining foods.

Since each individual's capacity for digesting is different, the potential impacts of "bad combinations" will vary as well (so don't worry). The effects of bad combinations can be lessened if:

- *You have a strong digestive fire. If your digestion is healthy and strong eating incompatible foods is less likely to cause issues.*

- *Suitable spices are added to foods in order to balance some of the intense or aggravating qualities*

- *Your body is accustomed to eating the incompatible combination.*

- *The incompatible combinations are eaten only occasionally.*

	Avoid combining it with:
Beans	Fruit, milk, cheese, yogurt, eggs, meat, fish
Cheese	Fruit, beans, eggs, milk, yogurt, hot drinks
Milk	Bananas, melons, sour fruits, yeasted breads, eggs, yogurt, meat, fish, starches)
Yogurt	Fruit, beans, milk, cheese, eggs, meat, fish, nightshades, hot drinks
Eggs	Milk, cheese, yogurt, fruit (especially melons), beans, kitchari, potatoes, meat, fish
Fruits	Any other food (aside from other fruit) *Exceptions: dates with milk, some cooked combinations
Lemons	Cucumbers, tomatoes, milk, yogurt Note: lime can be substituted for use with cucumbers and tomatoes.
Melons	Everything - Should be eaten alone or not at all.
Grains	Fruit
Nightshades *i.e. potatoes, tomatoes.*	Melon, cucumber, dairy

Ayurvedic Resources

Looking for up-to-date Ayurvedic resource information?

In order to give you access to the most up to date information possible I've put together a comprehensive list of providers of Ayurvedic foods, herbs, skin and beauty care products, books, services and education over on my website!

And unlike a book, this information is being updated regularly to ensure that it's current and relevant to your interests and needs!

Eat Like You Love Yourself
Ayurvedic Resources
Check out the website for up-to-date Ayurvedic resources information!
http://www.eatlikeyouloveyourself.com/ Ayurvedic-Resources

Food Qualities Guidelines:

The qualities of the foods we eat make a different to how they impact our state of balance and wellness. Understanding the actions and effects of the foods we eat isn't always intuitive but can be cultivated through awareness, presence and a little bit of study.

The purpose of this guide is to provide a foundation for your personal study of the impacts that your food has on your mind, body and doshas! Use it to confirm your experience and understanding OR to gain some insights into why your food makes you look and feel the way it does!

Overtime you'll gain a more intuitive approach to choosing the foods you eat every day and to new foods. So enjoy the process of discovery and take it on as a lifelong study of yourself and your food!

And for a more detailed guide to the foods in the list including their actions and medicinal properties jump over to my website to download the ***"Food as Medicine Reference Guide"***

Fruit

Fruit is generally sweet, sour and sometimes astringent. In general fruits tend to calm vata and pitta and increase kapha. Fruit can be eaten in many different ways to impact the doshas. Dry is best for kapha, cooked is best for vata and raw is best for pitta. The cooling and heavy qualities of fruit can be countered with appropriate warming spices like ginger, cinnamon and cardamom. **Combining:** Fruit is best eaten alone, but can be taken with whole grains. Sweet fruits, like apples, are fine with milk and yogurt.

Fruit	Rasa (taste)	Gunas	Actions
Amla	Sour, Astringent, Sweet	Cold, Light, Dry	**VPK**:Balances **K**:Moderation
Apples	Sweet, Astringent, Sour	Cold, Light, Dry	**P**: Balances **V,K**:Moderation (best cooked with spices for vata)
Apricot	Sweet, Sour	Cold, Light, Wet	**V,P**:Balances, **K**:Moderation
Banana	Sweet, Astringent	Cold, Heavy, Wet	**V,P**: Balances **K**:Moderation
Blackberry	Sweet, Sour, Astringent	Cold, Light, Wet	**VP**: Balances **K**:Moderation
Blueberry	Sweet, Astringent	Cool, Light, Wet	**VPK**: Balances
Cantelope	Sweet, Sour	Cool, Light	**PV**: Balances **K**:Aggravates
Cherry	Sweet, Sour	Cool, Light, Wet	**V**: Balances **P**:Aggravates
Coconut	Sweet	Cool, Heavy, Wet	**VP**: Balances **K**:Aggravates
Cranberry	Sour, Astringent	Cool, Light, Dry	**PK**: Balances **V**:Aggravates
Currant	Sweet, Sour	Cool, Light, Wet	**PK**: Balances **V**:Aggravates
Date	Sweet	Cool, Heavy, Wet	**VP**: Balances **K**:Aggravates
Elderberry	Sour, Bitter, Sweet	Cool, Light, Dry	**PK**: Balances **V**:Aggravates
Fig	Sweet	Cool, Heavy, Wet	**VP**: Balances **K**:Aggravates
Fig	Sweet	Cool, Heavy, Wet	**VP**: Balances **K**:Aggravates
Grapefruit	Sour, Sweet	Hot, Light, Wet	**K**:Balances **V,P**:Aggravates
Guava	Sweet, Sour	Cool, Light, Dry	**PK**: Balances **V**:Aggravates
Hoenydew (Rockmelon)	Sweet	Cool, Heavy, Wet	**VP**: Balances **K**:Aggravates

Fruit	Rasa (taste)	Gunas	Actions
Kiwi	Sweet, Sour	Cool, Light, Wet	**VP:** Balances **K:**Aggravates
Kumquat	Sweet, Sour	Hot, Light, Dry	**VK;** Balances **P:**Aggravates
Lemon	Sour, Bitter	Hot, Light, Wet	**KV:** Balances **P:**Aggravates
Lime	Sour, Bitter	Hot, Light, Wet	**PK:** Balances **V:** Neutral
Lychee	Sweet	Cool, Heavy, Wet	**V:** Balances **K,P:**Aggravates
Mango	Sweet	Cool, Heavy, Wet	**VP;** Balances **K:**Aggravates
Mulberry	Sweet	Cool, Light, Wet	**VP:** Balances **K:**Aggravates
Orange (Sweet)	Sweet, Sour	Hot, Light, Wet	**VP:** Balances **K:**Aggravates
Papaya	Sweet	Hot, Light,Wet	**VK:** Balances **P:**Aggravates
Passionfruit	Sweet, Sour	Cool, Light, Wet	**VP:** Balances; **K:** Neutral
Peach	Sweet	Cool, Light, Wet	**VP:** Balances **K:**Aggravates
Pear	Sweet	Cool, Light, Wet	**VP:** Balances **K:**Aggravates
Persimmon	Sweet	Cool, Heavy, Wet	**VP:** Balances **K:**Aggravates
Pineapple	Sweet, Sour	Hot, Light, Wet	**VP:** Balances **K:**Aggravates
Plum	Sweet, Sour, Bitter	Cool	**VP:** Balances **P:**(Moderation) **K:**Aggravates
Pomegranate	Sweet, Astringent	Cool, Light, Wet	**VP;** Balances; **K:** Neutral
Pomello	Sweet, Sour	Cool, Heavy, Wet	**VP:** Balances **K:**Aggravates
Quince	Sour, Sweet, Astringent	Cool, Light, Dry	**PK:** Balances **V:**Aggravates
Raspberry	Sweet, Sour	Cool, Light, Wet	**VP;** Balances **K:**Aggravates
Rhubarb	Sour, Sweet, Bitter, Astringent	Cool, Heavy, Wet	**VPK:** Balances
Strawberry	Sweet, Sour	Cool, Light, Wet	**V:** Balances **P:**Aggravates; **K:** Neutral
Tamarind	Sour	Hot, Light, Dry	**PK:** Balances; **V;** Neutral
Tangerines/ Mandarins	Sweet, Sour	Hot	**V:** Balances **P:**Aggravates **K:**Moderation
Watermelon	Sweet	Cool, Dry, Light	**VP:** Balances **K:**Aggravates

Vegetables

Vegetables tend to be pleasant and not too strong in flavor. They're a pretty diverse group and range from light and bitter (leafy greens, cruciferous veggies to heavy and sweet (root veggies), to pungent (chillies, onions, etc.). Vegetables are best in their appropriate seasons and the cold, rough nature of raw vegetables can be countered by cooking along with the use of appropriate warming spices like ginger, cayenne and oils. **Combining**: Vegetables combine well with grains, beans and most other foods, except fruit.

Vegetables	Taste (rasa)r	Qualities	Actions
Acorn Squash	Sweet	Cool	**VP**: Balances **K**:Aggravates
Alfalfa Sprouts	Astringent, Sweet, Pungent	Cool	**PK**: Balances **V**:Aggravates
Artichoke	Bitter, Sweet	Cool, Light, Wet	**KP**; Balances **V**:Aggravates
Arugula	Bitter	Cool, Light, Wet	**KP**: Balances **V**:Aggravates
Asparagus	Sweet, Bitter	Cool, Heavy, Wet	**VP**: Balances **K**:Aggravates
Avocado	Sweet	Cool, Heavy, Wet	**VP**: Balances **K**:Aggravates
Bamboo Shoot	Sweet, Bitter	Cool, Heavy, Wet	**VP**: Balances **K**:Aggravates
Bean Sprouts (Mung)	Astringent, Sweet	Cool	**PK**: Balances **V**:Aggravates
Beet Greens	Bitter	Cool, Light Wet	**KP**; Balances **V**:Aggravates
Beet Root	Sweet, Bitter	Cool, Heavy, Wet	**VPK**; Neutral
Bell Pepper (Capisicum)	Sweet, Pungent	Hot, Light, Wet	**VK**: Balances; **P**: Neutral
Bitter Gourd	Bitter	Cool, Light, Dry	**PK**: Balances **V**:Aggravates
Bok Choy	Bitter	Cool, Light, Dry	**KP**: Balances **V**:Aggravates
Broccoli	Bitter	Cool, Light, Dry	**KP**: Balances **V**:Aggravates
Brussels Sprout	Bitter	Cool, Light, Dry	**KP**: Balances **V**:Aggravates

Vegetables	Taste (rasa)r	Qualities	Actions
Cabbage	Bitter, Pungent	Cool, Light, Dry	**KP:** Balances **V:**Aggravates
Carrot	Sweet, Bitter	Hot, Light, Wet	**VK:** Balances; **P:** Neutral
Cassava	Sweet, Bitter	Hot, Heavy, Wet	**VPK:** Aggravates
Cauliflower	Bitter	Cool, Light, Dry	**KP:** Balances **V:**Aggravates
Celery	Salty	Cool, Heavy, Wet	**VPK:** Neutral
Chilies	Pungent	Hot	**KV:** Balances **P:**Aggravates
Chard	Bitter	Cool, Light, Dry	**KP:** Balances **V:**Aggravates
Chickweed	Bitter	Cool, Light, Dry	**KP:** Balances **V:**Aggravates
Chives	Pungent	Hot, Light, Wet	**K:** Balances **V,P:**Aggravates
Cilantro (Fresh Coriander)	Pungent	Cool	**P:** Balances **V:**Aggravates (in excess) **K:** Neutral
Collard Greens	Bitter	Cool, Light, Dry	**KP:** Balances **V:**Aggravates
Corn (Sweet)	Sweet	Cool, Heavy, Dry	**P:** Balances **VK:**Aggravates
Cucumber	Sweet, Bitter	Cool, Heavy, Wet	**VP:** Balances **K:**Aggravates
Daikon	Pungent	Hot, Light, Dry	**K:** Balances **VP:**Aggravates
Dandelion	Bitter	Cool, Light, Dry	**KP:** Balances **V:**Aggravates
Eggplant	Sweet, Pungent	Hot, Light, Dry	**VK:** Balances **P:**Aggravates
Endive	Bitter	Cool, Light, Dry	**KP:** Balances **V:**Aggravates
Gai lan	Bitter	Cool, Light, Dry	**KP:** Balances **V:**Aggravates
Garlic	Pungent, Sweet	Hot, Heavy, Wet	**VK:** Balances **P:**Aggravates
Ginger	Pungent	Hot, Light, Dry	**VK:** Balances **P:**Aggravates
Kale	Bitter	Cool, Light, Dry	**KP:** Balances **V:**Aggravates
Kohlrabi	Sweet, Bitter	Cool, Light, Dry	**KP:** Balances **V:**Aggravates

Vegetables	Taste (rasa)r	Qualities	Actions
Lambsquarters	Bitter	Cool, Light, Dry	**PK:** Balances **V:**Aggravates
Leek	Pungent, Sweet	Hot, Light, Wet	**VK:** Balances **P:**Aggravates
Lettuce	Bitter	Cool, Light Dry	**KP:** Balances **V:**Aggravates
Lotus Root	Sweet, Astringent	Cool, Light, Dry	**P:** Balances **VK:**Aggravates
Mushroom	Sweet	Cool, Heavy, Wet	**PV:** Balances **K:**Aggravates
Mustard	Pungent, Bitter	Hot, Light, Dry	**K:** Balances **VP:**Aggravates
Nettle	Bitter, Astringent	Cool, Light, Dry	**PK:** Balances **V:**Aggravates
Okra (Lady Finger)	Sweet	Cool	**PV:** Balances **K:**Aggravates
Onion	Pungent, Sweet	Hot, Heavy, Wet	**VK:** Balances **P:**Aggravates
Pak Choy	Bitter	Cool, Light, Dry	**PK:** Balances **V:**Aggravates
Parsley	Pungent, Astringent	Hot	**KV:** Balances **K:**(Aggravates in excess) **P:** Aggravates
Parsnip	Sweet, Bitter	Hot, Heavy, Dry	**K:** Balances **VP:**Aggravates
Peas/Snow Peas	Sweet, Astringent	Cool	**PK:** Balances **V:**Aggravates
Pea Sprouts	Bitter	Cool, Light, Dry	**PK:** Balances **V:**Aggravates
Potato	Sweet, Astringent	Hot, Heavy, Dry	**V:** Balances **PK:**Aggravates
Pumpkin	Sweet	Hot, Heavy, Wet	**V:** Balances **PK:**Aggravates
Purslane	Sour	Hot, Light, Dry	**PK:** Balances **V:**Aggravates
Radicchio	Bitter	Cool, Light, Dry	**PK:** Balances **V:**Aggravates
Radish	Pungent, Sweet	Hot, Light, Dry	**K:** Balances **VP:**Aggravates
Rutabaga, Turnip	Sweet, Pungent, Bitter	Cool, Light, Dry	**PK:** Balances **V:**Aggravates
Sea Vegetables	Salty	Hot, Heavy, Wet	**VK:** Balances **P:**Aggravates

Vegetables	Taste (rasa)r	Qualities	Actions
Shallot	Pungent, Sweet	Hot, Light, Wet	**VK;** Balances **P:**Aggravates
Sorrel	Sour	Hot, Light, Dry	**VK:** Balances **P:**Aggravates
Spinach/Chard	Sour, Bitter	Cool, Light, Dry	**P:** Balances **VK:**Aggravates
Sui Choy	Bitter, Sweet	Cool, Light, Dry	**PK:** Balances **V:**Aggravates
Sunflower Sprouts	Bitter, Sweet, Astringent	Cool, Light, Dry	**PK:** Balances **V:**Aggravates
Sweet Potato	Sweet	Cool, Heavy, Wet	**VP:** Balances **K:**Aggravates
Taro	Sweet, Pungent	Cool, Heavy, Wet	**PK:** Balances; **V:** Neutral
Tomatillo	Sour, Pungent	Hot, Light, Wet	**VK:** Balances **P:**Aggravates
Tomato	Sweet, Sour, Pungent	Hot, Light, Wet	**VK:** Balances **P:**Aggravates
Turnip Greens	Bitter, Pungent	Cool, Light, Dry	**PK:** Balances **V:**Aggravates
Water Chestnut	Sweet	Cool, Light, Wet	**P:** Balances **VK:**Aggravates
Winter Melon	Sweet	Cool, Light, Wet	**VP:** Balances **K:**Aggravates
Winter Squash	Sweet	Cool	**PV:** Balances **K:**Aggravates
Yam	Sweet	Cool, Heavy, Dry	**VP:** Balances **K:**Aggravates
Yu Choy	Bitter, Pungent	Cool, Light, Dry	**PK:** Balances **V:**Aggravates
Zucchini	Sweet, Bitter	Cool, Light, Wet	**VP:** Balances; **K:** Neutral

Grains

Grains tend to be sweet and somewhat neutral. They are calming to the mind, but can aggravate the doshas in excess. They are strengthening and pretty good for most vata conditions, although yeast can aggravate vata. Grains tend to be good for any time of the year. Although lighter, drier grains are better for kapha. Spices can make some grains easier to digest. **Combining:** Grains are somewhat neutral and combine well with many foods. When combining grains be careful not to combine them with foods that are incompatible with each other.

Grain	Taste	Qualities	Doshas
Amaranth	Sweet	Cool, Light, Dry	**VP**: Balances; **K**: Neutral
Barley	Sweet, Astringent	Cool, Light, Dry	**PK**: Balances; **V**: Neutral
Buckwheat	Sweet, Bitter	Cool, Light, Dry	**PK**: Balances; **V**: Neutral
Corn	Sweet, Pungent	Cool, Light, Dry	**PK**: Balances; **V**: Neutral
Einkorn	Sweet	Cool, Heavy, Dry	**PV**: Balances: **K**: Aggravates
Emmer	Sweet	Cool, Heavy, Dry	**PV**: Balances; **K**: Aggravates
Millet	Sweet, Astringent	Cool, Light, Dry	**VK**: Mildly Aggravates; **P**: Balances
Oat	Sweet	Cold, Heavy, Wet	**VP**: Balances; **K**: Aggravates
Quinoa	Sweet	Cold, Light, Dry	**VP**: Balances; **K**: Neutral
Rice	Sweet	Cold, Light, Dry	**VP**: Balances; **K**: Neutral
Rye	Sweet, Bitter	Cold, Heavy, Wet	**VP**: Balances; **K**: Aggravates
Sorghum	Sweet	Cold, Light, Dry	**V**: Aggravates; **PK**: Balances
Spelt	Sweet	Cold, Heavy, Wet	**VP**: Balances; **K**: Aggravates
Tef	Sweet	Cold, Heavy, Dry	**VP**: Balances; **K**: Aggravates
Wheat	Sweet	Cold, Heavy, Wet	**VP**: Balances; **K**: Aggravates

Legumes

Beans are a great source of protein. They tend to be heavy and dry and somewhat hard to digest (always good to soak them). They combine well with grains for energy, but not great with fruits and dairy. Spices like onions, cumin, asafoetida and salt are good for countering the heavy, drying, gas causing effects of beans and legumes. **Combining**: Beans combine best with vegetables or grains. They can be difficult to combine with dairy, fruit or sugars

Legume	Taste	Qualities	Doshas
Adzuki Bean	Sweet, Astringent	Cold, Heavy, Dry	**PK**: Balances; **V**:Neutral
Black-Eyed Pea	Sweet, Astringent	Cold, Heavy, Dry	**PK**: Balances **V**:Aggravates
Black Beans	Astringent	Cool,Heavy, Dry	**V**: Aggravates **PK**:Balances
Chickpea (Garbanzo Bean)	Sweet, Astringent	Cold, Heavy, Dry	**V**: Aggravates **PK**:Balances
Cowpea	Sweet, Astringent	Cold, Heavy, Dry	**V**: Aggravates **PK**:Balances
Fava Bean	Sweet, Astringent	Cold, Heavy, Dry	**V**: Aggravates **PK**:Balances
Flat Bean	Sweet, Astringent	Cold, Heavy, Dry	**V**: Aggravates **PK**:Balances
Horse Gram	Sweet, Astringent	Cold, Heavy, Dry	**V**: Aggravates **PK**:Balances
Kidney Bean	Sweet, Astringent	Cold, Heavy, Dry	**V**: Aggravates **PK**:Balances
Lentil	Sweet, Astringent	Cold, Heavy, Dry	**V**: Aggravates **PK**:Balances
Lima Bean	Sweet, Astringent	Cold, Heavy, Dry	**V**: Aggravates **PK**:Balances
Mung Bean	Sweet, Astringent	Cold, Heavy, Dry	**V**: Neutral; **PK**:Balances
Pea	Sweet, Astringent	Cold, Heavy, Dry	**V**: Aggravates **PK**:Balances
Pigeon Pea	Sweet, Astringent	Cold, Heavy, Dry	**V**: Aggravates **PK**:Balances
Soybean	Sweet, Astringent	Cold, Heavy, Dry	**V**: Aggravates **PK**:Balances
Split Peas	Sweet, Astringent	Cold, Heavy, Dry	**V**: Aggravates **PK**:Balances
Tofu	Sweet, Astringent	Cool, Heavy, Dry	**VK**: Neutral; **P**:Balances
Urad Dal	Sweet, Astringent	Cold, Heavy, Dry	**V**: Balances **PK**:Aggravates

Nuts & Seeds

Nuts are most often sweet, warm and heavy. They are great for vata, but tend to be aggravating for pitta and kapha. Nuts are strengthening and rejuvenative but can be difficult to digest, especially if they're roasted and salted, or eaten in the form of nut butter. Nut milks with added spices like ginger are much easier to digest and a great way to access the nourishing qualities of nuts without adversely impacting digestion. Seeds are similar to nuts but slightly lighter and less nourishing) so better for pitta and kapha. Nuts (particularly taken with sugar) are used as tonics in Ayurveda. And are a powerful medicine for countering fragility and supporting the process of recuperation.. **Combining:** Nuts combine best with grains, like rice, but do not combine well with beans, dairy or starchy vegetables

Nuts and Seeds	Taste	Qualities	Doshas
Almond	Sweet	Hot, Heavy, Wet	**V:** Balances **PK:**Aggravates
Coconut	Sweet	Cold, Heavy, Wet	**VP:** Balances **K:**Aggravates
Cashew	Sweet	Hot, Heavy, Wet	**VP:** Balances **K:**Aggravates
Chestnut	Sweet	Hot, Heavy, Wet	**VP:** Balances **K:**Aggravates
Pinenut	Sweet	Hot, Light, Wet	**V:** Balances **KP:**Aggravates
Pecan	Sweet	Hot, Heavy, Wet	**VP:** Balances **K:**Aggravates
Walnut	Sweet	Hot, Heavy, Wet	**V:** Balances **PK:**Aggravates
Hazelnut	Sweet	Hot, Light, Wet	**V:** Balances **PK:**Aggravates
Pumpkin Seed	Sweet, Bitter	Hot, Heavy, Wet	**VK:** Balances **P:**Aggravates
Sesame Seed	Sweet, Bitter	Hot, Heavy, Wet	**V:** Balances **PK:**Aggravates
Sunflower Seed	Sweet	Cold, Light, Wet	**V:** Balances **PK:**Aggravates
Hemp Seed	Sweet	Hot, Heavy, Wet	**V:** Balances **PK:**Aggravates
Flax Seed	Sweet, Bitter	Hot, Heavy, Wet	**V:** Balances **PK:**Aggravates
Peanut	Sweet	Hot, Heavy, Wet	**V:** Balances **PK:**Aggravates
Macadamia	Sweet	Hot	**V:** Balances **PK:**Aggravates
Brazil	Sweet	Heavy, Wet	**V:** Balances **PK:**Aggravates
Pistachio	Sweet	Hot, Heavy, Wet	**V:** Balances **PK:**Aggravates

Meats, Fish & Seafood

Meat is one of the most nourishing and building foods there is. It is one of the best foods for building immunity and lowering high vata. Most meats are sweet in taste and slightly warm or warming, which increases pitta and kapha. Meat is said to have a dulling effect on the mind (tamasic). It's heavy effects can be countered somewhat with raw, bitter vegetables and bitter herbs. **Combining:** Meat does not combine well with other foods (especially milk or dairy as is it somewhat challenging to digest as is. Bitter herbs, spices and raw vegetables can help with digesting meat.

Fish is salty, sweet and heating. It's a little more challenging to find good quality sources of fish as most of the commercially available fish is farmed and/or high in contaminants such as mercury, pesticides and or industrial chemicals. And the heaviness of fish can be balanced with spices like ginger, garlic, mustard or horseradish. **Combining:** Does not combine well with milk, sugars or meat.

Meat	Rasa (taste)	Gunas	Actions
Anchovy	Salty, Sweet	Hot, light, wet	**V:** Balances **P,K:**Aggravates
Beef	Sweet	Hot, heavy, wet	**V:** Balances **P,K:**Aggravates
Chicken	Sweet	Slightly warm, heavy, wet	**V:**Balances **P,K:**Moderation
Crab	Sweet	Slightly warm, heavy, wet	**V:** Balances **P,K:**Aggravates
Deer (venison)	Sweet	Slightly warm, light, wet	**V:** Balances **P,K:**Moderation
Duck	Sweet	Hot, heavy, wet	**V:**Balances **P,K:**Aggravates
Eggs	Sweet, salty	Hot, heavy, wet	**V:** Balance **P,K:**Moderation
Lamb/ Mutton	Sweet	Hot, heavy, wet	**V** Balances **P,K:**Aggravates
Oyster	Sweet, salty	Hot, heavy, wet	**V:**Balances **P,K:**Aggravates
Pork	Sweet	Slightly warm, heavy, wet/oily	**V,P:** Balances **K:**Aggravates (excessively)
Rabbit	Sweet, astringent	Hot, light, dry	**V:** Aggravates **P,K:**Moderation
Salmon	Sweet, salty	Warm, heavy, wet/oily	**V,P:** Balances **K:**Aggravates
Shrimp (prawn)	Sweet, salty	Hot, light, wet	**V:**Balances **P,K:**Moderation
Trout	Sweet	Cold, heavy, wet	**V:** Balances **P,K:**Moderation

Dairy

Most dairy products are sweet, cool and heavy (although sour products like yogurts and cheese can be slightly warming). Dairy products tend to be calming for the mind and building, strengthening and rejuvenating for the body. They don't combine well with other foods and are best taken warm or at room temperature owing to their heavy nature. Including spices like cumin, ginger, cardamom and cinnamon with dairy products can counter some of their mucus forming qualities. Combining: Combines best with grains and sugars. Does not do well with many other foods, i.e. nuts, sour fruits, meat, fish, yeasted breads and pickles, due to it's heaviness and tendency to ferment.

Dairy Product	Rasa (taste)	Gunas	Actions
Aged Cheese	Sweet, sour, pungent	Cold, heavy, dry	**V**: Balances **P,K**:Aggravates
Butter	Sweet	Cold, heavy, wet	**V,P**: Balances **K**:Aggravates
Buttermilk	Sour, astringent	Slightly warm, heavy, wet	**V**:Balances **P,K**:Aggravates
Cheese	Sweet	Cool, heavy, wet	**V,P**: Balances **K**:Aggravates
Cream	Sweet	Cool, heavy, wet	**V,P**: Balances **K**:Aggravates
Goat's milk	Sweet	Slightly warm, heavy, wet	**V,P**: Balances **K**:Moderation
Goat's cheese	Sweet	Slightly warm, heavy, wet	See Goat's milk
Ghee	Sweet	Cool, heavy, wet	**V,P**: Balances **K**:Moderation
Ice Cream	Sweet	Cold, heavy, wet	**P**: Moderation **V,K**:Aggravates
Kefir	Sour, sweet	Warm, heavy, wet	**V**: Balances **P,K**:Aggravates
Milk	Sweet	Cold, heavy, wet	**V,P**: Balances **K**:Moderation
Sour cream	Sweet, sour	Slightly warm, heavy, wet	**V**: Balances **P,K**:Aggravates
Yogurt	Sweet, sour	Slightly warm, heavy, wet	**V**: Balances **P,K**:Moderation

Herbs & Spices

Herbs and spices are one of the best tools we have for creating meals that balance and support our digestion. They play a key part in regulating the appetite and countering some of the adverse qualities and impacts of the foods we eat. In many ways, our herbs and spices provide the "glue" that makes the marriages between our food and our digestion work. Spices are also powerful medicines unto themselves, and are great for treating many issues that we commonly experience.

In general spices are balancing for vata and kapha and can aggravate pitta (there are exceptions!). They are wonderful tools for promoting everything from healthy skin to detoxification and more! When using spices it's best to buy them whole and grind them yourself in order to get the best quality and potency of their healing capabilities.

Spice	Rasa (taste)	Gunas	Actions
Ajwan	Bitter, pungent	Hot, light, dry	**V,K:** Balances **P:**Aggravates
Aloe	Bitter, sweet	Cold, heavy, wet	**V,P,K:** Balances
Anise	Pungent	Hot, light, dry	**VK:**Balances **P:**Moderation
Asafoetida	Pungent	Hot, heavy, wet	**V,K:** Balances **P:**Aggravates
Basil	Sweet, pungent	Warm, dry	**V,K:**Balances **P:**Moderation
Bay leaf	Pungent	Warm, dry	**V,K:** Balances **P:**Moderation
Black Pepper	Pungent	Hot, Light, dry	**V,K:** Balances **P:**Aggravates
Calamus	Pungent, bitter, astringent	Hot, light, dry	**V,K:** Balances **P:**Aggravates
Camomile	Pungent, bitter	Cool, light, dry	**V,P,K:** Balances
Caraway	Pungent, bitter	Warm, light, dry	**V,K:** Balances **P:**Moderation
Cardamom	Sweet, pungent	Cool, light, dry	**V,K:** Balances **P:**Moderation
Cayenne	Pungent	Hot, light, dry	**V,K:** Balances **P:**Aggravates
Cinnamon	Sweet, pungent	Warm, light, dry	**V,K:** Balances; **P:**Moderation
Clove	Pungent, bitter, sweet	Cool, light, wet	**V,P,K:** Balances
Coriander	Pungent, sweet, bitter	Leaves - Cool, light, wet | Seeds - Warm, light, wet.	**V,P,K:** Balances
Cumin	Pungent, bitter	Slightly warm, light, dry	**V,K:** Balances **P:**Moderation
Curry leaf	Pungent, bitter	Warm, light, dry	**V,K:** Balances **P:**Aggravates

Spice	Rasa (taste)	Gunas	Actions
Dill	Pungent, bitter	Seeds - Warm, light, dry | Leaves - cool, light, dry	**V,P,K:** Generally balancing;
Fennel	Sweet, pungent, bitter	Warming, Light, dry,	**V,P,K:** Balances
Fenugreek	Pungent, astringent, bitter, sweet	Warm, light, wet	**V,K:** Balances **P:**Aggravates
Garlic	Pungent, sweet, bitter, astringent, salty,	Warm, heavy, wet/oily	**V,K:** Balances **P:**Aggravates
Ginger	Pungent, sweet	Fresh - Warm, heavy, wet; Dry - Hot, light, dry	**V,K:** Balances **P:**Aggravates
Holy Basil (Tulsi)	Pungent, bitter	Hot, light, dry	**V,K:** Balancing **P:**Aggravating
Horseradish/ Wasabi	Pungent, bitter	Hot, light, dry	**V,P:** Aggravates **K:**Balances
Lemongrass	Pungent, bitter, sour	Cool, light, dry	**V,P,K:** Balances
Lemon Balm	Pungent, sweet,	Cool, light, dry	**V,P,K:** Balances
Licorice	Sweet, bitter	Cool, heavy, wet	**V,P,K:** Balances
Long Pepper (pippali)	Pungent, sweet	Hot, light, wet/oily	**V,K:** Balances **P:**Aggravates
Marjoram	Pungent, bitter	Warm, light, dry	**V,K:** Balances **P:**Moderation
Mint	Sweet, pungent, bitter	Cool/Hot, light, dry	**V,P,K:**Balances
Mustard	Pungent, bitter	Hot, light, dry	**V,K:** Balances **P:**Aggravates
Nutmeg	Pungent, bitter, astringent	Warm, light, wet/oily	**V,K:** Balances **P:**Aggravates
Oregano	Pungent, bitter	Warm, light, dry	**V,K:** Balances **P:**Aggravates
Orange peel	Sweet, pungent, bitter	Warm, light, dry	**V,K:** Balances **P:**Aggravates
Parsley	Pungent, bitter	Warm, light, dry	**V,K:** Balances **P:**Moderation
Pink Salt (sanchal)	Salty, sweet,	Cool, heavy, wet	**V,P,K:** Balances (in moderation)
Poppy seed	Pungent, astringent, sweet	Hot, light, dry	**V,K:** Balancing **P:**Aggravates

Spice	Rasa (taste)	Gunas	Actions
Rosemary	Pungent, bitter	Hot, dry, light	**V,K:** Balances **P:**Aggravates
Rose	Bitter, pungent, astringent, sweet	Cool, dry, light	**V,P,K:** Balances
Saffron	Pungent, bitter, sweet	Warm, light, wet/oily	**VPK:** Balances
Sage	Pungent, bitter, astringent	Cool, light, dry	**V,K:** Balances **P:**Aggravates
Sea salt	Salty, sweet, pungent	Hot, heavy, wet	**V:** Balances **P,K:**Aggravates
Star anise	Pungent, sweet	Hot, light, dry	**VK:**Balances **P:**Moderation
Tarragon	Pungent, bitter	Hot, light, dry	**V,K:** Balances **P:**Aggravates
Thyme	Pungent, bitter	Hot, light, dry	**V,K:** Balances **P:**Aggravates
Turmeric	Pungent, bitter, astringent	Hot, light, dry	**V,P,K:** Balances (can aggravate **V,P** if used excessively)

Ayurvedic Kitchen Pharmacy

What are the most important spices to have in your kitchen and why?

Check out this video tutorial to find out!

http://www.eatlikeyouloveyourself.com/ ayurvedic-kitchen-pharmacy

Oils

Most oils are sweet and warming. They decrease vata and can aggravate pitta and kapha with the exception of ghee. Oils are VERY useful for massage and they soothe, lubricate and rejuvenate muscles, joints and skin. They're often used in Ayurveda for dissolving toxins.

Oil	Rasa (taste)	Gunas	Actions
Almond	Sweet	warm, heavy, wet/oily	**V:**Balances **P,K:**Aggravates
Avocado	Sweet astringent	Warm, heavy, wet/oily	**V:** Balances **P:**Moderation **K:**Aggravates
Canola	Sweet, pungent, astringent	Hot, light, wet/oily	**V:**Aggravates **P,K:**Balances
Castor	Bitter, sweet, pungent	Hot, heavy, wet/oily	**V,P,K:** Moderation
Cocoa butter	Sweet	Cold, heavy, wet/oily	**V,P:**Balances **K:**Aggravates
Coconut	Sweet	Cold, heavy, wet/oily	**V,P:** Balances **K:**Moderation
Fish	Sweet, salty pungent	Hot, heavy, wet/oily	**V:** Balances; **P,K:**Aggravates
Flaxseed linseed	Pungent, sweet	Warm, heavy wet/oily	**V,P:** Balancing; **K:**Moderation
Ghee	Sweet	Heavy, cold, wet/oily	**V:** Balancing **P,K:**Moderation
Hemp	Sweet	Hot, heavy, wet/oily	**V,P:** Balances **K:**Aggravates
Lard	Sweet, sour	Heavy, wet/oily	**V:** Balances **P,K:**Aggravates
Mustard	Pungent, Sweet	Hot, light, wet/oily	**V,K:** Balances **P:**Moderation
Olive	Sweet, bitter	Hot, heavy, wet/oily	**V,P:** Balances **K:**Moderation
Peanut	Sweet	Hot, heavy, wet/oily	**V:** Balancing **P,K:** Moderation
Safflower	Sweet, pungent	Hot, heavy, wet/oily	**V,K:** Balances **P:**Aggravates
Sesame	Sweet, pungent	Hot, Wet/oily	**V:** Balances **P,K:**Moderation
Soy	Sweet, astringent	Slightly tCool, heavy, wet/oily	**P,K:** Balances **V:**Moderation
Sunflower	Sweet, astringent	Slightly Cool, heavy, wet/oily	**P,K:** Balances **V:**Moderation
Walnut	Sweet	Hot, heavy, wet/oily	**V:** Balancing **P,K:**Aggravating

Sweeteners

Since most of the food we eat is sweet AND our cells use sugar for fuel, it's important to ensure that we get enough, but not too much of the right kinds of sweetness in our diet. Most pure sugars are highly refined and can cause issues and the formation of toxins. Sugar (sweet taste) typically balances vata and pitta and aggravates kapha. It has a tonic effect on the tissues and in the right quantities (and quality) a rejuvenative effect on the mind and body. Sugar can be used topically to soothe burns, rashes, wounds and sores.
Combining: Can be difficult to combine with other foods. The addition of spices can help with this.

Sweetener	Rasa (taste)	Gunas	Actions
Agave	Sweet, astringent	Cold, heavy, wet	**V,P:** Balances **K:** Aggravates
Barley Malt	Sweet	Cold, heavy, wet	**V,P:** Balances **K:** Aggravates
Brown sugar	Sweet astringent	Cold, heavy, wet	**V,P:** Balances **K:** Aggravates
Fructose - Fruit Sugar	Sweet	Cold, heavy, wet.	**V,P:** Balanced **K:** Aggravates
Honey	Sweet, astringent, pungent	Warm, heavy, wet	**V,K:** Balances **P:** Moderation
Jaggary *Indian raw natural sugar*	Sweet	Warm, heavy, wet	**V:** Balances **P,K:** Moderation
Maple Syrup	Sweet	Cool, heavy, wet	**V,P:** Balances **K:** Moderation
Molasses	Sweet	Warm, heavy, wet	**V:** Balances **P,K:** Moderation
Maltose	Sweet	Cold, heavy, wet	**V,P:** Balances **K:** Moderation
Stevia	Sweet, astringent, bitter	Cool, Heavy	**V,P,K:** Balances all
White Sugar	Sweet, astringent	Cold, heavy, wet	**V,P:** Balances **K:** Aggravates
Yacon Syrup	Sweet, astringent	Cold, heavy, wet	**V,P:** Balances **K:** Aggravates

Condiments

Condiments are prepared foods that in many ways are treated like a single ingredient. And like the ingredients list above, they have effects on the doshas that in some cases reflect their combination of constituent parts. It makes sense to consider how the condiments you use can change the energetic balance of your dishes and you. Here are a few of the most common condiments in use.

Condiment	Taste	Qualities	Doshas
Carob	Sweet, Astringent	Warm, Heavy, Wet	**VPK:** Balances (Can aggravate V in excess)
Chocolate	Pungent, Bitter	Hot, Light, Dry	**VK:** Balance; **P:** Aggravates
Chutney (sweet mango)	Sweet, Sour	Hot, Heavy, Wet	**V:** Balances; **PK:** Mildly aggravates
Ketchup	Sweet, Sour	Hot, Heavy, Wet	**V:** Balances; **P:**Aggravates; **K:** Mildly aggravates
Mayonnaise	Sweet, Sour	Hot, Heavy, Wet	**V:** Balances; **PK:** Aggravates
Miso	Sweet, Salty, Sour	Hot, Heavy, Wet	**V:** Balances; **PK:** Aggravates
Mustard	Pungent, Bitter	Hot, Light, Dry	**VK:** Balances; **P:** Aggravates
Vinegar	Sour	Hot, Light, Wet	**V:** Balances; **PK:** Aggravates
Pickles	Sweet, Sour, Pungent	Hot, Heavy, Wet	**V:** Balances; **PK:** Aggravates
Soy Sauce	Salty, Sweet	Hot, Heavy, Wet	**V:** Balances; **P:** Mildly aggravates; **K:**Aggravates
Tahini	Sweet, Bitter	Hot, Heavy, Wet/Oily	**V:** Balances; **PK:** Aggravates
Tamari	Salty, Sweet	Hot, H	**V:** Balances; **PK:** Mildly aggravates

HOW TOXIC ARE YOU?
Check your ama quotient

To get a general idea of your current ama levels complete the questionnaire below answering between 1 and 5 in for each question.

1	=	NEVER
2	=	RARELY
3	=	SOMETIMES
4	=	OFTEN
5	=	VERY OFTEN

A score between 0-15 indicates a low level of ama; 16-35 indicates a moderate amount of ama; and 36-50 indicates a high level of ama.

ISSUE	RATING
My body feels blocked (as in constipation) or congested.	
My digestion is slow or challenged	
I wake up feeling tired, slow or foggy	
I'm fatigued and weak, but am not sure why.	
My motivation has left me and I feel lethargic	
I catch a cold several times a year.	
I'm rarely actually hungry for anything	
I frequently feel depressed.	
I become easily exhausted, both mentally and physically.	
I feel the need to cough regularly.	
TOTAL	

Other questions to consider in order to get a sense of your levels of ama?

Physical Ama:

- Is my breathing slow and steady, deep and unrestricted?
- Is my appetite keen?
- Do I experience thirst at regular intervals?
- Is my waste (urine, stool, sweat) output normal?
- Are my five senses (sight, hearing, taste, touch and smell) performing well?
- Is my skin lustrous and supple?
- Am I generally free of ulcers, lumps, and bumps?
- Do I feel active and energetic?
- Is my breath fresh and are my teeth strong?
- Are my joints well-lubricated and healthy?
- Is my sexual urge normal?
- Do I sleep well?

Mental & Emotional Ama

- Am I happy at work?
- Do I have a stable family life and strong support system?
- Am I happy with my partner?
- Do I have a strong relationship with my co-workers and friends?
- Is my ability to rest – both physically and mentally – adequate?
- Do I handle difficult situations calmly?
- Do I have enough leisure time and do I make positive use of it?
- Do I usually feel calm inside?

Dosha Test

Dosha Questionnaire Instructions:

For each category, please circle the option that best describes you. If you feel you can equally relate to more than one of the descriptions, circle all that apply to you.

When taking the questionnaire, select the description that best fits how you've been MOST of your life (Not just how you feel in the moment or have been most recently).

After finishing a profile: For each column, tally up how many descriptions you circled. This number goes in the Subtotal row at the bottom of each profile.

After finishing the profiles, record all your profile totals in the Totals Chart on the last page.

Note the column you have the most points in, and then find the corresponding Dosha Type. You can read a little about your Dosha in the Doshic Summaries information.

MENTAL

CATEGORY	VATA	PITTA	KAPHA
Mental activity	Quick mind, restless	Sharp intellect, aggressive	Calm, steady, stable
Memory	Short-term best	Good general memory	Long-term best
Thoughts	Constantly changing	Fairly steady	Steady, stable, fixed
Concentration	Short-term focus best	Better than average mental concentration	Good ability for long-term focus
Ability to learn	Quick grasp of learning	Medium to moderate grasp	Slow to learn new things
Dreams	Fearful, flying, running, jumping	Angry, fiery, violent, adventurous	Include water, clouds, relationships, romance
Sleep	Interrupted, light	Sound, medium	Sound, heavy, long
Speech	Fast, sometimes missing words	Fast, sharp, clear-cut	Slow, clear, sweet
Voice	High pitch	Medium pitch	Low pitch
Mental subtotal:			

BEHAVIORAL

CATEGORY	VATA	PITTA	KAPHA
Eating speed	Quick	Medium	Slow
Hunger level	Irregular	Sharp, needs food when hungry	Can easily miss meals
Food and drink	Prefers warm	Prefers cold	Prefers dry and warm
Achieving goals	Easily distracted	Focused and driven	Slow and steady
Giving/donations	Gives small amounts	Gives nothing, or large amounts infrequently	Gives regularly and generously
Relationships	Many casual	Intense	Long and deep
Sex drive	Variable or low	Moderate	Strong
Works best	While supervised	Alone	In groups
Weather preference	Aversion to cold	Aversion to heat	Aversion to damp, cool
Reaction to stress	Excites quickly	Medium	Slow to get excited
Financial	Doesn't save, spends quickly	Saves, but big spender	Saves regularly, accumulates wealth
Friendships	Tends toward short-term friendships, makes friends quickly	Tends to be a loner, friends related to occupation	Tends to form long-lasting friendships
Behavioral subtotal:			

	EMOTIONAL		
CATEGORY	VATA	PITTA	KAPHA
Moods	Change quickly	Change slowly	Steady, unchanging
Reacts to stress with	Fear	Anger	Indifference
More sensitive to	Own feelings	Not sensitive	Others' feelings
When threatened, tends to	Run	Fight	Make peace
Relations with spouse/partner	Clingy	Jealous	Secure
Expresses affection	With words	With gifts	With touch
When feeling hurt	Cries	Argues	Withdraws
Emotional trauma causes	Anxiety	Denial	Depression
Confidence level	Timid	Outwardly self-confident	Inner confidence
Emotional subtotal:			

	PHYSICAL		
CATEGORY	VATA	PITTA	KAPHA
Amount of hair	Average	Thinning	Thick
Hair type	Dry, coarse, curly	Normal, fine, soft	Oily, lustrous, wavy
Hair color	Light brown, blonde	Red, auburn	Dark brown, black
Skin	Dry, rough, or both	Soft, normal to oily, acne	Oily, moist, cool
Skin temperature	Cold hands/feet	Warm	Cool
Complexion	Darker, dull, brown	Pink-red, flushed, smooth, rosy, freckles	Pale
Eyes	Small, sunken, dry	Medium, irritated, sensitive to light	Large, calm, lucid, wide, prominent
Whites of eyes	Blue/brown	Yellow or red	Glossy white
Size of teeth	Very large or very small	Small-medium	Medium-large
Shoulder	Thin, small, flat, hunched	Medium	Broad, thick, firm
Weight	Thin, hard to gain	Medium	Heavy, gains easily
Appetite	Variable, erratic, scanty	Strong, sharp	Constant, slow & steady
Elimination	Dry, hard, thin, gas, easily constipated	Many during day, soft to normal	Heavy, slow, thick, regular
Sweat & body odour	Scanty, no smell	Profuse, strong smelling	Moderate, pleasant smell
Veins and tendons	Very prominent	Fairly prominent	Well covered
Physical subtotal:			

FITNESS			
CATEGORY	VATA	PITTA	KAPHA
Exercise tolerance	Low	Medium	High
Endurance	Fair	Good	Excellent
Strength	Fair	Better than average	Excellent
Speed	Very good	Good	Not so fast
Competition	Doesn't like competitive pressure	Driven competitor	Deals easily with competitive pressure
Walking speed	Fast	Average	Slow and steady
Muscle tone	Lean, low body fat	Medium, with good definition	Brawny/bulky, with higher fat percentage
Body size	Small frame, lean or long	Medium frame	Large frame, fleshy, stocky, well-developed
Reaction time	Quick	Average	Slow
Fitness subtotal:			

Totals

Your Primary Dosha Type is the column you scored highest in.

Profile	VATA	PITTA	KAPHA
Mental			
Behavioral			
Emotional			
Physical			
Fitness			
TOTAL:			

One-Day Detox Guide

Why Detox...?

The primary purpose of this day of detoxification is to refocus your mind, body and spirit, to revisit what you're committed to in your life, and to align yourself with the cycles of nature. Doing so will allow you to clear away some of what's between you and your most powerful expression of yourself. It will also amplify your gifts and allow you to dedicate more of you to what really matters.

What's possible in 1-Day?

Transformation can happen in an instant. And so what's possible in this 1 day will be entirely up to you! It is my hope that you use this day to re-examine your physical, mental and emotional levels of balance and perhaps even dedicate yourself to making small changes today and every day after that will leave you feeling cleaner, clearer and more alive.

Here's what to do:

MAKE THIS DAY ABOUT... Tuning in to where your attention goes throughout the day. They say "energy flows where our attention goes". Where does your attention go most?

ASK YOURSELF... What's the priority in your life right now? (Be honest).

Morning

- Get up early
- Breathe for 2 mins
- Warm water w/lemon
- Slow yoga practice OR 3-5 Sun Salutations
- 5 - 15 minutes of meditation

Breakfast

- *Tune in to your level of hunger. Choose a bowl of oats, Yogi breakfast, or a cup of tea, based on how hungry you are right now.*
- *Finish breakfast by 8:30am.*

Day

- Breath for 2 mins
- Eat lunch between 11 - 2pm

Lunch

- *Tune in to your level of hunger. Enjoy a bowl of mung bean soup or kitchari - eat only enough to just satisfy your hunger.*
- *Take a walk after lunch*

Evening

- Start winding down by 6pm
- Eat dinner before 7pm

Dinner

- *Tune in to your level of hunger. Enjoy a bowl of mung bean soup or kitchari - eat only enough to just satisfy your hunger.*
- Turn off screens at least 1 hr before bed.
- Take some time to journal or reflect on the day and let go.
- Get to be no later than 10:30pm

Glossary

Agni - The fire of digestion

Amla - Sour taste

Apana - Downward moving energy

Dinacharya - The Ayurvedic daily routine.

Dosha - A sanskrit word meaning "That which can be deranged", another term for Prakriti, or one of the functional/biological energies.

Guna - The Ayurvedic qualities or characteristics of substances or things. There are twenty

Guru - Heavy quality

Kapha - The functional/biological energy of cohesion and structure

Karma - Action or characteristic effect/impact of a thing or substance.

Kashay - Astringent taste

Katu - Pungent taste

Kitchari - Ayurvedic cleansing dish made of basmati rice and moong dhal.

Laghu - Light quality

Lavana - Salty taste

Madhura - Sweet taste

Mahagunas - The three qualities of the mind.

Manda agni - Slow digestion or indigestion

Panchamahabhutas - The five great elements, said to be the building blocks of all of everything in the material world.

Pitta - The functional/biological energy of transformation and metabolization

Prakriti - True nature, sometimes referred to as your "dosha". It is your unique combination of biological energies.

Rajas - The dynamic, aggitated, active, and controlling quality of the mind.

Rasa - Taste or essence

Ritu Sandhi - The period of between seasons, during which we can be at our most vulnerable. Typically is occurs over the period marked by the last two weeks of one season and the first two weeks of the next.

Ruksha - Rough or dry quality

Sadhana - Rituals, or self created sacred practices.

Saindhava - Pink salt or rock salt

Sama agni - Balanced digestive fire

Sattva - The pure, calm, creative, and compassionate quality of the mind.

Shita - Cold quality

Snigda - Moist or oily quality

Tamas - The disconnected, dull, slow and ignorant quality of the mind.

Tikshna agni - Sharp digestion or a situation where the digestive fire burns too hot.

Tikta - Bitter taste

Upakarma - The first six of the Ayurvedic qualities or gunas; namely - hot, cold, light, heavy, wet/oily, dry.

Ushna - Warm or hot quality

Vata - The functional/biological energy of movement

Vikriti - Current state of imbalance. It is the combination of biological energies which represents your current state of mind - body balance or imbalance.

Vishama agni - Variable digestion

Bibliography

Ayurveda A life of Balance, Maya Tiwari, Healing Arts Press 1995

Ayurvedic cooking for Westerners, Amadea Morningstar, Lotus Press 1995

Modern Ayurvedic Cookbook,Healthful, Healing recipes for life, Amrita Sondhi, Arsenal Pulp Press 2006

Food as Medicine: The theory and practice of food, Todd Caldecott, 2012

Ayurvedic Medicine, Sebastian Pole, Singing Dragon 2006, 2013

Ayurveda The Science of Self Healing, Vasant Lad, Lotus Press 2004

The Ayurvedic Guide to diet and weight loss, Scott Gerson M.D., Lotus Press 2002

The Yoga of Herbs, David Frawley, Vasant Lad, Lotus Press 1986

Perfect Health: The complete mind body guide, Deepak Chopra, Three Rivers Press 1991, 2000

Textbook of Ayurveda : General Principles of Management and Treatment, Vasant Lad M.A. Sc.

Ayurvedic Healing: A comprehensive guide, Dr. David Frawley, Lotus Press 2000

The three season Diet: Eat the way nature intended. Lose Weight. Beat food cravings. Get fit, John Douillard, Three Rivers Press 2000

Ayurvedic Curative Cuisine for Everyone, Light Miller, Lotus Press 2011

The Complete Book of Ayurvedic Home Remedies, Vasant Lad, B.A.M.S., M.A.Sc., Three Rivers Press 1998

The Yoga Body Diet, Slim and Sexy in 4 weeks (without the stress), Kristen Schultz, John Douillard, DC, PhD. Rodale Inc. 2010

Acknowledgements

A big thanks to all of my teachers for their inspiration and wisdom, and without whom this book would not have been possible. To my ever patient and enthusiastic family for your support on the good days and the not so good days. And to my students past, present, and future for your interest in and dedication to discovering the simple secrets of a beautiful life.

Thanks also to the many photographers whose work has been included within:

Wanda Chin - instagram.com/wandertrail_

Donatella Parasini - www.donatella.com.au

Shantanu Starick - shantanustarick.com

Aaron Burden - aaronburden.com

Christine Siracusa - christinesiracusa.net

Hannah Pemberton - thekitchenalchemist.co.uk

Annie Spratt - mammasaurus.co.uk/store

Neha Deshmukh - alamodetheblog.com

Goran Vučićević - facebook.com/goranv.photos

Karsten Würth - instagram.com/inf1783

Viktoria Hall-Waldhauser

Gaelle Marcel - gaellemarcelphotography.com

Daniel Norris - danielnorris.com

Luis Paico - luispaico.com

Kristina Tripkovic - tinamosquito.com

Ehud Neuhaus - society6.com/photolion/prints

Florian Pérennès - instagram.com/florian.perennes

Gabriel Gurrola - gabrielgurrola.com

Nathan Dumlao - nathandumlaophotos.com

Heather Schwartz - themodernlifemrs.com

David Mao - instagram.com/itsdavo

Chloe Ridgway - picturetakermemorymaker.co.uk

Kira auf der Heide - instagram.com/kadh.photography

Taylor Kiser - foodfaithfitness.com

Al Kawasa

Jess Watters - designedbyjess.com

Matt Seymour - mattseymour.co.uk

Colter Olmstead - youtube.com/theskinnyfilmer

Brooke Lark - brookelark.com

Kowit Phothisan

Magdalena Raczka - sweetspoon.pl

Index

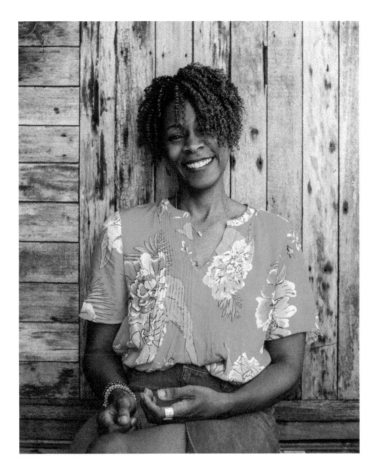

Chara Caruthers is a passionate and outspoken voice for the power of living your truth. An international teacher, speaker, advocate and mentor for women's wellness, she has inspired and motivated a global community of women of all ages to live juicier and more connected lives by embracing the enduring principles of yoga and Ayurveda.

Chara is a long-time practitioner and student of yoga, a senior yoga teacher (E-RYT 500) and a certified Yoga Therapist (C-IAYT). She has studied and practiced Ayurveda in the United States, Australia and India and is a graduate of the American Institute of Vedic Studies (USA), the International Academy of Ayurveda (Pune, India), and Kerala Ayurveda Academy (Kerala, India). Her work is focused on sharing these ancient principles in a modern context empowering wellness seekers of all backgrounds and cultures to boldly embrace the everyday challenges of knowing and loving ourselves.

As a writer (Huffington Post, DoYouYoga.com, Elephant Journal), presenter (Wanderlust Yoga Festivals, FoodMatters TV), and creator of outreach and educational programs aimed at helping folks "get real" about what's keeping them stuck, Her unique voice and soulful approach have been celebrated as a galvanizing force for the future of authentic wellness. **For information about her unique approach, free goodies and details of how to join her blissful community of wellness seekers, check out www.blissbodyandsoul.com**

CPSIA information can be obtained
at www.ICGtesting.com
Printed in the USA
LVHW071959150421
684634LV00024B/921